PENGUIN BOOKS

Natural Health fo

Dr John Briffa is a qualified doctor and leading practitioner and author
in the field of complementary medicine. He was formerly the natural
health columnist for the *Daily Mail* and is currently the nutrition and
well-being columnist for the *Observer*. He has contributed to over fifty
publications and has authored several books in the field of nutrition
and natural medicine, including *Ultimate Health – 12 Keys to Abundant
Health and Happiness*. He runs two hospital-based practices in London,
where he specializes in the natural management of health and disease.
Dr Briffa lectures extensively across the UK, Europe, South Africa,
America and Canada, and is a regular guest on TV and radio.

700030777333

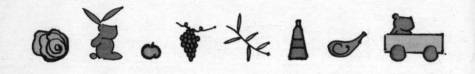

Natural Health for Kids

How to give your child the very best start in life

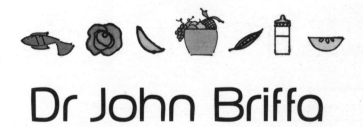

Dr John Briffa

Penguin Books

For children, everywhere

PENGUIN BOOKS

Published by the Penguin Group
Penguin Books Ltd, 80 St[rand, London WC2R 0RL, England]
Penguin Group (USA) Inc. [375 Hudson Street, New York, New York 10014, USA]
Penguin Group (Canada), [90 Eglinton Avenue East, Suite 700, Toronto, Ontario, Canada M4P] 2Y3
(a division of Pearson Pen[guin Canada Inc.])
Penguin Ireland, 25 St St[ephen's Green, Dublin 2, Ireland]
(a division of Penguin Bo[oks Ltd])
Penguin Group (Australia[) Pty Ltd, 250 Camberwell Road, Camberwell, Victoria 3124, Australia]
(a division of Pearson Au[stralia Group]
Penguin Books India Pvt [Ltd, 11 Community Centre, Panchsheel Park, New Delhi - 110 017, I]ndia
Penguin Group (NZ) Ltd, [67 Apollo Drive, Rosedale, North Shore, New Zealand]
(a division of Pearson Ne[w Zealand Ltd)]
Penguin Books (South Afr[ica (Pty) Ltd, 24 Sturdee Avenue, Rosebank, Johannesburg 2196, S]outh Africa

Penguin Books Ltd, Registered Offices: 80 Strand, London WC2R 0RL, England

www.penguin.com

First published by Michael Joseph 2004
Published in Penguin Books 2007
1

Copyright © John Briffa, 2004

Designed and typeset by Smith & Gilmour, London
Printed in Great Britain by Clays Ltd, St Ives plc

ISBN: 978-0-141-01338-1

*Every effort has been made to ensure that the information in this book is accurate.
The information in this book will be relevant to the majority of people but may not
be applicable in each individual case, so it is advised that professional medical
advice is obtained for specific information on personal health matters. Neither the
publisher nor the author accept any legal responsibility for any personal injury or
other damage or loss arising from the use or misuse of the information and advice
in this book.*

Contents

Acknowledgements

First and foremost, I would like to thank Anna Kowal, who did a wonderful job of unearthing and organising a great deal of the research contained in this book. Anna's tireless efforts were a major factor in *Natural Health for Kids* coming into being. A big thank you goes to Ingrid Yngstrom, my brother Joe and assistant Debbie Vandepeer, for reading through the manuscript and offering such constructive criticism and advice. My appreciation also goes to my parents, Dorothy and Joe, for so many things, but especially for their love, support and belief in my work (despite their conventional medical training!). I would also like to thank Louise Moore and Kate Adams at Michael Joseph, as well as Robert Kirby, my agent, who is always such a pleasure to work with and be around. I am also grateful to Linda Valins, for her invaluable advice on breast-feeding. Last, but not least, I would like to express my enormous gratitude to my patients, young and old, past and present. My honest belief is that the experience and learning they have given me over the years were essential ingredients in the writing of this book.

Part one

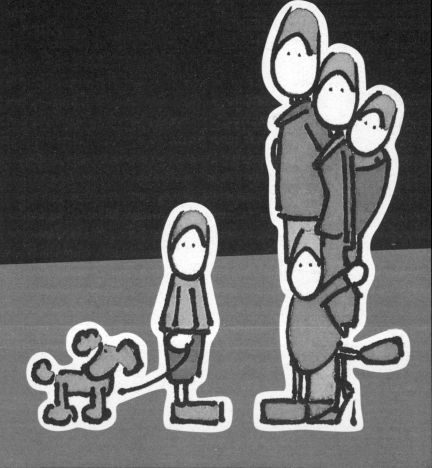

Foreword

Few would deny that having and bringing up children can be a uniquely rewarding experience. However, as many parents will testify, it can be an intensely challenging one too. Parents have an inherent concern for the welfare of their children, including a desire to feed them well and look after their health and wellbeing. If you are a parent yourself, you might have picked up this book in a search for a natural solution to some health issue that is affecting your child. Perhaps your child is struggling with physical or behavioural issues, and you suspect diet may be playing some part in this. You may be concerned about your child taking potentially toxic conventional medicines, and are seeking a gentler alternative. Or perhaps you are simply looking for some guidance on how to ensure your child gets all the nutrients needed for healthy growth and development. Whatever you and your child's specific needs are, *Natural Health for Kids* is here to help.

The bulk of this book contains information and advice about how to manage specific health issues using natural approaches such as nutrition, nutritional supplements, herbal remedies and flower essences. About 150 of the most common conditions are dealt with, from relatively minor problems, such as cuts and colds, right through to issues that can cause considerable suffering for children and their families, including hyperactivity, autism, dyslexia and eating disorders. For each condition, practical advice is given on how to address it using safe, effective, natural therapies.

The main natural approaches

Part one includes an introduction to the main natural approaches, which form an important part of the treatment strategies for the individual conditions. This section contains information on nutritional supplementation and offers advice on the specific types of products that are likely to provide a real advantage to children in the long term. I also give a guide to the major medicinal herbs, and have included information on their safe and effective use in children. In this section, I have also included a description of flower essences. These particular natural remedies are very gentle, but I have found them to be very useful in practice in helping resolve emotional and behavioural issues in children, as well as physical issues too. The major flower essences, and the specific conditions for which they are indicated, are also covered.

What is a healthy diet?

Many of the natural approaches to specific conditions involve some form of dietary adjustment. There is now considerable evidence that nutritional factors can play key roles in the development of disease and illness, and that the diet can often hold the key to overcoming health issues. My experience is that while many parents are keen to feed their children a nutritious, balanced diet, there is considerable confusion about what this actually means. For instance, while some advocate full-fat milk as a wholesome and nutritious drink for children, many nutritionists see it as nothing short of poison. And while starches such as bread and pasta are often emphasised in a child's diet, there are also reports that these foods may be helping to drive the epidemic of childhood diabetes and obesity we are seeing in the West. In the world of nutrition, it seems as though confusion reigns.

To this end, I have dedicated Chapters 1, 2 and 3 to an in-depth look at what it really means to feed a child healthily. Chapter 2 examines the health effects of the key components in the diet, including sugar, starch, protein, fat (in its various forms), water, salt, additives and artificial sweeteners. This chapter is about the science of food and looks at the evidence for what is healthy (and what is not) in our diet. While the thrust of the core information in this chapter is geared towards ensuring good health in childhood, I have also kept one eye on the longer-term benefits (and mention this where relevant) too.

Once the major nutritional foundation stones have been laid, in chapter three I turn my attention to specific foods, discussing their relative merits. Here, the pros and cons of all the most common foods, including meat, fish, eggs, grains, dairy products, sweets, soft drinks and breakfast cereals, are explored. The information here is then used as the basis for suggestions for healthy, balanced meals for kids, together with ideas for nutritious snacks and lunch-box items too.

As many parents will know, making healthy foods available to children is one thing, but getting them to eat them is another. Some children can be picky eaters, and may be quite resistant to change. The evidence suggests that using strong-arm tactics is likely to compound problems here, which means more subtle tactics are usually called for. To this end, Chapter 4 contains information and advice on how to improve and upgrade your child's diet with the minimum of fuss. In this chapter, I also explore eating culture and the benefits to be had from regular breakfasts and family meals. For those looking for a quick guide to healthy eating for kids, I have summarised Chapters 1, 2 and 3 in the form of ten principles entitled 'Primer on Nutrition for Kids', which appears on pages 7–10.

Health issues

The ailment section of the book frequently refers to specific health issues that I find are commonly at the root of so many childhood conditions. In Chapter 4, I explore these imbalances in depth. I start by looking at the area of blood sugar balance, a topic of critical importance to the short- and long-term health of our children. The other major issues covered in this chapter are those of food sensitivity, yeast overgrowth and a deficiency of certain healthy fats in the diet. Questionnaires are included to help you identify these core issues in your child, along with practical advice about what to do if you have identified a problem.

And something for mothers and babies

I have found dietary strategies, along with other natural approaches, to be highly effective in the treatment of childhood illnesses. However, it is also true that the value of a healthy diet doesn't just start in childhood. Nutritional factors have been shown to be of critical importance during pregnancy. Chapter 5 examines these in depth, and offers advice about what to eat during these critical times. In Chapter 6 I go on to explore the theory and practicalities of infant feeding and weaning.

One central theme of the nutritional component of this book is the value of keeping the diet as natural and unprocessed as possible. Food processing generally detracts from the nutritional attributes of a food, and often adds to it things that are far from healthy. For many of us, the idea of preparing every meal from fresh ingredients seems unrealistic and arduous. You can take heart from the fact that you really don't need to make sweeping changes to your child's diet for him or her to get benefit. One thing that I have learned over the years is that relatively small improvements can reap big dividends. Weaving a bit more fruit into a child's diet, easing off the soft drinks in favour of water, and being more conscious of additives in the diet, for instance, is likely to pay off handsomely in the long term. Also, I do believe that it's better to start by making little changes and to build on these over time. Children generally acclimatise well to this sort of approach. Attempting a complete dietary revamp overnight is more likely to elicit resistance from your child, which can create unwanted stress and conflict.

Throughout the book, I have included scientific evidence for the information and advice I have given. There is now a wealth of research on nutrition and natural therapies, and I have drawn on this wherever relevant. However, at least as important as this, is that the recommendations in this book are based on what I have found to work *in practice*. For more than a decade I have had the privilege of treating countless children with a wide variety of problems. I think it is this experience, perhaps aided and abetted by the science, which has allowed me find what works and what doesn't. By distilling literally thousands of hours' worth of clinical experience with kids into this book, my sincere hope is that you will find the answers you are looking for much more quickly than it took me find them for myself.

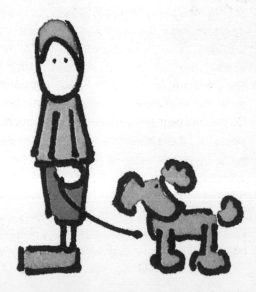

PRIMER ON NUTRITION FOR KIDS

You may intend to use this book primarily as a guide to the natural management of childhood health issues. In my experience, a healthy, balanced diet will generally go a long way to preventing and treating many of the conditions covered in the A–Z section of this book. Because of this, I have summarised here the fundamental nutritional information found in much greater detail in the second part of this book. Bearing these principles in mind will almost certainly help in the management of your child's specific problem, whatever it may be. Also, putting into practice at least some of these concepts is likely to help in the growth and development of your child, and should help to prevent many of the conditions that are common in childhood.

1 Base your child's diet on natural, unadulterated foods

Food provides the raw materials for a child's growth and development and has the capacity to protect against health issues and disease. There is a wealth of evidence that shows the most nutritious diet is one based on whole, unprocessed foods. Some of the foods that should form the basis of a child's diet include:

- Meat
- Fish
- Seafood
- Eggs
- Fruit
- Vegetables
- Nuts
- Seeds
- Beans
- Lentils

These foods are 'primal' foods that are believed to have been in the human diet for very long periods during our evolution and are therefore the foods to which the human body is best adapted.

Standard dietetic advice recommends that foods rich in saturated fat such as red meat should be avoided because they can increase the risk of conditions such as heart disease and obesity. However, the evidence shows that dietary fat is not a cause of excess weight, and there is little or no relationship between saturated fat and heart disease (see pages 154–5). Meat, fish and eggs are all valuable sources of protein that is important for normal growth and development.

Fruits, vegetables, nuts and beans are highly nutritious foods that all have a potential role to play in a healthy balanced diet for kids. These foods have a variety of health-promoting properties. Dairy products are often emphasised for children. However, these are a relatively recent addition to the human diet (see page 177–8), and foods such as milk, cheese and yoghurt quite frequently cause problems associated with what is known as food sensitivity. Common childhood health issues associated with dairy sensitivity include eczema, asthma, nasal congestion and catarrh, tonsillitis, ear infection and glue ear. See page 211 for more information on the diagnosis and treatment of food sensitivity.

Meal and snack suggestions based on the best foods for your child can be found on pages 187–91.

2 Avoid giving your child too much in the way of fast and processed food

Fast and processed foods tend to be rich

in dietary elements that can have adverse effects on health, including refined sugar (see page 149), salt (see page 161) and food additives (see page 159).

Other common ingredients in fast and processed foods are types of fats known as partially hydrogenated and 'trans' fatty acids. These fats have only been in the human diet in significant quantities for a few decades and the human body is therefore not well adapted to them. There is evidence that trans fatty acids may increase the risk of many chronic conditions, including heart disease and diabetes (see page 157–8). Trans fats are found in a wide range of foods, including commercial baked goods (biscuits, cakes, doughnuts, crackers), fast foods (e.g. burgers, fries, fried chicken) and processed foods (such as pies and ready meals). Another common source of trans fats is margarine. Butter, which is in contrast to margarine a natural and relatively unprocessed food, is a healthier option (see page 180).

3 Keep the balance towards healthy foods in your child's diet and don't worry about the occasional treats and slip-ups

It is easy to become neurotic about the range and extent of dietary hazards that your child will inevitably run into. It is nigh-on impossible to get all unhealthy foods out of a child's diet. Also, attempting to ban certain foods often leads to a child wanting them more. The key here is *balance.* In among a generally healthy diet, there is room for treats and occasional dietary indiscretions! It is worth bearing in mind that it's what children eat most of the time, not some of it, that determines the overall effect of the diet on their health.

4 Ensure your child eats regular meals, perhaps with healthy snacks in between

The main function of food is to nourish your child and ensure healthy growth and development. Regular meals help to ensure a child does not go short on key nutrients. Breakfast eating seems to be of particular importance here, with evidence showing that it is associated with better nutrition in kids, as well as improved school attendance and academic performance (see page 196). Studies have also found that the more family meals a child eats, the better his or her diet tends to be (see page 195). Family meals also appear to foster greater nutritional awareness in children, which helps them make healthy food choices for themselves.

While snacking between meals is often frowned upon, there is good evidence that it may have significant health advantages. Eating between meals provides an opportunity for children to eat health-giving foods, such as fruit and nuts, which they may not eat at other times. Snacking may also quell the appetite and help to maintain levels of sugar (the body's primary fuel) in the bloodstream. This helps to prevent over-eating at mealtime and may also reduce the risk of behavioural problems. Pages

196–7 contain more information on the benefits of snacking. Fresh fruit and nuts (see pages 169 and 175) make healthy and convenient snacks for children. Other ideas for healthy snack items can be found on pages 190–1.

5 Emphasise foods rich in healthy fats such as oily fish, nuts, seeds, olive oil and avocado

Some foods are especially rich in healthy fats known as essential fatty acids. These healthy fats in the diet come in what are known as polyunsaturated and monounsaturated forms (see page 155). Polyunsaturated fats themselves come in two main forms, known as omega-6 and omega-3 fatty acids (see page 156). There is evidence that the modern diet is generally deficient in omega-3 fats and that consuming more of them can have considerable health benefits (see page 156).

Oily fish such as salmon, trout, mackerel, herring and sardine are especially rich in omega-3 fats, which are believed to be important for brain development and may help to treat or protect against problems such as hyperactivity, dyslexia and depression. The omega-3 fats also seem to have a vital role to play in the healthy development of the foetus (see page 262). Monounsaturated fats have been linked with health effects, too, particularly with regard to the health of the heart and circulation (see page 155). Good sources of monounsaturated fats include olives, olive oil, nuts, seeds and avocado.

6 Avoid basing your child's diet on potato and refined grains such as white bread, pasta, white rice and many breakfast cereals

One strong conventional dietetic theme is for the diet to be based on starchy carbohydrates such as bread, potatoes, rice, pasta and breakfast cereals. These foods primarily provide carbohydrate for the body, which is an important source of energy. However, many starchy carbohydrates give rapid release of sugar into the bloodstream (see page 151), which can upset the body's chemistry. The consumption of these foods is increasingly being linked with a wide variety of health issues, including excess weight and diabetes (see page 204).

While there is room for potato and grains in the diet, over-emphasis of these appears to be contributing to the rising rates of obesity and diabetes in children. Refined grains, such as white bread and other foods based on white flour, white rice and pasta, are also stripped of much of their fibre and nutrients. Also, like dairy products, grains are a relatively recent addition to the human diet and are therefore foods to which we are not particularly well adapted. Wheat, the most widespread grain in the diet (it is the base ingredient in most bread, pasta, crackers, biscuits, cakes, and breakfast cereals), is a common cause of food sensitivity reactions, a health issue that is discussed in more depth on pages 211–22.

When grains are eaten, these are best had in their unrefined forms such as wholemeal bread, wholewheat pasta, brown rice and whole oats. These release sugar more slowly into the bloodstream than their refined versions, and are higher in fibre and nutrients too. Other good sources of carbohydrates in the diet include fruit, vegetables, nuts, seeds, beans and lentils.

7 Make water the principal drink for your child

Water makes up about 70 per cent of a child's body, and its consumption is important for general wellbeing (see page 158) as well as helping to prevent major illness in the long term (see pages 181–3). Some of the chemicals in tap water have been associated with significant health issues (see page 182), so it is best to filter tap water before drinking. Mineral water, which is water in its most natural and unprocessed form, is the healthiest option.

Milk is a reasonably nutritious drink, and in particular provides calcium and vitamin D for growing bones and teeth. However, a significant percentage of children do not react well to cow's milk (see pages 178–9), which may lead to a variety of problems linked with food sensitivity, including eczema, tonsillitis and ear infections. Other good sources of calcium for children include calcium fortified rice milk, nuts, green leafy vegetables and tinned fish such as sardines and salmon.

Fruit juices are not as healthy as whole fruit, partly because some healthy elements get left behind as a result of the juicing process. Also, the juicing of fruit makes the fruit sugar fructose very accessible to the body. While fructose is often thought of as a 'healthy' form of sugar, there is evidence that its excessive consumption can lead to the sorts of health issues associated with other forms of sugar in the diet (see page 150–1). Even freshly squeezed fruit juice is best diluted (about half-and-half) with water to reduce its sugariness.

Fruit drinks and fruit-flavoured drinks have very low fruit juice content and tend to be laden with refined sugar, which has been linked with a range of health issues, including tooth decay, behavioural problems and immune system suppression (see pages 149–50). Another common ingredient in these drinks is artificial sweetener. Evidence in the scientific literature has linked the most commonly used artificial sweetener – aspartame – to symptoms such as headaches and mood disturbance (see page 161). Fruit drinks and fruit-flavoured drinks may also contain other additives, some of which have been linked with health issues, including hyperactivity (see page 159).

8 Use natural methods of cooking when preparing food

Traditional methods of cooking, including baking, grilling, poaching and frying, all heat food from the outside in, in a way that has remained the same since man discovered fire tens of thousands of years ago. In contrast, microwave ovens heat food in a very different way to conventional cooking methods. Microwave is what is known as an alternating current, the effect of which is to cause food molecules to vibrate in an unnatural way. Microwaves appear to have the capacity to change the molecular structure of food. There is also some evidence that consuming microwaved food can cause undesirable changes in the blood, including a tendency to anaemia and an increase in the overall number of immune cells in the bloodstream (see page 186). Convenient though they are, it is probably wise to avoid using microwaves in the cooking and heating of food.

9 Use stealth tactics when encouraging your child to eat healthily

Many parents are keen to see their children eat healthy foods such as fruit and vegetables. However, research shows that attempting to coerce a child into eating a food tends to lead to resistance to that food (see page 200). Also, giving a food (such as chocolate or cake) as a reward tends to cause a child to want that food more in the long term (see page 198). There is also the risk that this tactic can upset a child's own internal messages that signal when he or she is full. In general, it seems that subtle tactics work best when encouraging a child to eat and enjoy a wide variety of healthy foods.

It seems to help to lead by example. Evidence suggests that when parents eat healthily, the children are more likely to follow suit and tend to need minimal encouragement to do so (see page 199). Putting some emphasis on family meals will also help to have children eat healthy foods (see page 195). When introducing a new food, it is generally best offered in small amounts and cut up small. Also, don't be put off making available to a child a food that has previously been rejected. Repeated offering, without cajoling, often gets there in the end (see page 287). You can also take heart in the fact that picky eating rarely persists for long.

10 Supplementation with nutrients is likely to have benefits for your child in the long term

Conventional dietetic wisdom dictates that children have all of their nutritional needs met by eating a healthy, balanced diet. However, ensuring a child gets the range and levels of nutrients he or she needs for optimum health and development is easier said than done. There is evidence that the levels of nutrients in the diet have declined significantly in the last 50 years. Government statistics show that many children are getting inadequate levels of key nutrients, including iron and zinc (see page 12). Nutritional supplementation can help plug any nutritional gaps left by the diet and is likely to help ensure your child's healthy growth and development. More details about supplements designed specifically with children's needs in mind can be found on pages 14–17.

Introduction

The last few years have seen an explosion of interest in natural medicine and, increasingly, parents are seeing this as a safer, gentler and more effective alternative to conventional approaches to health. In my experience, natural remedies can be a very useful adjunct to a healthy diet for many children. At the very least, vitamin and mineral supplementation can help plug the nutritional gaps that may be left by our diet and help ensure the optimum health of your child. In children with specific health issues, natural remedies have particular value. Vitamins and minerals often have their part to play here, as do therapeutic herbs. In this chapter I look at how to administer these natural therapies to your child.

This chapter also contains information about flower essences. These have traditionally been used to help correct a range of emotional issues that may trouble individuals and may also be a factor in physical illnesses. Flower essences are very gentle remedies, yet they can have a profound effect on a child's wellbeing. We'll be looking at what flower essences are and how to use them later on.

To supplement or not to supplement?

A lot of parents wonder whether they should give their child a multivitamin and mineral supplement each day. Most dieticians take the line that children will get all the nutrients they need from a healthy balanced diet. This is true in theory, but the reality may be quite different. Evidence suggests that many children do not eat ideal diets and therefore their intake of essential nutrients can fall seriously short.

The most recent data on what children eat are contained in a Government study known as the National Diet and Nutrition Survey (NDNS) conducted in 1993. This study found that, in general terms, pre-school children tend to eat a preponderance of unhealthy foods. For instance, 70 per cent of them consumed relatively unhealthy foods such as biscuits, white bread, soft drinks and savoury snacks (including crisps and cereal-based snacks), chocolate, sweets and chips during the four-day period in which they were assessed. Vegetable consumption was poor, with peas and carrots being the only cooked vegetables consumed by more than half the children. Leafy green vegetables were eaten by only 39 per cent of the children, and in fairly small quantities. And only 24 per cent ate raw vegetables or salad. Some fruit appeared in the diets of most children, but it was limited to apples, pears and bananas, and in relatively small quantities too. More detailed results are given in the box, below.

RESULTS OF THE NDNS SURVEY

A less-than-ideal diet was reflected in the children's nutrient intake.

- **Vitamin A:** About half of the children had average daily vitamin A (required, among other things, for bone growth and vision) intake below RNI (recommended nutrient intake) – 8 per cent of children aged under four years and 7 per cent of children aged four had intakes of vitamin A below the lower recommended nutrient intake (LRNI) – considered a sort of bare minimum intake level for a nutrient.
- **Vitamin D:** The average daily intakes of vitamin D (especially important for bone growth) from foods were also low. The RNI for those aged one to three years was only met by 5 per cent of the children.
- **Minerals:** These were also in short supply. The average daily intakes were well below the RNI for iron, which plays a variety of roles in the body, including as a blood builder and energy giver. 84 per cent of those under four years of age and 57 per cent of those aged four to four-and-a-half were found to have intakes of iron below the RNI. Zinc, too, was missing from the diets of many children. 72 per cent of those under four and 89 per cent of those aged four to four-and-a-half had intakes of zinc lower than RNI.

The NDNS results for older children do not make any better reading, unfortunately.

- The most commonly consumed foods by individuals aged 5–18 were white bread, savoury snacks, crisps, biscuits, boiled/mashed/jacket potatoes and chocolate confectionery – 80 per cent of children ate these foods over the week-long assessment period.
- Less than 50 per cent of boys and girls ate raw and salad vegetables. While 40 per cent ate cooked leafy green vegetables and 60 per cent ate other cooked

vegetables, a staggering 88 per cent of the sample ate chips at least once during the assessment period.

- Fizzy drinks were the most popular beverage – 75 per cent of young people drank standard carbonated soft drinks and 45 per cent drank low calorie versions.
- Up to a fifth of older girls and 12 per cent of older boys had vitamin A intakes below the 'bare minimum' LRNI.
- One fifth of older girls had intakes of riboflavin (vitamin B2) below LRNI.
- Other assessments found that there was some evidence that some children were deficient in vitamin D, vitamin C, folic acid, riboflavin and thiamine (vitamin B1). Intakes for many minerals in those aged over seven years were below the RNI, especially for zinc, potassium, magnesium, calcium, iron, iodine and copper. These are all crucial minerals required for proper growth, immunity, development and learning.

The validity of RNIs

The fact that so many children seem not to make the RNIs for one or more nutrients is an argument for supplementation in itself. However, some even question whether the RNIs are enough. Increasing numbers of nutritionists and scientists now claim that the RNIs are set too low. What the RNIs represent is the level of nutrients needed to prevent deficiency diseases and maintain normal nutrition. For instance, 60 mg of vitamin C is deemed to be the amount of this nutrient that we need to consume each day to keep us from getting scurvy. However, what may be enough to keep an obvious problem with deficiency at bay may not be what might be regarded as the amount required for *optimum* health and wellbeing.

Over the last 20 years, there has been growing evidence of the role nutrients play in preventing chronic disease. In general, the doses of nutrients that seem to be required to prevent these diseases are significantly higher than the standard RNIs. For instance, there is evidence that supplementation with 200 mcg of selenium (in adults) can dramatically reduce the risk of cancer.[1] However, in comparison, the RNI for selenium is a mere 60 mcg per day. Another problem with the RNIs is that they simply do not exist for some key nutrients, including beta-carotene, chromium, copper and manganese.

Suitable supplements for children

All-in-all, it seems that there is a good argument for giving children a supplement that contains *at least* the RNI of the key nutrients together with other nutrients for which there is no RNI. Finding a good supplement for children is not always easy, however. The ones that I use in practice are made by a company called BioCare. This company has a very good mail order service (next day delivery). (For more details, see Useful contacts and information – under BioCare.)

For children old enough or capable of taking supplements, BioCare make a very good multivitamin and mineral capsule called Kids' Complete Capsule. For children aged five or over, two capsules of this supplement each day will provide useful but safe levels of the major nutrients. This supplement does not contain calcium because this is a very bulky nutrient, and tends to make capsules too big for children to swallow comfortably. However, BioCare also make a separate calcium supplement called Kids' Calcidophilus, which also contains healthy gut bacteria. It comes in capsules that can be opened into a drink. One capsule per day provides a useful dose for most children, though those who are not having much in the way of dairy products are generally better off taking two capsules a day.

For children who are not old enough or simply won't take capsules, BioCare make a multivitamin and mineral powder that can be mixed into a drink. The base ingredient in this product, known as Kids' Complete Complex, is freeze-dried banana. Add one scoop to some milk, soya milk or rice milk each day to make a very nourishing and tasty drink. This dose is safe for all children under the age of five. Kids' Complete Complex contains calcium, so unless there's a particular need, it is not necessary to give a child a separate calcium supplement.

Kids' Complete Complex can also be used by older children who prefer not to take capsules. For children aged five or older, give two scoops a day. (For more details, see Useful contacts and information – under BioCare.)

Taking supplements

One of the concerns many individuals who take supplements have is that they may overdose on certain nutrients. This concern is often based on the assumption that the RNIs in some way represent what are deemed to be the 'safe' levels of nutrient intake. Actually, the RNIs are not intended to encompass safety issues at all. There is now a wealth of scientific literature that seeks to determine the levels of nutrients safe for human consumption. Generally, the safe daily intake for a nutrient is much higher than the RNI. Multivitamin and mineral supplements provide a good nutritional safety net, but have no potential for toxicity as long as they are taken as directed.

Specific nutrients are recommended for many of the individual ailments covered in this book. Often, the dose will be significantly higher than the RNI. Again, while the RNI may be enough to prevent an obvious deficiency of a nutrient, it may not be enough to reverse or treat an existing symptom and medical condition. The dosages recommended in this book are known to be safe over the time periods recommended (if specified).

Dosages do need to be adjusted according to the weight of the child.
- Where a treatment may apply to children of many different ages (and therefore weights), dosages are specific for a child weighing 40 kg (about 6 stones).
- If your child is say, about 20 kg (3 stones), then the recommended dose needs to be halved.
- If your child is 60 kg (just over 9 stones), then the dose needs to be multiplied by one-and-a-half.

Precise adjustment of dose is not important, as treatment with nutrients (and herbs) is generally very safe and has quite a wide margin of error.

Essential fatty acid supplements

In addition to a good quality multivitamin and mineral, another useful everyday supplement for kids is an omega-3 fat supplement. Studies suggest that these have important health effects and are particularly important for brain development and for reducing the risk of problems such as hyperactivity and depression. Omega-3 fats are generally deficient in the Western diet, and this is very likely to be the case in children who are not consuming much in the way of oily fish such as salmon, trout, mackerel, herring and sardine. More details about the importance of omega-3 fats in the diet and the problems that can ensue if a child is deficient in them can be found on page 245.

BioCare makes a supplement for kids that contains the two most important omega-3 fats, eicosapentaenoic acid (EPA) and docosahexaenoic acid (DHA). The supplement is child-friendly in that it comes in capsules much smaller than regular fish oil supplements. Children old enough to take capsules should take two capsules a day. For younger children, two capsules may be opened into food each day. EPA and DHA come from fish and (not surprisingly, therefore) have a fishy odour. For this reason, it is best to add the contents of the omega-3 capsules to a strong tasting food such as a soup, stew or casserole. (For more details, see Useful contacts and information – under BioCare.) More details about essential fatty acid supplements, including those suitable for vegetarians, can be found on page 232.

Probiotics

Probiotics are supplements of healthy gut bacteria. I find them some of the most useful supplements in practice, and offer support in a wide range of conditions, including digestive and allergic problems. One particular indication for probiotics is if a child has taken antibiotics. Antibiotics can kill healthy bacteria in the gut, which can lead to an imbalance in the ecosystem there. This, in turn, can lead to various problems, including an overgrowth of yeast organisms such as *Candida albicans* (see page 223), an increased risk of food sensitivity (see page 211) and irritable bowel syndrome (see page 103). Taking a probiotic supplement after antibiotics can help restore bacteria in the gut, and reduce the risk of these and other complications.

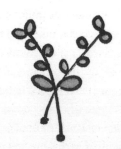

Probiotics for children under the age of 2

The bacteria in the gut come in many different forms. In early life, before the age of about two, one of the predominant and most important strains of bacteria is known as *Bifidobacterium infantis*. The product INT B1 contains this organism and is ideal for children under the age of two. It should be given at a dose of ½ tsp (about 1 g) in water, each day for one to two months. (For more details, see Useful contacts and information – under BioCare.)

For older children

Over the age of two years, organisms by the name of *Lactobacillus acidophilus* and *Bifidobacterium bifidum* are the predominant organisms in the gut. The product Strawberry Acidophilus contains both these strains of bacteria in a base of freeze-dried strawberry. This can be added to water or milk, soya milk or rice milk at a dose of ½ tsp a day. This should be given for one to two months. (For more details, see Useful contacts and information – under BioCare.)

Herbal remedies

Herbal remedies have been growing in popularity in the UK over the last decade or so, and for good reason. Plant extracts very often offer cheap, safe and effective alternatives to conventional drugs. One important quality medicinal herbs have is that they contain literally dozens, possibly hundreds, of different substances. This means they generally have a broader-ranging and more balanced effect in the body than conventional drugs (that normally contain only one active ingredient), and are less likely to have side effects too.

Herbal remedies come in a number of different forms, including tinctures (alcoholic extracts), tablets and capsules. My preference is always to use tinctures, if possible. Part of the reason for this is that not all children like or are able to take tablets or capsules. Also, the plant components in tinctures are generally more accessible to the body than they are in tablets and capsules.

Good quality herbal remedies are normally available in health food stores. Independently-owned health food stores often have good supplement sections and someone on hand who is knowledgeable about remedies. Alternatively, advice may be sought from a qualified herbal medicine practitioner. (For more help, see Useful contacts and information.)

COMMON HERBS AND THEIR USES

Herb name	What's it for?	Side effects and cautions	Standard dose for 40 kg child
Agnus castus	Pre-menstrual syndrome	None known	40 drops of tincture taken in the morning
Echinacea purpurea and Echinacea angustifolia	As an immune stimulant for the treatment of infections such as cold, flu, bronchiolitis, sore throats and croup	Should not be used in children who have an allergy to flowers in the daisy family	15–20 drops of tincture, every two to three hours on the first day of the illness, followed by dosing three to four times a day for the next 10–14 days
Feverfew (*Tanacetum parthenium*)	Migraine headaches	Should not be used in children under the age of two years	125 mcg of parthenolide (one of fever-few's active ingredients) in the morning
Garlic (*Allium sativum*)	Antimicrobial action and immune support	Not to be used around the time of surgery because of its anti-blood-clotting activity	Variable
Ginger (*Zingiber officinale*)	For nausea and vomiting and as a natural anti-inflammatory	May cause indigestion	For nausea, 125 mg, taken every three hours or 5 drops of 1:2 tincture taken in water, three times a day
Ginkgo biloba	Circulatory stimulant	May cause mild stomach upset or headaches	20–40 mg of standardised extract, taken three times a day
Gotu kola (*Centella asiatica*)	Wound healing	None known	30 mg of standardised extract 1–2 times a day or 2–3 mls of tincture 3 times a day
Gymnema sylvestre	Diabetes and general blood sugar balance issues	In diabetes, to be used under the supervision of a doctor	200 mg of extract per day
Oregon grape (*Mahonia aquifolium*)	Blepharitis, conjunctivitis and psoriasis	Long term use should be under the supervision of a herbalist	15 drops of tincture, three times a day
Milk thistle (*Silybum marianum*)	Liver support and general detoxification	None known	140 mg of silymarin (the main active ingredient in milk thistle) per day
St John's wort (*Hypericum perforatum*)	Depression and anxiety	Should not be taken with other anti-depressant drugs unless under the supervision of a doctor	150 mg of extract, three times a day
Valerian (*Valeriana officinalis*)	Insomnia	None known	150–250 mg of extract, 30–60 minutes before bedtime

Flower essences

Flower essences, or flower remedies, as they are more commonly known, are usually made by putting a specific flower or plant in a bowl of water and exposing that to sunlight. It is believed that subtle energies from the plant are 'imprinted' on the water, which then can exert a healing effect in the body if taken as a remedy. In this way, many therapists believe that flower remedies contain the energy or 'memory' of the plant from which it was made and work in a similar way to homeopathic remedies – on a subtle level. In practice, flower essences are primarily used to dissolve negative emotions and thought patterns. This may have very positive effects on the psychological wellbeing of a child, though it can also be reflected in better physical health too.

Flower remedies are ideal for home use and are simple to use. They are made in water and preserved in alcohol. Some parents are concerned about using a remedy preserved in brandy or another alcohol, but the amount of alcohol that is taken with a remedy is tiny. Another option is to rub the remedy into the skin (the front of the wrists near where the pulse can be felt is a good site) or put the remedy in the bath.

The Bach flower remedies

Some of the most commonly used flower essences are known as the Bach (pronounced 'batch') flower remedies. Back in the 1930s, Dr Edward Bach developed 38 individual remedies, which are really a cornerstone of flower essence therapy. They are widely available in health food stores and pharmacies and are an excellent starting point for any parent keen to use flower essences in their child.

Dr Bach developed his 38 remedies with a view to supporting every conceivable personality, attitude and negative state of mind. They were developed as a complete system and, before his death, Bach gave instructions that no more remedies were to be added to the set. The remedies were devised for self-help and most users find their simplicity appealing.

Flower remedies can complement other types of therapies such as herbalism and nutritional therapy, or can be used alone. In general terms, the remedies can be used to:

- Address a particular reoccurring emotional or behavioural pattern

- Give support in times of crisis
- Treat the emotional symptoms produced by illness
- Help prevent or treat illness by identifying negative emotional states that may be underlying factors in that illness.

THE BACH FLOWER REMEDIES AND THEIR INDICATIONS

Bach flower remedy	Emotional state
Agrimony	For those who hide their feelings behind humour and put on a brave face.
Aspen	For fear of the unknown. Vague, unsettling fears that cannot be explained.
Beech	For the perfectionist who tends to be intolerant of other people's methods and experience.
Centaury	For those who find it impossible to say no to others' demands and thus exhaust themselves by doing too much.
Cerato	For those who lack confidence in themselves and are constantly seeking the advice of others.
Cherry Plum	For the fear of losing the mind and having irrational thoughts or behaviour.
Chestnut Bud	For those who find it hard to learn from life and keep making the same mistakes.
Chicory	For the self-obsessed, mothering type who is overprotective and possessive.
Clematis	For the absent-minded day-dreamer who needs to be awake and have the mind focused on the here and now.
Crab Apple	For those who feel unclean or polluted on any level, physical, emotional or spiritual. For those who need a purification ritual.
Elm	For those who suffer temporary feelings of inadequacy brought on by their high expectations of themselves.
Gentian	For despondency and those who are easily discouraged and set back in life. Pessimism.
Gorse	For those who suffer hopelessness and despair after a long struggle and who are stuck in a negative pattern.
Heather	For those who like to be the centre of things and talk constantly about themselves. Poor listeners.
Holly	For those who develop the victim mentality and suffer bouts of anger, jealously and envy.
Honeysuckle	For those who suffer from nostalgia or who dwell in the past to escape a painful future.
Hornbeam	For those who are stuck in a rut and exhausted so that work which used to be fulfilling is now tiresome.

Bach flower remedy	Emotional state
Impatiens	For impatience and irritability. For those who are always in a rush and are too busy to slow down.
Larch	For those who feel worthless and who are suffering from lack of confidence or low self-esteem.
Mimulus	For the fear of known things. For the strength to face everyday fears and all fears that can be named, for example the fear of flying.
Mustard	For depression and those who feel they are under a dark gloomy cloud, for no apparent reason.
Oak	For the fighter who never gives in and is exhausted by being too narrow minded in the same old fight.
Olive	For those who are exhausted on all levels. Fatigued and drained of further optimism and spirit.
Pine	For those who suffer self-reproach and guilt. For those who say sorry, even if things are not their fault.
Red Chestnut	For those who are overanxious for the welfare of family or friends.
Rock Rose	For those who feel helpless and experience terror or panic. There may or may not be a reason but the feeling is real.
Rock Water	For perfectionists who are hard on themselves and demand perfection in all things.
Scleranthus	For those who suffer from indecision and who cannot make up their mind.
Star of Bethlehem	For shocks of all kind, accidents, bad news, sudden startling noise and trauma.
Sweet Chestnut	For utter despair and hopelessness, for when there seems no way out.
Vervain	For over-straining and stress. For the perfectionist, hard on themselves and over-strained by trying to meet their own exacting ideals.
Vine	For the over strong and dominating leader who may tend towards tyranny. For bullying.
Walnut	For change. For breaking links so that life may develop in another direction.
Water Violet	For people who are aloof, self-reliant and self-contained. To relax the reserved and enable sharing.
White Chestnut	For tiresome mental chatter and the overactive mind, full or persistent and unwanted patterns of thought.
Wild Oat	For those who need help in deciding on their path and purpose of their life.
Wild Rose	For those who drift through life resigned to accept any eventuality. Fatalists.
Willow	For those who feel they have been treated unfairly. For pessimism and self-pity.

Making and taking flower remedy blends

You'll need:

- 30 ml amber glass dropper bottle
- 30 ml spring water or 10 ml brandy and 20 ml spring water
- Bottles of the remedies you have chosen

Put 4 drops of each individual remedy into a clean dropper bottle and fill with clean spring water. The remedies should be used within a week or so, and kept in the refrigerator. If you want to keep the personal blend for longer, you can add 10 ml of brandy before filling with spring water as this helps preserve the mixture.

Dosing

Flower essences are generally best taken direct from the dropper, under the tongue. The standard dose is 2–3 drops, given four to six times each day for four to six weeks. After this, or even before, it is a good idea to review your child and see if you think a change to the remedies is in order. Don't be afraid to experiment – remember, flower essences are very gentle remedies and perfectly safe for children of all ages.

RESCUE REMEDY

In addition to the 38 remedies outlined above, Dr Bach also developed something called Rescue Remedy (also called Five-Flower Essence). This is made from equal amounts of the five following essences:

- Cherry plum – for feelings of desperation
- Rock rose – to ease terror, fear or panic
- Impatiens – to soothe irritability and tension
- Clematis – to counteract the tendency to drift away from the present
- Star of Bethlehem – to address the mental and physical symptoms of shock

Rescue Remedy is generally used for occasions when there is acute stress, injury, shock or trauma.

HOW TO CHOOSE REMEDIES

If you are new to flower essences, then a good starting point is simply to scan the list of indications on pages 20–1 for individual remedies. As you do this, make a note of any characteristics that seem to match your child's mood and/or behaviour. At the end of this, it may seem that one remedy seems perfect for your child. However, it is also likely that you will have a list of two or more remedies that seem appropriate. This is fine, because it is perfectly OK (in fact, encouraged) to administer a blend of remedies made up for an individual child's specific needs. Many individuals will settle on three to five remedies that seem to be most suitable for a child's needs. You do not need to concern yourself about toxicity or potential interactions between remedies. Flower essences are not like drugs: they have no side effects and are non-toxic. The very worst that can happen is that they don't work.

A FEW POINTERS
While choosing flower essences is an individual affair, some emotional problems are quite common in children. Here is a list of some of the more frequent emotional issues and some suggestions for remedies.

- For a child who is **afraid of something 'known'** such as the dark, cats or school, try Mimulus. This is also a good remedy for stage fright, fear of public speaking or exam nerves.
- For a child who seems **afraid, but seems not to know why,** try Aspen.
- For a child who seems unduly **concerned about the safety of others,** such as her parents or siblings, try Red Chestnut.
- If your child has been unwell and now seems **rundown, and lacking in energy and enthusiasm,** try Olive.
- If your child is experiencing (and perhaps struggling with) **change,** such as a new school or teachers, a parental divorce or a friend moving away, offer Walnut.
- For an **impatient** child, who cannot seem to accept life's pace, his own shortcomings or those of others, try Impatiens.
- For a child who seems to have a **problem with finishing things,** including homework, projects, or even a board game, try Chestnut Bud.
- For a child who likes to be the centre of attention, but may be a **poor listener,** try Heather.
- For a hysterical child who seems to be **seeking attention,** try Chicory.
- For a child who seems unduly **angry or aggressive,** try Holly or Vine.
- For a child who seems **critical and judgmental,** try Beech.
- For a child prone to **temper tantrums,** try Cherry Plum.
- For a **homesick** child, try Walnut and Honeysuckle.
- For a child who has **difficulty getting up in the morning,** try Hornbeam.

- For a child who is **upset by the prospect of going to school,** try Honeysuckle.
- For a child who is prone to **nightmares,** try Rescue Remedy and Rock Rose.
- For a **distracted child** who seems to have his head in the clouds, try Clematis.
- For a child who appears to be **lacking interest,** try Wild Oat and Wild Rose.
- For a child who is **envious,** and seems to want to emulate other children, try Cerato.
- For a **jealous** child, try Holly.
- For a child who is **jealous and also possessive,** try Chicory.
- For a child who is **afraid of failure** and has adopted a pessimistic attitude, try Larch.
- For a child who seems to be **traumatised by recent failure,** try Gentian.
- For a child who seems to have **not recovered from a past failure,** try Star of Bethlehem.

OTHER FLOWER ESSENCES

The 38 Bach flower essences are only 38 of hundreds of remedies available from all over the world, including Australia, Africa, Brazil and Japan. The Bush flower essences (from Australia) are now widely available here in the UK and I tend to use quite a lot of them (in addition to the Bach remedies) in practice. Throughout the book, I have recommended flower essences for specific conditions where appropriate.

AVAILABILITY

The Bach flower essences are readily available in health food stores and many pharmacies. Other ranges, including the Australian Bush flower essences, are also becoming increasingly available. A very wide selection of flower remedies can be had from The International Flower Essence Repertoire. (For more details, see Useful contacts and information.)

OTHER RESOURCES

There are many books on the subject of flower remedies. However, my personal favourite because it is written in such a clear and useful way is *The Lazy Person's Guide to Emotional Healing* by Dr Andrew Tressider (Newleaf).

Key points

- Natural remedies are often effective in the prevention and treatment of physical and emotional problems.
- Supplementation with a multivitamin and mineral (as an adjunct to a healthy diet) is likely to help ensure a child gets the nutrients needed for optimum health.
- Essential fatty acid supplements, particularly those rich in omega-3 fats, may also help maintain health and wellbeing.
- Supplements of healthy gut bacteria (probiotics) have a variety of uses, but are particularly useful if a child has been treated with antibiotics.
- Herbal remedies often offer safer and gentler alternatives to conventional medication.
- Flower essences can be very useful in the treatment of emotional and behavioural problems, and have a role to play in the treatment of physical illness too.

Part
two

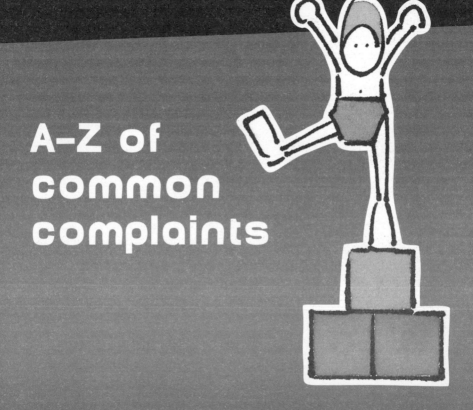

A–Z of common complaints

Acne

Acne is caused by blockages in the glands responsible for making a skin-waterproofing agent called sebum. Acne is common in adolescence, when surges in hormones (especially testosterone) can bring on spots by increasing sebum secretion. In some adolescent girls, acne can be the result of a condition known as polycystic ovarian syndrome (PCOS). In this situation, the acne may be associated with other symptoms, including irregular periods and hirsutism (excess hair growth on the face or body). See 'Polycystic Ovarian Syndrome' for more details about this condition.

Diet
Carbohydrates
Traditionally, the risk of acne is said to be related to the over-consumption of fat in the diet. However, there is emerging evidence that the high prevalence of acne in the West is related to a high intake of refined sugars and starches in foods such as sweets, cakes, chocolates, biscuits, muffins, white bread and many breakfast cereals. These tend to cause the body to secrete copious quantities of the hormone insulin. Studies suggest that insulin and hormones related to insulin can increase the levels of 'male' hormones that predispose to acne.[1] Reducing the carbohydrate content of the diet, particularly those foods that tend to cause excessive amounts of insulin to be secreted, may therefore help to control acne in time. More details about this dietary approach can be found on pages 149–51.

Fats and other components
In natural medicine, acne is often viewed as a problem of excess toxicity within the body. For this reason, sufferers are often advised to eat as 'clean' a diet as possible. This means avoiding foods that contain significant quantities of fat (particularly what are known as 'partially hydrogenated' and 'trans fatty acids' found in many margarines and most fast, baked and processed foods). Other food components to avoid include artificial colourings, flavourings, preservatives and sweeteners. More information on the fundamentals of eating a diet low in chemical and potentially toxic ingredients can be found on pages 159–61.

Yeast
A common factor in acne is overgrowth of yeast organisms such as *Candida albicans*. Identification and successful treatment of this problem almost always leads to a significant improvement in skin condition. More information about the diagnosis and treatment of yeast overgrowth can be found on pages 223–48.

Supplements
Zinc
Certain nutrients may be useful in controlling acne. The mineral zinc has been found to help acne sufferers.[2] One study found that zinc therapy worked as well as antibiotic medication.[3] I generally recommend acne sufferers take 30 mg of zinc, twice a day for three to four months, after which the dose can be reduced to once a day. Studies show that zinc therapy takes time to work, with 12

weeks being the amount of time generally needed to see good results. My preference is to use a form of zinc that is readily absorbed by the body such as zinc citrate or zinc picolinate. Because zinc can induce copper deficiency, 1 mg of copper should be taken for every 15 mg of supplemental zinc.

Pre-menstrual acne and Agnus castus

Some girls find their acne tends to flare-up before a period, a condition that is often referred to as 'pre-menstrual acne'. This sort of acne is often helped by taking 50 mg of vitamin B6 each day.[4] The herb *Agnus castus,* probably through its hormone-balancing effects, has also been found to be of benefit.[5]

Flower essences

• The Bach flower essence Crab Apple is useful for children who feel **'unclean' or 'dirty'** as a result of their acne.

Allergy

See 'Anaphylactic shock', 'Asthma', 'Bites and stings', 'Eczema' and 'Hives'

Anaemia and iron deficiency

Oxygen is transported around the body by a substance called haemoglobin contained in the red blood cells. If the level of haemoglobin in the blood falls, oxygen may not be delivered efficiently to the tissues. A shortage of haemoglobin – the medical term for which is 'anaemia' – can give rise to potentially debilitating symptoms, including fatigue, easy tiring on exercise, mental sluggishness and depression.

The most common cause of anaemia is iron deficiency. Iron is essential for the manufacture of haemoglobin and actually makes up 60–70 per cent of the haemoglobin molecule. Statistics show that iron deficiency is one of the more common nutritional deficiencies in children. Vegetarian and vegan children are at increased risk of anaemia (their intake of iron is generally lower than that of meat-eaters). Menstruating girls are also at risk of anaemia due to the loss of blood each month.

Blood testing for anaemia and iron deficiency

The conventional test for anaemia is a blood test known as the full blood count. The full blood count measures the haemoglobin level (a lower than normal level of this indicates anaemia) along with other measurements, including the average size of the red blood cells and the average amount of haemoglobin they contain. These measurements can be useful in determining the precise nature of an anaemia problem. Individuals with iron deficiency anaemia tend to have smaller than normal red blood cells that contain lower than normal amounts of haemoglobin.

Sometimes, it can be useful to take a direct measurement of the amount of iron in the body. Doctors often use a test known as the serum iron for this, which is basically a measure of the amount of iron circulating in the bloodstream. This test, though commonly used, is not thought to provide a good measure of overall amount of iron in the body. It is generally recognised that the best test to gauge iron stores is to measure the level of a substance called 'ferritin'. Low ferritin levels strongly suggest that the body is deficient in iron.

It is important to bear in mind that a child may be iron deficient but not anaemic. However, iron deficiency, even without anaemia, can cause problems with fatigue and low mood. This means that checking ferritin levels is important as part of any investigations for anaemia. Even when haemoglobin levels are normal, individuals with a low ferritin level will generally benefit from treatment with iron.

Diet
Iron
Individuals with iron-deficiency anaemia generally do well to increase their consumption of iron-rich foods. The iron found in animal products such as red meat, liver (this is best eaten in an organic form), oysters and fish is what is called haem-iron. This form of iron is bound to protein and tends to be well absorbed and utilised by the body. While non-animal foods such as green leafy vegetables and dried fruit contain iron, the form that is found in these foodstuffs (non-haem iron) does not appear to be especially useful for the

body. Sufferers of iron deficiency should avoid coffee and tea, as these can reduce the amount of iron absorbed from the diet and/or supplements.

Supplements
Iron
Supplementation with iron can often be very beneficial for individuals suffering from iron deficiency or iron deficiency anaemia. The recommended daily allowance for iron is 14 mg per day, though higher doses are generally recommenDed for individuals attempting to correct a specific deficiency. Dosages of 25–100 mg per day are not uncommon, though these need to be adjusted according to a child's circumstances, clinical symptoms and the ferritin level (see box, on left).

Different forms of iron supplements
The most commonly prescribed form of iron is iron sulphate (ferrous sulphate), which is not very well absorbed and notorious for giving rise to gastrointestinal symptoms such as nausea and constipation. More absorbable and less troublesome forms of iron include iron fumarate, iron citrate, iron picolinate and iron gluconate (the form of iron found in the most popular over-the-counter liquid iron preparations).

Caution with iron
Iron is what is known as an oxidising agent, having quite the opposite effect of antioxidant nutrients such as vitamins C and E, which protect against disease. Some research suggests that high doses of iron

induce changes that, at least theoretically, would increase the risk of heart disease. Also, a small percentage of the population suffer from a condition known as haemochromatosis in which iron tends to accumulate in the body, depositing itself in various organs. More common in males than females, haemochromatosis can lead to problems with diabetes, cirrhosis of the liver and heart rhythm abnormalities. Before supplementing with significant doses of iron, it is important to have ferritin levels checked first (see box, opposite).

Anaphylactic shock

Anaphylactic shock is a severe and violent allergic response that may occur as a result of exposure to a provoking agent such as a food (e.g. peanuts), food additive, medicine, chemical, or insect bite or sting.

Anaphylactic shock may cause severe breathing problems, swelling in the throat and very low blood pressure, and can be life-threatening. It should always be treated as a medical emergency. Conventional medical treatments for anaphylactic shock centre around adrenaline, antihistamines (anaphylactic shock is caused by the secretion of histamine in the body) and sometimes steroids. Children who are prone to this condition are often advised to have an adrenaline injection near to hand for use in emergencies.

Supplements
Vitamin C

There is some evidence that high doses of vitamin C can treat anaphylactic shock. A number of studies have shown that vitamin C has antihistamine action. Some naturally-oriented doctors have reported that giving several grams of vitamin C at the first sign of a severe allergic reaction can reduce its severity or stop it altogether. The best way to administer this is to dissolve 5–10 g of vitamin C powder in water before drinking. This might possibly cause some stomach upset (diarrhoea and bloating), but this generally passes quite quickly.

Vitamin C should not be considered as an alternative to conventional medical treatments. It is, nonetheless, a potentially useful treatment that may be administered in addition to conventional treatment, and may help start the healing process even before there is access to appropriate medical care. It is a good idea to ensure that a small bottle of water with 5–10 g of vitamin C dissolved in it is ready to hand if your child has suffered from a severe allergic reaction in the past.

Angular stomatitis

Angular stomatitis is a condition characterised by cracking at the corners of the mouth. It is often a painful condition that can make talking and eating quite uncomfortable. Angular stomatitis is usually caused by a deficiency in one or more nutrients. Sometimes, it is associated with iron deficiency. The best test for iron deficiency is a blood test for a substance known as 'ferritin'. Because iron can have damaging effects in the body at high levels, it is advisable for any child or adolescent to have a ferritin test before supplementing with significant quantities of iron (see pages 29–30).

Diet
B-complex

Another factor that seems to be common in angular stomatitis is a deficiency in the B group vitamins, particularly vitamins B2 and B6. In general, the diet should be rich in foods that contain vitamins B2 and B6, such as wholemeal bread, green leafy vegetables, eggs and fish.

Supplements
B-complex

It may also help to take a B-complex supplement each day containing about 25 mg of the major B vitamins B1, B2, B3, B5 and B6 (for a 40 kg child). On this regime, angular stomatitis usually clears within a few weeks.

Anorexia nervosa

Anorexia nervosa is a form of eating disorder characterised by extreme weight loss, an intense fear of becoming fat and an altered body image. Typically, anorexics are painfully thin, but actually perceive themselves to be overweight. Anorexia may be related to emotional issues such as problems with relationships in the family, feelings of deprivation and abuse. However, physiological and biochemical factors appear to play their part too.

Supplements
Multivitamins and minerals

It comes as no surprise that anorexia can lead to severe deficiencies of dietary elements such as protein, iron, calcium, B vitamins, folic acid and vitamin C. Taking a potent multivitamin and mineral supplement is one simple thing that sufferers can do to correct these deficiencies. Details of specific supplements can be found on pages 14–17.

Zinc

One nutrient that appears to have particular benefit in anorexia is the mineral zinc. Zinc has many important functions in the body, and one of these appears to be the normalisation of brain function and perception. In one study, a daily dose of 45–90 mg of zinc led to weight gain in 17 out of 20 anorexics after periods ranging between eight and 56 months.[6] In a double-blind study, 14 mg of zinc per day doubled the speed of weight increase in a group of anorexic women.[7]

I generally recommend that in addition to a good quality multivitamin and mineral, anorexics also take 45–90 mg of zinc per day. Because zinc can induce copper deficiency, 1 mg of copper should be taken with each 15 mg of supplemental zinc. Once improvement is seen, the dose of zinc may be reduced, and more emphasis may be placed on a nutritious, varied diet as outlined on pages 187–91.

Flower essences
• Loquat essence (a South African flower remedy) is indicated for anorexia.

Anxiety

Many kids, like adults, can be prone to bouts of anxiety or nervousness. While these may be a natural response to the ups and downs of growing up, they might also be caused by specific pressures at home or school such as sibling rivalry or bullying. Encouraging a child to talk about what it is that's troubling them, and offering support and comfort, is a good first step in overcoming problems with anxiety. However, while emotional factors and specific events or situations in a child's life may be causing anxiety, it is also true that biochemical and nutritional factors can also play a part. Dietary and other natural approaches can often be very effective in restoring a state of calm to an anxious child.

Diet

Caffeine

Caffeine is well known for its stimulant effects and its ability to provoke anxiety. In adults prone to anxiety, it seems that as little as one cup of coffee can increase feelings of anxiety. While children may not be regular drinkers of double espresso, they can nonetheless get a fair dose of caffeine from fizzy drinks such as cola and, to a lesser degree, from chocolate. Some evidence suggests that small doses of caffeine taken throughout the day can have as much effect on anxiety as a single large dose.[8] Another study found that even a small intake of caffeine can exaggerate the response to stressful events of normal daily life.[9] The bottom line is that children who are anxious are generally better off without caffeine.

Cutting out caffeinated fizzy drinks is a good starting point. Decaffeinated carbonated drinks are not a particularly healthy alternative, however, because they may contain other potentially harmful ingredients, including sugar and aspartame (see page 161). Tea and coffee both contain caffeine and other stimulants, and are therefore best avoided too.

Hypoglycaemia and anxiety

One of the hormones responsible for feelings of anxiety and nervousness is adrenaline. While this may be secreted in the body in response to emotional stress, certain physiological changes will tend to stimulate this too. A major cause of adrenaline release in the body is low levels of sugar in the bloodstream, also known as hypoglycaemia. When blood sugar levels are very low, adrenaline is secreted, which helps restore blood sugar levels by stimulating the conversion of a substance called glycogen (a form of starch) in the liver into sugar. While adrenaline can help pick up blood sugar levels, it can also induce feelings of anxiety, nervousness or even panic. One study found that symptoms of hypoglycaemia could include trembling, palpitations, anxiety, sweating and hunger.[10]

If your child is prone to mood swings and cravings for sweet foods, this suggests a problem with blood sugar imbalance. The steps that may be taken to stabilise blood sugar levels are covered in detail on pages 204–10. In brief, however, the diet

---

should be based on foods that give relatively sustained releases of sugar into the bloodstream such as meat, fish, eggs, fruit, vegetables, beans, pulses and wholegrain starches. Regular meals and healthy snacks such as fresh fruit and nuts taken between meals are likely to help too.

Supplements

Magnesium

Magnesium plays a particularly important role in the regulation of mood and excitability and seems to have a calming and soothing effect on the nervous system. Many children have lower-than-ideal intakes of magnesium and a deficiency of this mineral can worsen feelings of anxiety. There is some evidence that our need for magnesium increases under stress.[11] Other research also points to magnesium as a valuable agent in the treatment of panic attacks, sleep disturbance and anxiety states.[12]

Given the increasing stress that many children seem to be under and the fact that magnesium tends to be deficient in the diet, making sure a child gets adequate amounts of this precious nutrient is of prime importance, especially in children prone to anxiety. In addition to eating plenty of magnesium-rich foods such as green leafy vegetables, nuts, seeds, beans and pulses, supplementation may also be useful. I recommend 150–250 mg of magnesium per day (for a 40 kg child).

Selenium

The mineral selenium seems to have an important effect on mood, with one study finding that supplementation with this nutrient on a daily basis brought about a general elevation of mood and a decrease in anxiety.[13] Unfortunately, most of the UK population have selenium intakes that are well below the recommended amount (see page 165). To help ensure your child gets enough of this nutrient, it helps to include some Brazil nuts, wholegrains (e.g. wholemeal bread and brown rice) and broccoli in their diet. Supplementation, as part of a multivitamin and mineral preparation, is also likely to ensure a child gets adequate amounts of selenium.

Multivitamins and minerals

While sometimes there is a need for supplementation with specific nutrients in kids, a better approach might be to use a good quality multivitamin and mineral. This is generally simpler and more cost-effective than supplementing a range of single nutrients and also helps to ensure a child gets enough of the whole complement of vital nutrients. Supplementing with a multivitamin and mineral has been found to bring broad benefits for children. For instance, one study found that adolescent boys given a multivitamin had consistent reductions in anxiety and perceived stress. Not only that, but they also tended to rate themselves as less tired and better able to concentrate following treatment.[14] A good multivitamin and mineral is quite likely to reduce a child's tendency to anxiety by helping to put blood sugar levels on an even keel. See pages 14–17 for information on specific supplements.

Flower essences

Flower essences were first developed with emotional issues in mind, so it's no wonder that several of them seem to offer significant benefits for those prone to anxiety. A guide to a range of flower essences and their indications can be found on pages 20–7. Some of the most commonly used flower essences for anxiety are:

• Elm for **anxiety** accompanying feelings of being unable to cope
• Mimulus for a child who is **anxious** because of something 'known', such as the dark, cats or school. This is also a good remedy for stage fright, fear of public speaking or exam nerves
• Aspen if there is **no apparent reason for the anxiety** (perhaps it's just an emotion that a child can't attribute to any one cause)
• Rescue Remedy for times of **extreme stress** (e.g. an examination or visit to the dentist), or if anxiety seems unbearable.

Appendicitis

Appendicitis is a condition caused by infection and inflammation in the appendix – a thin, tube-shaped structure that protrudes from the first section of the large intestine. The symptoms of appendicitis usually begin with pain around the belly button, which generally becomes worse over several hours and then tends to move to the lower right-hand side of the abdomen. This area is likely to be very tender, even to light pressure, and a child will usually try to protect it by lying on one side and drawing the knees up towards his or her chest.

An inflamed appendix can burst, causing a life-threatening infection of the abdominal wall (peritonitis). Appendicitis is a medical emergency and will usually require an operation under general anaesthetic. If you suspect your child has appendicitis, it is important to seek medical attention. Avoid giving your child anything to eat or drink, as this may delay an operation if this is deemed necessary. After the operation, natural approaches may help the healing process and prevent scarring. See 'Surgery – recovery from' and 'Scarring'.

Preventing appendicitis

There's an old adage: an ounce of prevention is worth a pound of cure, and this is certainly true for any condition that may require emergency surgery. Plenty of fibre in a child's diet is important for the prevention of appendicitis. It is thought that many blockages of the appendix are caused by hardened faeces. Keeping children 'regular', and avoiding constipation by increasing fibre in the diet can help to prevent anything from being lodged in the appendix. According to research, a lower fibre intake may be the cause of appendicitis in 70 per cent of cases.[15] This study also found that children who had suffered from appendicitis were more likely to be constipated. Apart from a diet rich in fibre (fruits and vegetables, wholegrains, beans, pulses and nuts and seeds), the other essential ingredient for bowel regularity is water (dehydration can cause faeces to stick in the colon like a cork in the neck of a wine bottle). For more information about natural approaches to bowel regularity, see 'Constipation'.

Flower essences

Because constipation increases the likelihood of appendicitis occurring, it's worth looking at some of the emotional reasons why it can occur. Some children, for example, are embarrassed by bowel movements and find the whole process 'unclean', thereby holding movements for as long as possible.
• In this case, you might try the Bach flower remedy Crab Apple in your child, as this can help to dissolve feelings of **uncleanliness.**

Asthma

Asthma is a chronic (long-term) lung condition characterised by recurrent attacks of breathlessness, often accompanied by wheezing. Asthma is caused by inflammation in the air passages of the lungs. These passages will then tend to become constricted (known as 'bronchospasm'), which makes breathing difficult. Asthma can be classified into two main types: extrinsic, in which attacks are triggered by an allergy, and intrinsic, in which there is no obvious external cause for attacks. Extrinsic or 'allergic' asthma

tends to come on during childhood, while intrinsic asthma usually develops later in life. However, either condition can appear at any age.

Diet
Food sensitivity

Allergic asthma is often set off by an inhaled trigger such as animal fur, dust, feathers and air pollutants. However, there is also good evidence that asthma attacks can be linked to certain foods, especially in childhood. One study showed that 90 per cent of children with asthma or allergic rhinitis (runny nose due to allergy) improved on a food elimination programme.[16] The most common offenders in this respect are dairy products, eggs, chocolate, wheat, corn, citrus fruits and fish. More information about the detection and elimination of problem foods can be found on pages 211–22.

Fatty acids

It is well known that certain foodstuffs may promote inflammation in the body, which can then perhaps contribute to asthma and other allergic conditions such as eczema. Some of the foods that may do this are what are known as the omega-6 fatty acids. Omega-6 fats are generally found in quantity in margarine and vegetable oils such as sunflower, safflower and corn oil. They are also found in processed and fast foods. Omega-6 fats are known to be converted in the body into substances that tend to encourage inflammation in the body. On the other hand, fats of the omega-3 type, such as those found in oily fish, appear to have the ability to reduce inflammation in the body.

Some scientists have suggested that an increased consumption of omega-6 fats, coupled with a decreased consumption of omega-3 fats, might increase the risk of asthma. One study noted that the increasing rates of asthma in Australia appeared to be mirrored with a five-fold increase of intake of polyunsaturated fats, particularly of the omega-6 type.[17] This research also drew attention to the increased consumption of these fats in New Zealand, the United States and the UK, all places where asthma rates are rising significantly. In contrast, countries where consumption of omega-3 fatty acids is high and omega-6 fats is low (such as Mediterranean and Scandinavian nations) have low rates of asthma. Research has also found that asthma symptoms appear to be better controlled in children who consume oily fish.[18] Avoidance of margarine and vegetable oils, and the inclusion of oily fish, such as salmon, trout, mackerel, herring and sardine, in the diet may possibly help control asthma symptoms in time.

Salt

There is also some evidence linking salt consumption with asthma. Salt appears to heighten the airways' response to histamine, causing increased constriction.[19] Asthmatics should therefore avoid adding salt to their food during cooking or at the table and minimise their consumption of processed foods, which tend to have a lot of salt already added. Other substances that seem to have the ability to provoke asthma include tartrazine (a yellow colouring found in some processed foods) and sulphites (used as a preservative in many alcoholic drinks and processed foods). More details about food additives can be found on pages 159–60.

Supplements

Magnesium

The mineral magnesium can be a useful supplement for asthmatics. Magnesium can help prevent the bronchi going into spasm and might also help to prevent histamine release.[20] Giving 150–250 mg per day for a 40 kg child is a good dose.

Vitamin B6

Vitamin B6 is often deficient in asthmatics and in one study the supplementation with this nutrient has been found to be beneficial in children.[21] The dose in the study in children was 200 mg per day. Because there is a slight risk of neurological symptoms at this dose, I recommend children on this regime be monitored by a medical practitioner.

The Buteyko Method

The Buteyko Method is a specific breathing exercise that was developed in the 1940s. It is based on the principle that many of us breathe more quickly than we should (hyperventilation). This lowers levels of carbon dioxide in the blood, which actually reduces the delivery of oxygen to the body's tissues. The Buteyko Method teaches individuals how to slow their breathing, and this can be highly effective in combating asthma. While classes in the Buteyko Method are available, the company LifeSource offer a very good self-help package based on CD-roms. (For more details, see Useful contacts and information.)

Athlete's foot

Athlete's foot, also known as *tinea pedis,* is a fungal infection that normally causes cracking and itching of the skin between the toes. The fungal organism that causes athlete's foot thrives in warm, moist environments. The condition is common in children, partly because they are likely to subject their feet to damp or wet environments, such as changing rooms, swimming pools and sweaty socks, but also because they may not show a huge amount of interest in drying their feet properly after bathing or showering. As a general rule, a child with athlete's foot should be encouraged to dry his feet carefully, particularly between the toes after bathing or showering. This is especially important if he has been swimming or has spent some time in a changing room. Ensure that he wears clean socks (no matter how much resistance he offers)!

Topical treatments
Garlic
Garlic is a powerful fungicide (yeast-killing agent), and many studies back this up. One study found that 27 of 34 individuals were completely cured after seven days of treatment with an extract of garlic used topically.[22] Rubbing some garlic oil (from a pierced garlic oil capsule) into the affected area twice each day for a week or two may help to clear an athlete's foot infection.

Tea tree oil
Another natural anti-fungal agent is tea tree oil. One study found that using diluted tea tree on the affected area for a period of four weeks brought about significant improvement in about 70 per cent of sufferers.[23] Soak your child's feet in warm water, with 10 drops of tea tree essential oil twice a day, or apply undiluted oil twice a day if your child won't sit still long enough to soak. If undiluted oil causes discomfort or a rash, dilute it in a little olive oil or almond oil before applying.

Persistent athlete's foot
Some children experience a problem with persistent athlete's foot, which often recurs and is maybe resistant to simple treatment. This generally means a child is harbouring too much yeast in the body, especially the gut. More details about this, and what to do about it, can be found on pages 223–8. Purging the body of yeast, combined with topical treatments, is usually very effective for getting on top of a problem with persistent athlete's foot.

Attention deficit hyperactivity disorder and Hyperactivity

Some children exhibit extreme mood and behaviour disruption indicative of a condition known as attention deficit hyperactivity disorder (ADHD). More and more children are coming to be diagnosed with ADHD, which is characterised by hyperactivity, mood swings and lack of focus and concentration. Sleep disturbance, bedwetting and excessive thirst are other common symptoms. The diagnosis of ADHD is usually made by an educational psychologist and treatment revolves around behavioural therapy and drugs such as Ritalin (methylphenidate hydrochloride). Even though Ritalin is an amphetamine (a form of 'speed'), it can have the paradoxical effect of calming the nervous system in some children. However, Ritalin does not work for a significant proportion of hyperactive children and is also linked with a variety of side effects, such as insomnia and restlessness.

Behavioural approaches

There is some thought that a child's seemingly unruly behaviour may have some root in how that child is dealt with on a behavioural level. When a child misbehaves, for whatever reason, there is a natural tendency for parents (or carers) to tell their children to stop. As many parents find, however, children tend not to respond to being told what and what not to do, especially when they are upset and/or angry. Attempting to force a child to change his or her behaviour often leads to a worsening of the situation, which can cause things to spiral out of control.

A better approach appears not to be not to attempt to control the behaviour, but to control the *consequences* of that behaviour. Some sort of reward and forfeit system that is connected to a child's behaviour often reaps dividends. The goal is to make clear to a child what will happen if he or she behaves inappropriately. A warning needs to be given each and every time the child exhibits the behaviour, which gives him an opportunity to change. The consequences of continued misbehaviour need to be acted upon immediately. Some parents may find a time-out session (for example, five minutes alone on his own in a room) is an effective deterrent. Another option is to give a child a set number of penny coins each day, and remove one coin each time a child misbehaves (after the warning). Whatever you choose, it needs to be consistent, and all carers need to apply the same rules.

The beauty of this approach is that it tends to stop the cycle of parents feeling that they can't control their children. The critical thing is that it puts the emphasis on factors that parents can control, which can take a lot of angst out of difficult situations that can arise within families. More details about this approach to behaviour modification can be found on the website www.behaviourchange.com.

Diet

ADHD is very often amenable to a nutritional approach. Certain foodstuffs and food ingredients do seem to be associated with an increased risk of mood and behaviour disturbance. Recent evidence suggests that certain colourings and preservatives may be particularly problematic. These are outlined in the box, below.

Colouring and preservatives that effect mood
Colours
- Tartrazine E102
- Sunset Yellow E110
- Carmoisine E122
- Ponceau 4R E124

Preservative
- Sodium Benzoate E211

More details about the research that has linked these particular additives to mood and behavioural problems can be found on pages 159–60. In brief, though, the scientists that conducted this study estimated that the removal of these chemicals from the diet would lead to a reduction in the number of children suffering from ADHD by about two-thirds. Another additive that children with ADHD are best to avoid is the artificial sweetener aspartame. There is evidence that this chemical can upset the brain's chemistry, which is unlikely to help a child prone to behavioural problems. Caffeine (a known stimulant) and sugar also seem to have the capacity to upset a child's behaviour and should be avoided.

Food sensitivity

Not uncommonly, ADHD is related to food sensitivity.[24] Here, one or more foodstuffs may provoke an unwanted reaction in the body, giving rise to symptoms typical of ADHD. Children suffering from food intolerance often have dark circles or bags under their eyes and may exhibit very red cheeks and/or ears during fits of uncontrollable behaviour or screaming. While any food may give rise to these sort of unwanted reactions, the most common problems are wheat, milk, cheese, ice cream, chocolate, citrus fruits and egg. Children quite often crave the foods that they are sensitive to, so it is wise to be especially suspicious of a child's favourite foods. Information about the identification of individual food sensitivities can be found on pages 211–22.

Sugar levels

Another quite common feature in children with ADHD is fluctuations in the level of sugar in the bloodstream. The body generally keeps blood sugar levels within relatively narrow parameters and this is especially important for normal brain function. The brain tissue uses a large proportion of the sugar in the bloodstream and, if fuel supply stalls, it can provoke significant problems with mood. Many children suffer from episodes of low blood sugar throughout the day, which may manifest as mood swings, tantrums and uncontrolled behaviour. This problem is quite likely if the child craves sweet foods or gets very irritable if he or she does not eat regularly and on time. These children will often respond to a diet designed to stabilise blood sugar levels. More details about this can be found on pages 204–10.

Essential fatty acids

Children with ADHD are often found to have nutrient deficiencies, especially in healthy fats known as essential fatty acids (EFAs).[25-7] The most important EFAs for mood maintenance appear to be the omega-3 fats found in oily fish such as salmon, trout, mackerel, herring and sardine, as well as some nuts and seed oils. Physical symptoms suggestive of EFA deficiency (which may accompany the behavioural ones associated with ADHD) include:

• Excessive thirst
• Frequent urination
• Dry skin
• Dry hair
• Soft or brittle nails
• Dandruff
• Follicular keratosis (a skin condition characterised by what look like permanent goosebumps, usually at the back of the upper arms).

More details about the role of EFAs (including the omega-3 variety) in health can be found on pages 229–32.

Supplements
Fish oils
Omega-3 fats in the form of fish oils may help children with ADHD. The omega-3 fat eicosapentaenoic acid seems to be particularly important in this respect.[28–9] A good dose is generally 2–3 g of a concentrated fish oil supplement per day for a 40 kg child.
Magnesium
Magnesium is another nutrient that may help in ADHD. Some children with ADHD have low levels of magnesium in their bodies and supplementation with this mineral has been shown to help reduce hyperactive behaviour.[30] I recommend 150–250 mg of magnesium per day for a 40 kg child.
Flower essences
Flower essences may be very useful for treating hyperactivity. Some of the more common indications and their remedies include:

• For an **impatient** child, who cannot seem to accept life's pace, his own shortcomings or those of others, try Impatiens
• For a child who likes to be the **centre of attention,** and tends to be a **poor listener,** try Heather
• For a **hysterical** child who seems to be seeking attention, try Chicory
• For a child who seems **unduly angry or aggressive,** try Holly or Vine
• For a child prone to **temper tantrums,** try Cherry Plum
• For a child who is **envious,** and seems to want to emulate other children, try Cerato
• For a **jealous** child, try Holly
• For a child who is **jealous and also possessive,** try Chicory.

Autism and Asperger's syndrome
Autism is a disorder characterised by problems with social communication and understanding and affected children often have problems with speech and language. Autism affects the way a person communicates and relates to people around them. Children with autism generally have problems relating to others in a meaningful way. Their ability to develop friendships is generally impaired, as is their capacity to understand other people's feelings. People with autism tend to have difficulty making sense of the world, and may have learning difficulties too.

Linked with autism is a condition known as Asperger's syndrome. This is similar to autism, but tends not to be as severe. Children with Asperger's syndrome share many of the same characteristics as autism, such as difficulty with social relationships and communication, limitations in imagination and need for routine. In contrast to children with autism, those with Asperger's syndrome tend to have normal language skills.

Autism and Asperger's syndrome are included under the umbrella term autistic spectrum disorders (ASD).

Diet
Food sensitivity

There is considerable evidence that children affected by an ASD may have abnormal reactions to specific foods. Some foodstuffs appear to have the ability to convert into what are known as 'opioid-type peptides' – essentially, small protein molecules that may have a drug-like influence on the functioning of the brain. Studies suggest that the foods most likely to give problems with opioid-type peptides are gluten containing foods (wheat, oats, rye and barley) and those containing casein (a protein found in dairy products such as milk and cheese).[31–2] These studies have found that the elimination of gluten and casein from the diet tends to reduce autistic behaviour and increase social and communicative skills. More details about food elimination and alternative foods can be found on pages 211–22.

Supplements
Multivitamins and minerals

A range of nutritional supplements may be of benefit in children with ASD, including magnesium, vitamin B6 and omega-3 fish oils.[33]

I suggest a combined approach of a good quality multivitamin and mineral, magnesium (150–250 mg magnesium per day for a 40 kg child) and a concentrated fish oil supplement (2–3 g a day for a 40 kg child).

Flower essences

Flower essences may help in the treatment of autism and Asperger's syndrome.

• For a child that seems to have a problem with **finishing things,** including homework, projects, or even a board game, try Chestnut Bud
• For a **distracted** child who seems to have his head in the clouds, try Clematis
• For a child who appears to be **lacking interest,** try Wild Oat and Wild Rose.

Bad breath

Bad breath (halitosis) can obviously be caused by problems in the mouth with poor oral hygiene and/or dental decay. However, a significant number of cases of bad breath are caused by internal imbalance, creating toxicity in the body, which then comes out in the breath. This problem may be linked with food sensitivity and/or toxicity caused by food additives. In one study, researchers found that removing problem foods from the diet of hyperactive children reduced a tendency to halitosis.[34] More details about food sensitivity and suitable replacement foods can be found on pages 211–22. Because generalised toxicity seems to be a common factor in halitosis, it makes sense to keep the diet as natural as possible with as little in the way of processed and fast foods as possible. More details about this can be found on page 184.

Supplements
Breathies
One natural supplement that may prove a simple but effective remedy for bad breath is Breathies. Based on spearmint and parsley seed oils, this supplement helps combat bad breath by neutralising odour and toxicity within the digestive tract. Breathies are available in good health food stores.
Probiotics
Healthy gut bacterial supplements (also known as probiotics) can be helpful for reducing toxicity in the gut. More details about suitable probiotic supplements can be found on pages 16–17.

Flower essences
• Crab Apple is recommended for children who **feel unclean** as a result of their bad breath.

Bedwetting
Bedwetting, the medical term for which is 'enuresis', affects about one in ten five-year-olds. However, the problem is also known to persist after this age, even into a child's teens. Sometimes, bedwetting is associated with stressful events such as a house move, trouble at school, or the birth

of a new sibling. This is normal and usually short-lived. However, giving your child a little more attention and encouraging the child to express what the problem is is likely to help resolve the issue.

Sometimes, bedwetting can be related to urinary infections and these can go undiagnosed for some time. Symptoms to look out for include fever and abdominal pain. Cloudy and/or pungent urine may be other signs of infection. If you suspect an infection, then it is generally best to get a medical opinion. Information and advice about urinary tract infections can be found on page 141.

Diet
Food sensitivity
Food sensitivity seems to be a common and frequently missed factor in bedwetting. While the mechanism for this is unclear, it does appear that unwanted reactions to certain foods and drinks in the diet can cause bedwetting.[35–6] Symptoms to look out for that suggest food sensitivity include the presence of dark bags under the eyes (sometimes referred to as 'allergic shiners'), red ears, behavioural problems and frequent colds or other infections. Some of the most common problem foods are milk, cheese, wheat, egg and citrus fruits. However, it is also worth bearing in mind that children tend to crave the foods to which they are most sensitive. Information and advice on food sensitivity can be found on pages 211–22.
Fluids
Parents of children who are prone to bedwetting are often advised to limit their fluid intake. However, one study

shows there is some evidence that many children who suffer from enuresis do not consume enough fluid.[37] The authors of this study recommended that while perhaps only about 20 per cent of a child's fluid consumption should come in the evening, there should be no overall restriction of fluid. Caffeine, however, should be avoided, as experience shows that this is likely to increase the risk of bedwetting.

Constipation and bedwetting
Research indicates that constipation can be a cause of bedwetting in children, perhaps due to the added pressure this puts on the bladder.[38–9] Even mild constipation can cause problems in susceptible children. *See* 'Constipation' for advice on dealing with this problem.

Supplements
Magnesium
Magnesium supplementation can often help in cases of bedwetting. Magnesium is thought to be especially important for the normal function of the muscle in the bladder that is involved in urination. In adults, magnesium deficiency seems to be a common factor in symptoms such as urinary incontinence, frequent urination and the need to get up at night to pass water. Also, supplementation with magnesium has been shown to help these symptoms in many sufferers. Children seem to be prone to magnesium deficiency and it is possible that this is an important factor in bedwetting. Foods rich in magnesium to

emphasise in a child's diet include green leafy vegetables, nuts, seeds, beans and pulses. In addition, it may help to give a child additional magnesium at a dose of about 150–250 mg each day for a 40 kg child.

Flower essences
• The Australian Bush flower essences Red Helmet and Dog Rose are specifically indicated for bedwetting.
• The Bach flower remedy Pine is good for children who **feel guilty** about their bedwetting and may be suffering from some self-reproach.

Bites and stings
Bites and stings are common complaints in childhood. Even if a repellent is used, it's easy for this to lose its effect after some dipping in and out of the swimming pool or sea. Mosquitoes, gnats and fleas are the most common bites and cause itchy welts on the affected parts. Bees, wasps and hornets can cause swelling and stinging at the site and, if your child is susceptible, can cause a serious condition known as anaphylactic shock (see page 31).

Preventing mosquito and other insect bites
Covering up is the best prevention, and using a good repellent is essential. Many conventional repellents may not be safe for children because they are insecticides and the chemicals they contain can be absorbed through the skin in doses that may be particularly toxic to younger children. DEET (diethyl

toluamise) is a very effective repellent, but because of its high potential toxicity, I don't particularly recommend it for children (or adults, for that matter).

Natural repellents

Natural insect repellents do seem to work very well. In fact, one study found that natural repellents are actually more effective than DEET.[40] In particular, a eucalyptus-based repellent gave over 96 per cent protection for four hours, while DEET offered 85 per cent protection over the same period. Natural repellents based on eucalyptus oil are generally available in health food stores.

Garlic

Garlic is another natural insect repellent. It appears that insects are none-too-keen on the scent of fresh garlic in the bloodstream. A Swedish study showed that ticks were much less likely to bite those who took daily doses of garlic (in the form of capsules) than those taking a placebo.[41] Although this study was undertaken with ticks, it is likely that garlic has a similar effect on other biting insects, such as mosquitoes. Fresh garlic is your best bet, as heat destroys many of its active ingredients. However, if your child is reluctant to eat fresh garlic (e.g. as a salad dressing ingredient), an alternative is to stir it into a sauce (e.g. pasta sauce) just before serving. Another alternative, of course, is to use garlic capsules or pills. A good dose for a 40 kg child is 500 mg of garlic each day.

Citronella

Citronella candles are also effective, although they are best used in conjunction with a good natural repellent on the skin. One study found that citronella candles can prevent bites by up to 42 per cent, although citronella incense appears to be only half as effective.[42] Interestingly, a plain, unscented candle also appeared to be effective in preventing at least some of the bites.

Allergies to stings

About one in every hundred people is allergic to wasp and/or bee stings. It is believed that once a sensitivity occurs, it almost always increases in severity with each following sting. The more quickly symptoms appear after the sting, the more severe the reaction. The problem occurs when susceptible people produce excessive quantities of antibodies in their immune system. The excess antibody production usually follows the initial sting to which there is no reaction. However, when the person is stung again, the insect venom entering the body combines with the antibody, produced by the first sting, which triggers a series of internal reactions, resulting in severe allergic symptoms.

When a bee or wasp stings, it injects a venomous fluid under the skin. Honey bees have a barbed stinger that is left (with its venom sac attached) in the skin of its victim. Since it takes two to three minutes for the venom sac to inject all its venom, instant removal of the stinger and sac usually reduces harmful effects. Scrape away with a sideways movement (one quick scrape) with a fingernail or the back of a knife blade. It's best not to try to pick out the stinger using fingers or tweezers, as this tends to force more venom from the sac down into the wound.

Most children who have been stung will experience a local reaction with redness, pain, swelling and some itching only at the sting site. However, if a child starts to have difficulty breathing, begins to choke or swell up, then it is likely that they may be suffering from a generalised allergic reaction, which may develop into anaphylactic shock. This condition requires urgent medical treatment (see page 31).

General treatment for wasp and bee stings

After removing the sting if appropriate (see box, pages 45–6), wash the area carefully to help remove any more venom. Applying some tissue or cotton wool soaked in cold water to the area can help to reduce the spread of histamines and other chemicals that cause itching and swelling. I suggest giving a child vitamin C, if possible, as this has natural antihistamine and anti-inflammatory effects in the body. Give 500–1000 mg every few hours. If this causes diarrhoea or discomfort in the stomach, cut back the dose.

General treatment for mosquito and insect bites

Apply witch hazel neat to the sting to help prevent itching. Vitamin C can also be taken to reduce the itching and the inflammation (see above).

Flower essences

• Rescue Remedy is good for all types of bites and stings. It is best to use this as soon as possible; it can be taken orally and/or rubbed directly into the bite or sting.

Blepharitis

Blepharitis is a condition characterised by redness, irritation and scaliness around the edges of the eyelids. Sometimes the roots of one or more lashes may become infected or the surface of the eye itself may become inflamed. Blepharitis can be complicated by bacterial infection (often by the organisms *Staphylococcus epidermidis* or *Staphylococcus aureus*) or seborrhoeic dermatitis (see page 134), or a mixture of the two. The precise cause of blepharitis is not known, though it does seem to be more common in children who have dandruff, skin allergies or eczema, suggesting that it might be related to problems such as food sensitivity and excess yeast (candida) in the body. For more details about these conditions, and how to treat them, see pages 211–22 and 223–8.

Supplements
Oregon grape

A natural remedy that may well help to reduce symptoms is the herb Oregon grape (*Mahonia aquifolium*). This plant extract has traditionally been used to treat a variety of eye disorders, including blepharitis and conjunctivitis. [43] Oregon grape contains a substance called berberine, which has antimicrobial action and can therefore help to combat the bacterial infection that is often a feature in blepharitis. Oregon grape is also thought to strengthen delicate membranes around the body, including the eyelids.

Oregon grape should be applied topically and taken internally for best effect. To make a soothing eyewash, simmer 10 g of the herb in 600 ml of water for 20 minutes. Strain the resulting fluid and allow to cool. Apply the mixture via an eye bath or cotton wool balls, bathing the eyes for ten minutes, twice a day, wiping gently from the corner of the eye to the outside. In addition, it usually helps to take a tincture (alcoholic extract) of Oregon grape internally. For a 40 kg child, give 15 drops of tincture, three times a day.

Vitamin A and beta-carotene

There is some evidence that chronic (long-term) or recurring blepharitis can be a symptom of vitamin A deficiency.[44] Vitamin A can be found in foods such as fish, eggs and liver, though it is also made in the body from beta-carotene. Beta-carotene-rich foods to emphasise in the diet include carrots, sweet potato and red peppers. It may also help a child with blepharitis to take a good quality multivitamin and mineral preparation that contains beta-carotene and/or vitamin A.

Boils

Also called furunculosis, boils are bacterial infections that begin deep in a hair follicle or a sebaceous gland (responsible for producing the oil that keeps the skin moist). The infection gradually works its way to the surface of the skin, where it becomes swollen, red and normally hard and painful to the touch. Boils most commonly appear on the neck, face, underarms or buttocks.

Any parent faced with a boil should resist the urge to burst or squeeze it, as this might spread the infection deep into the tissues and even the bloodstream. Your child's doctor may cut open the boil to allow the pus to drain, perhaps followed by a topical antibiotic. You can, however, work on treating the boil yourself, both from the inside and the outside.

Medical attention should be sought for a child with persistent and/or recurrent boils, as this may be a sign of some underlying problem such as diabetes.

Supplements

Vitamin C

Vitamin C has natural anti-inflammatory and immune-stimulating properties that may help in the treatment of boils. A good dose would be 1–2 g of vitamin C each day (for a 40 kg child) for a week or two.

Zinc

Zinc can help support the immune system and heal skin tissue. In one study, zinc was found to help individuals with chronic (long-term) boils.[45] A good dose of zinc is 30–45 mg of zinc for a 40 kg child each day for a month. Long-term zinc supplementation can, in theory, lead to a deficiency in copper. However, there is very little chance of this happening if relatively high dose zinc is taken for a month only.

Echinacea

The herb echinacea, which can be taken in tablet or tincture (alcoholic extract) form can improve immunity and encourage your child's body to fight infection. The recommended dose is 15 drops of tincture in a little juice or water each day for one to two weeks.

Topical treatments

Oregon grape

The herb Oregon grape (*Mahonia aquifolium*) contains a substance called berberine, which is known to have a natural antibacterial action.[46] Applying a tincture of Oregon grape to the boil twice each day should help keep the area clean and may help resolve the infection too.

Tea tree oil

Tea tree oil is another natural antiseptic. It can be used undiluted, applied to the boil twice a day.

Ginger tea

A warm ginger tea compress may help bring a boil to a head. Grate some fresh root ginger into some boiling water and allow to steep for ten minutes. Once it has cooled sufficiently, soak some tissue or cotton wool in the tea and leave on the boil for half an hour or more. This can be repeated if necessary.

Flower essences

• Crab Apple is good for feelings of **uncleanliness.**

• Mountain Devil (an Australian Bush flower essence) can be used for general internal cleansing purposes.

Breath-holding attacks

Breath-holding attacks are most common between the ages of one and two years of age and are often accompanied by an expression of pain, anger or frustration. Often, a child will go red or blue in the face during an attack and may even faint if it is very severe. Fortunately, an instinctive reflex invariably restarts the breathing mechanism. Although breath-holding attacks are thought to be harmless, they can nonetheless be disturbing for parents and child. It is not clear what causes breath-holding attacks, but one theory is that children unconsciously bring on the attacks as an attention-seeking mechanism.

Some research casts some doubt on the thought that children bring on breath-holding attacks themselves. However, there is some evidence that the condition may be caused by a deficiency in the mineral iron. In one study, almost 90 per cent of children treated with iron suffered no more attacks or had the frequency of attacks cut by at least half.[47] While iron may be effective for controlling breath-holding attacks in many children, too much iron can be hazardous to health. Before a child is treated with iron, he should be assessed for iron levels in his body. The best blood test for this is something known as 'ferritin'. If this is low or on the low side of normal, iron supplementation may be tried. For more details about iron deficiency and iron supplementation see page 30.

Broken bones

Intrepid children are always at risk of a bone fracture, and many will suffer broken bones in their childhood. If this does occur, there are numerous ways to encourage healing and to ensure that the bone returns to a healthy, strong state. More importantly, however, ensuring that your children's bones are strong to begin with will not only prevent fractures, but also help to ensure that they do not suffer from weak and brittle bones later in life.

Diet

Wide and varied

Diet is crucial to healthy bones, and there are many studies into which nutrients have the best effect. Overall, however, the general consensus is that a varied diet, with plenty of fresh fruit and vegetables, good quality protein, fibre in the form of wholegrains and cereals, and beneficial fats is important.[48] Fruit and vegetables seem to be particularly important for the bones, and a number of studies over the last decade have suggested a positive link between their consumption and bone health.[49] Fruit and vegetables tend to make the body less acidic, an effect that makes it less likely that calcium will be lost from the bone. While dairy products are often emphasised for their bone-building potential, fruit and vegetables are clearly important in this respect and have a whole host of other health benefits besides.

Calcium

One of the most important nutrients for bone health is calcium. Calcium is the main constituent of hydroxyapatite – the principal mineral in bones and teeth. An adequate calcium intake is vital to bone health, particularly when the bone is growing during childhood and adolescence. Good sources of calcium include milk, oily fish (such as salmon, sardines and pilchards), sesame seeds, watercress, okra, spinach, tofu, dried figs, currants and dried apricots. In addition, green leafy vegetables all contain good levels of calcium. Ensuring that your child eats plenty of these foods is important. However, there is evidence that even when a child gets enough calcium from their diet, supplementation can be beneficial. One study found that even in children getting the daily requirement of calcium, additional calcium in supplement form improved bone density.[50]

Vitamin D

Vitamin D is required for optimal absorption of calcium from the gut and is believed to play a key role in bone health of children and adults. Most of the vitamin D in the body is made as a result of the action of sunlight on the skin, but some also comes from the diet. Until recently, vitamin D deficiency was considered a problem only in those children from cultures where skin exposure to sunlight is limited. However, evidence is emerging that a relative lack of vitamin D is more prevalent in children and adolescents than previously thought. In fact, 90 per cent of Europeans have dietary vitamin D intakes below the recommended levels and are potentially insufficient in vitamin D for significant parts of the year.[51] The latest Government statistics found that some 11 per cent of boys and girls aged between 11 and 14 as well as 16 per cent of boys and 10 per cent of girls aged between 15 and 18 years were deficient in vitamin D.

Oily fish is a good source of vitamin D, though supplementation as part of a good multivitamin and mineral complex may prove the most practical way of ensuring a child gets enough of this nutrient in their diet.

Exercise and healthy bones
Exercise builds stronger bones, and being physically active on a regular basis is therefore important for bone strength. Encouraging physical activity and exercise in your child is likely to bring a range of health benefits, including stronger, more fracture-resistant bones.

Supplements
Multivitamins and minerals
Other nutrients that are believed to have an important role to play in bone health include magnesium, zinc, copper and vitamin K, and these are available in a good quality multivitamin and mineral formulation.

Vitamin C
When bone heals, it requires nutrients to do this. If your child has been unfortunate enough to break a bone, then supplementing with a range of nutrients may help. Vitamin C seems to be especially important as it appears to accelerate the rate at which the bone rebuilds itself.[52–3] Children may take 500–1000 mg of vitamin C per day for four to six weeks. In addition, more speedy bone healing can be expected if a child is supplemented with a good quality multivitamin and mineral and 200–300 mg of calcium each day.

Bronchiolitis
Bronchiolitis is a lower respiratory tract (lung) infection that occurs most commonly in infants under the age of 12 months. The condition is characterised by widespread inflammation in the smallest airways (the bronchi and bronchioles), which causes them to become swollen, produce mucus and perhaps also to go into spasm. The condition may be accompanied by an ear infection or pneumonia. Over half of the cases of bronchiolitis are caused by a virus called the respiratory syncitial virus (RSV).

Bronchiolitis typically develops after a few days of cold symptoms, often beginning with a harsh cough, fever, wheezing and some difficulty in eating and breathing. A few days after the cough and breathing difficulty start, the illness tends to worsen. There may be increased difficulty in breathing, anxiety, fatigue due to inability to sleep, and problems with eating or drinking. Children exhibiting these symptoms should receive medical attention immediately. Although standard medical treatment for bronchiolitis is limited, some children with this condition are hospitalised so that they can be supported and watched closely. The main reason for this is that there is a danger that inadequate oxygen and exhaustion can lead to serious and possibly life-threatening breathing problems.

Prevention

Children who are weaned early or not breast-fed appear to be at increased risk of contracting bronchiolitis.[54] The best advice is to leave weaning until at least six months (see pages 280–5) and to breast-feed for as long as possible (see page 249–77). Premature babies also appear to be more at risk and breast-feeding or bottle-feeding with breast milk may have particular protective benefits for these children. Generally speaking, exposure to tobacco smoke should also be avoided, especially in children who have a history of chest infections and/or asthma.

Topical treatments
Thyme or eucalyptus oil

It is important to ensure a child suffering from bronchiolitis gets enough fluid. Rapid breathing and a fever can dehydrate a little body quite quickly. Water or perhaps some dilute fruit juice is best. Formula milk or milk is best avoided as these may increase mucus production, which is unlikely to help matters. Certain essential oils are believed to open up the airways and help breathing. Mix 5 drops of either thyme or eucalyptus oil in a small cup of olive or almond oil, and rub this mixture along your child's spine, particularly the upper back over the lungs.

Supplements
Vitamin C

Vitamin C has immune-stimulating and anti-viral properties and giving this to your child may just help get control of the infection at the root of many cases of bronchiolitis. Put 250 mg of vitamin C (as vitamin C powder or the contents of a capsule) in some water or juice, and give this two to three times a day (for a 40 kg child).

Flower essences

• Rescue Remedy may help to reduce the fright and upset that your child might be feeling.

• After the infection, you might like to give your child the Bach flower remedy Olive as this may help to resolve the **fatigue** that is common after a serious infection.

Bronchitis

Bronchitis is an inflammation of the trachea (the windpipe) and the large airways (bronchi) of the lungs. There are many causes for bronchitis, but it often comes after a viral infection such as a cold or flu. There are two main types of bronchitis: acute and chronic.

Acute bronchitis

Symptoms of acute bronchitis (the result of infection) begin with a runny nose, fever, a dry cough and possibly wheezing. This is often followed with the production of mucus (phlegm), which may be clear at first, but then turns yellow – generally a sign that a bacterial infection has set in. If this happens, particularly if a child is quite unwell, antibiotics may be deemed the best thing. However, if a course is taken, it is a good idea to give the child a supplement of healthy gut bacteria (also known as a probiotic) to replace organisms likely to have been killed by the antibiotic. More details about this can be found on page 16.

For a child in the throes of an infection, it can help to take steps to enhance immune system function. Two of the most important agents in this respect are vitamin C and the herb echinacea, both of which have immune-stimulating properties. There's plenty of evidence that vitamin C, in particular, is effective for treating lung infections. For example, researchers have found that even low doses of vitamin C (around 200 mg per day) improve the body's ability to fight off respiratory infections by improving immune function.[55] Another study found that low doses of vitamin C are as effective as antibiotics in treating acute bronchitis.[56] Try putting 250 mg of vitamin C (as vitamin C powder or the contents of a capsule) in some water or juice, and giving this to your child two to three times a day. This dose is suitable for a 40 kg child.

Echinacea, which has a wide spread reputation as an immune-enhancer, may also be able to help to control an infection. One study found that it significantly reduced symptoms of bronchitis in subjects with colds and other respiratory infections.[57] There are two main species of echinacea used therapeutically – purpurea and angustifolia. Because each form of echinacea has slightly different properties, it is probably a good idea

to combine them for maximum effect. Give 15–20 drops of tincture, every two to three hours on the first day of the illness, followed by this dose three to four times a day for the next 10–14 days.

Chronic bronchitis

Chronic bronchitis, which can be the result of allergies or prolonged contact with cigarette smoke or other irritants, is generally characterised by a persistent dry cough without the other symptoms that tend to be characteristic of acute bronchitis.

A diet based on whole, unrefined foods will help ensure your child gets all the nutrients they need to support the immune and respiratory systems. Fruit and vegetables seem to be particularly important in this respect, as there is evidence that increased intake of these can reduce the risk of all sorts of lung conditions, including chronic bronchitis. Dairy products are not the best foods for children with chronic bronchitis, perhaps because they tend to increase mucus production in the body. For more details about identifying potential problem foods in your child, see pages 211–22.

In addition to a healthy diet, supplements may also help a child prone to chronic bronchitis.

Supplements for chronic bronchitis
N-acetyl cysteine

The nutritional agent N-acetyl cysteine (NAC) has the ability to break up and 'loosen' the secretions that commonly cause problems in chronic bronchitis. One study showed NAC had real benefit at a dose of 600 mg per day, three days per week.[58] For a child weighing 40 kg, 300 mg of NAC should be taken three times a week.

Multivitamins and minerals

Individuals with chronic bronchitis tend to be lower in certain nutrients, including vitamin C and zinc.[59] Giving a child a good quality multivitamin and mineral preparation each day may counter any nutritional deficiencies and may help improve a child's resistance to respiratory problems. More details about this can be found on page 14.

Bruises

Bruises are caused by injury to blood vessels, causing blood to leak into the surrounding tissues beneath the skin. Bruising is a natural event, but very occasionally signals a problem with the blood's ability to clot normally. A child prone to what seems to be unusual or very severe bruising may benefit from medical tests designed to assess clotting ability.

Diet
Vitamin C

Children prone to bruising are often helped by having more vitamin C in their diets. Vitamin C is important for the strength of blood vessels and there's evidence that low levels of this nutrient can cause children (particularly infants) to bruise more easily.[60] Plenty of fruit and vegetables in a child's diet, particularly vitamin C-rich ones such as citrus and kiwi fruits, will generally help them to be less prone to bruising. These foods also may give a child more in the way of substances called bioflavonoids that

appear to help vitamin C do its job in the body, and also seem to help improve the strength of blood vessels in the body. For speedier results, supplementation with these nutrients may be considered. Give 500 mg of vitamin C and 250–500 mg of bioflavonoids each day (for a 40 kg child).

Homeopathic treatments
Arnica

The homeopathic treatment Arnica may help limit the extent and duration of a bruise. Homeopathic remedies come in a variety of strengths (dilutions). Give the 6 or 30 C dilution every hour or two for the first couple of days after the injury, and then once or twice daily until the bruising has gone. In addition, arnica cream can be rubbed gently into the affected area two to three times a day.

Flower essences

• Rescue Remedy may be used immediately after a fall or injury, as this may help to aid a child over the shock associated with this.

Bulimia nervosa

Bulimia nervosa, also known as just 'bulimia', is an eating disorder characterised by bouts of food bingeing, after which sufferers may make themselves sick or take excessive amounts of laxatives. The condition is generally thought of as a predominantly psychological condition. However, there is good evidence that physiological and/or nutritional factors often underlie the condition and that dietary management can be very effective in controlling symptoms.

Blood sugar imbalance seems to play an important role in the condition. In one study, a group of bulimic women were put on a diet that was designed to maintain a stable level of sugar in the bloodstream.[61] The diet excluded all alcohol, caffeine, refined sugar, white flour products, monosodium glutamate and flavour-enhancers. All the women in the study stopped bingeing while they were on this regime, and were still binge-free two-and-a-half years later. More information about the management of blood sugar instability can be found on pages 204–10.

Another factor that may be at play in bulimia is low levels of the brain chemical serotonin. Serotonin generally induces happy, feel-good emotions. It is manufactured in the brain from an amino acid called 'tryptophan', which is found in foods such as meat, tofu, almonds, peanuts, pumpkin seeds, sesame seed and tahini (sesame seed paste). Tryptophan is absorbed into the brain more efficiently when there is carbohydrate present. This might explain why certain individuals gravitate towards sweet or starchy foods when upset or stressed. In one study, bulimic women were treated with tryptophan (3 g per day) or a placebo for about a month.[62] Those taking tryptophan were also given vitamin B6 (45 mg per day) as this nutrient is thought to help the conversion of tryptophan into serotonin. Those taking the tryptophan/B6 combination were found to have significantly improved measures of mood, eating behaviour and feeling about eating compared to those taking a placebo. Unfortunately, tryptophan is not available over-the-counter in many countries, including the UK and the US. However, 5-hydroxytryptophan (5-HTP) – the substance tryptophan is converted into before it is made into serotonin – is a good alternative. Children aged 16 or more may benefit from taking 50 mg of 5-HTP, two to three times a day.

Burns

Most children will suffer from a burn at some point in their lives – anything as simple as sunburn (see 'Sunburn') to something more serious, such as an electrical burn, or a burn caused by corrosive chemicals. The key is to establish the severity as soon as the burn occurs and seek the appropriate treatment immediately.

Degrees of burn

• *A first-degree burn* involves only the upper layer of the skin. The area is hot, red and painful but without swelling or blistering. Sunburn is usually a first-degree burn, as would be a burn caused by a brush against a radiator or another hot surface.

• *A second-degree burn* involves the upper layer of the skin and part of the underlying skin layers. This type of burn tends to be very painful and the area will usually be pink or red, mottled and moist, as well as moderately swollen and blistered.

• *A third-degree burn* involves injury to all layers of the skin – and is therefore also referred to as a 'full-thickness' burn. This severe burn destroys the nerves and blood vessels in the skin. Because the nerves are damaged there is little or no pain at first. The affected area may be white, yellow, black or deep red. The skin may appear dry and leathery.

What to do

The most important thing to do after a burn sustained by contact from something hot like boiling water, a naked flame or a kitchen utensil is to run cold water over it. This will take much of the heat out of the burn and is likely to help limit its severity. For maximum benefit, the burn should be kept under cold running water for several minutes and ice should be applied if possible. While minor burns can be treated at home, large or severe burns should be looked at by a doctor just in case there is a need for medical treatment. Keep the ice on the burn while your child waits for treatment.

Topical treatments
Lavender, aloe vera and vitamin E
A few natural agents can be beneficial for helping burns to heal and to reduce scarring. Pure essential oil of lavender, aloe vera gel and vitamin E squeezed from a soft gelatine capsule are all good for this. Applying one or more of these soothing and healing agents several times each day does seem to reduce discomfort and often seems to have a dramatic effect on the speed at which a burn heals. Aloe vera in particular seems to be much more effective than emollient creams (such as Vaseline), and almost halves the time for healing to take place.[63]

Supplements
Vitamin C
Vitamin C and zinc are both important for skin healing. For a 40 kg child, give 1000 mg of vitamin C and 30 mg of zinc each day for two weeks.

Flower essences
• Rescue Remedy is always the first essence to offer, and it can be taken immediately following the burn to calm and help to reduce the trauma (both emotionally and physically).

Cancer

Childhood cancers are rare, with about 600 new cases occurring in the UK every year (compared to 250,000 in adults). Of all the forms of cancer in children, brain tumours and leukaemia (cancer of the white blood cells) are the most common and account for about half of all cases. Natural medicine may help in the treatment of cancer, including as an adjunct to conventional approaches. A useful resource for individuals looking to use natural approaches is *How to Prevent and Treat Cancer with Natural Medicine: A Natural Arsenal of Disease-fighting Tools for Prevention, Treatment and Coping with Side Effects* by Joseph Pizzorno, Tim Birdsall, Paul Reilly and Michael Murray (ISBN: 1573222224).

Other support may be had from CLIC (Challenging Cancer and Leukaemia in Childhood). This national charity offers support to families in a variety of forms, including care grants and crisis breaks. (For more details, see Useful contacts and information.)

Car sickness

See 'Motion sickness'

Chickenpox

Chickenpox is a contagious childhood disease that is caused by what is known as the varicella-zoster virus, a member of the herpes family. Chickenpox typically begins with a headache, fatigue, loss of appetite and fever. A day or two later, this will be followed by a rash of flat red dots, which usually begin on the chest, stomach and back and spread a day or two later to the face and scalp. The red dots of the rash come together to form clusters of tiny pimples, which then progress to small clear blisters. These blisters will continue to erupt over the next three to five days. Scabs will eventually form about five days after the blisters develop and they last for up to two weeks before falling off. The skin beneath is usually tender and freshly healed, so ensure that your child stays out of bright sunlight for a few weeks and avoid any clothing that might cause irritation.

The worst part of chickenpox is the discomfort. The rash is intensely itchy and it can be difficult to prevent children from scratching, which increases the likelihood of scarring and infection. The good news is that one bout of chickenpox usually provides complete immunity from further attacks. However, the infection can lie dormant in the body and erupt again as a bout of something known as shingles.

Supplements

Vitamin A and beta-carotene

Supplementing with vitamin A and/or beta-carotene seems to help skin healing and reduce the risk of complications.[64] There is also research that indicates that when given before symptoms manifest themselves (in other words, to siblings, or when you know that your child has been in contact), these nutrients may dramatically reduce the severity of the condition. Give 10,000 IU of vitamin A each day for two weeks. This dose is absolutely safe to be taken in the short term.

Multivitamins and minerals

There is evidence that taking a multivitamin and mineral tablet each day can help protect children from chickenpox. A study of nursery children found that when children who had been given multivitamins and minerals came into contact with chickenpox, only 11 of the 37 vitamin-treated children contracted this disease.[65] Normally, about 90 per cent of children would be expected to contract the disease in these circumstances. Regular supplementation with a multivitamin and minerals is likely to reduce the risk of chickenpox, and perhaps other infections too.

Topical treatments

Calendula cream

Calendula cream applied topically to the affected area can ease itching.

Chilblains

Chilblains are itchy, purple-red swellings that usually occur on the toes and are related to problems with circulation. They are caused by excessive narrowing and constriction of blood vessels, usually as a result of exposure to cold.

Supplements
Vitamin E and magnesium
There are several natural agents that may reduce the tendency to suffer from chilblains. Vitamin E seems to help, which may work by reducing the stickiness of blood components called platelets, effectively thinning the blood and thereby improving circulation. Give 200 IU of vitamin E each day to a 40 kg child. A supplement of the mineral magnesium may also help because it has a relaxant effect on blood vessels. A good dose is 150–250 mg per day.
Ginkgo
The herb *Ginkgo biloba* is also likely to provide some relief as it is well known to enhance circulation. For a 40 kg child, I recommend 40–60 mg of standardised extract, given twice a day.

Chondromalacia patellae

Chondromalacia patellae is a knee condition that most commonly affects adolescents and young adults. The condition is caused by a degeneration of the cartilage that covers the back of the kneecap, causing pain in the front of the knee, often after running or when walking down stairs. Some sufferers of chondromalacia patellae may need to

have an operation, which involves either scraping the inside of the kneecap and/or re-alignment of the knee cap so that it is less prone to damage.

Supplements
Glucosamine sulphate
One nutrient that may well help heal this is glucosamine sulphate. This nutrient is an essential building block for cartilage formation in the body and speeds up cartilage regeneration. Take 500 mg three times a day. Once symptoms have improved this dose may be reduced to 500 mg, once or twice a day.
Selenium and vitamin E
Two other nutrients that experience shows may be very useful in combating chondromalacia patellae are selenium and vitamin E. Take 200–300 mcg of selenium and 400–800 IU of vitamin E each day until a month after the symptoms are under control.

Chronic fatigue syndrome
See also 'Fatigue'
Chronic fatigue syndrome (CFS) is characterised by severe, usually disabling fatigue, which has lasted for at least six months. Symptoms are almost always made worse by physical or mental exertion, sometimes even when this is only moderate in nature. Despite considerable research, there does not appear to be a single adequate medical explanation for this condition. It's likely that multiple factors are at play.

Some of the most common underlying features in chronic fatigue are nutrient deficiency (especially iron deficiency), blood sugar imbalance, food sensitivity and weakness in the adrenal glands. These factors are discussed more fully in the section on fatigue, and are certainly worth exploring. In addition, specific nutritional supplements may help combat CFS.

Supplements

Essential fatty acids

Healthy fats in the diet known as essential fatty acids (EFAs) play a wide variety of roles in the body, including the regulation of the action of hormones, nervous system activity and immune function. Low levels of EFAs are associated with CFS.[66-7] Some research suggests EFA supplementation may be effective for the treatment of CFS. One study, in adults, involved a group of 63 patients who had had post-viral fatigue syndrome (a form of chronic fatigue) for at least one year. Tests revealed that the blood levels of EFAs in these sufferers tended to be low. The subjects were then treated with a mixture of evening primrose oil and fish oil, or a placebo for three months. At the end of the study, 85 per cent of patients treated with the EFAs rated themselves as better, compared to 17 per cent of those on the placebo. Individual symptoms, such as fatigue, aches and pains and depression, all tended to improve on the EFA treatment.[68]

Children with CFS may benefit from EFA supplementation. Hemp seed oil is a good all-round supplement as it contains essential fats of both the omega-3 and omega-6 type (see page 247 for more details). I recommend 10

ml (2 tsp) a day for a 40 kg child. Children may be reluctant to take this oil off a spoon, so it may be best to put it in a soup, stew, sauce or casserole.

Carnitine

Low levels of the nutrient carnitine (related to the B-vitamin group) appear to play a role in some cases of CFS.[69-70] Carnitine's main function is to help transport nutrients known as long-chain fatty acids into the parts of the body's cells that can burn them for energy. Carnitine can be manufactured by the body, but only if sufficient amounts of nutrients such as iron, vitamin B1, vitamin B6, vitamin C and the amino acids (building blocks of protein) lysine and methionine are available. Getting your child on a good quality multivitamin and mineral might help to provide them with the nutrients they need to make carnitine. The two studies quoted above have found that taking carnitine can often be effective in combating the symptoms of chronic fatigue. For a 40 kg child, give 500–1500 mg of carnitine a day.

B-complex vitamins

Several studies show that a deficiency in one or more of the B vitamins may be a factor in CFS.[71] Vitamin B12 deficiency seems to be a particular problem and this is more likely to be a factor in vegan children as B12 is found in useful quantities in animal foods only. Supplementation with a B-complex supplement that contains about 25 mg of the major B-vitamins B1, B2, B3, B5 and B6 may help restore energy levels in children with CFS.

Magnesium

Magnesium is a key nutrient in the body, and certainly plays a very important part in the processes that generate energy in the body. However, it is also one of the nutrients that tend to be in short supply in the diet, and there is evidence that many children and adolescents simply do not get enough magnesium from their food. Magnesium deficiency seems to be a common factor in CFS. Researchers have found that many of the symptoms of CFS are similar to those of magnesium deficiency.[72] Other evidence suggests that magnesium levels tend to be low in people suffering from CFS.[73–4] One study of several hundred CFS patients discovered that half of them were magnesium-deficient.[75]

Magnesium is found naturally in foods such as green leafy vegetables, fish, meat, beans, pulses and nuts and seeds. Ensuring your child is getting enough of these foods will help him or her get a decent amount of magnesium. However, in practice, magnesium supplementation often works well in children with CFS. A good dose for a 40 kg child would be 150–250 mg of magnesium per day.

Coenzyme Q10

Coenzyme Q10 (CoQ10) is a vitamin-like substance that participates in the reactions within the body's cells that produce something called ATP (adenosine triphosphate) – the basic unit of energy in the body. Some practitioners use CoQ10 in the treatment of CFS and there is some evidence that it can help. One study found that supplementing with CoQ10 for three months improved symptoms in 90 per cent of patients studied.[76] I recommend 30–60 mg per day for a 40 kg child.

Flower Essences

• The Bach flower essence Olive is good for **overall fatigue**.
• For feelings of **low self-esteem** (common in CFS), try larch.
• For **depression**, mustard is generally good.
• If **stress** is a major component in your child's fatigue, vervain is a good remedy.

Coeliac disease

Coeliac disease is a condition caused by an inability to tolerate gluten, a protein found in wheat, oats, rye and barley. In individuals with coeliac disease, gluten is seen by the body as foreign and this results in an immune reaction in the lining of the gut. This reaction leads to the loss of finger-like projections in the bowel wall that are important for the absorption of nutrients from digested food. The condition also causes a reduction in the amount of enzymes found naturally in the bowel wall, which may impair digestive ability.

Symptoms of coeliac disease (when gluten is consumed) include diarrhoea, flatulence, abdominal bloating and a feeling of weakness and/or fatigue. There may also be behavioural changes. In the long term, the problems with nutrient absorption and digestion can lead to a range of conditions, including slowed growth and development. In the longer term, coeliac sufferers may have problems with anaemia and osteoporosis.

Coeliac disease is usually diagnosed before a child is two years of age, though the condition may be missed and should be considered in any child with suggestive symptoms.

Diet
Gluten-containing foods
Conventional wisdom dictates that coeliac sufferers must avoid all gluten-containing foods such as wheat, oats, rye and barley. However, recent research suggests that the majority of coeliac sufferers do not have adverse effects from eating oats. One five-year study found no ill effects from oat eating in coeliac sufferers.[77] It is worth testing oats in a child with coeliac to see if this has any effect. The chances are that oats will be tolerated, which does open up a few food possibilities (e.g. oat muesli, porridge, oat cakes) that are traditionally outlawed in the coeliac diet. Foods such as buckwheat (buckwheat is not wheat), rice and corn-based pasta, rice noodles, rice cakes and polenta (corn) are other options for coeliac sufferers.

Supplements
Multivitamins and minerals
It's extremely important that your child has good levels of all key nutrients, in particular calcium and vitamins D, A and B12, not just for growth, but also to help prevent chronic conditions such as anaemia and osteoporosis. A good healthy diet will go a long way to achieving this, though it probably makes sense for children to take good quality multivitamin and minerals each day too. (See page 14 for more details about suitable supplements.)

Digestive enyzmes
Supplements of digestive enzymes may be useful for children with coeliac disease. One particular supplement, which goes under the name of Glutenzyme, is specifically designed to help with the digestion of gluten. It is handy to have this supplement around for when a child may have difficulty controlling his diet or may not be sure what is in the food he is eating. Take one capsule after any suspect food. This supplement is available from the manufacturers BioCare. (For more details, see Useful contacts and information.)

Cold sores
Cold sores are caused by the herpes simplex virus (HSV). Once it has infected the body, the virus lies dormant but may reactivate and cause a cold sore at any time, especially when the immune system is weak or run-down. Cold sores typically last between seven and ten days, are unsightly, and can cause considerable discomfort. Before a full-blown cold sore erupts, your child may notice symptoms such as tingling or burning in or around the lip. Used early enough, nutritionally-oriented treatments can help to stop a cold sore in its tracks.

Supplements
Lysine
The amino acid lysine inhibits the growth and replication of the herpes simplex virus. Most studies have found that lysine has the ability to reduce the frequency and severity of cold sore attacks.[78] Before or during a cold sore attack, I recommend giving your child 500 mg of lysine, two to three times a day (for a 40 kg child). This can be continued for several days. The earlier this treatment is started, the better.

Prevention

While lysine inhibits HSV, another amino acid – arginine – encourages it. Arginine is found in high concentration in nuts, especially peanuts and cashews, chocolate and grains. Limiting these foods in the diet might help prevent cold sore attacks. These foods should be particularly avoided at the first signs of an eruption.

Vitamin C and bioflavonoids
A combination of vitamin C and bioflavonoids (plant-derived nutrients related to vitamin C) has also been found to reduce the duration of symptoms by more than half.[79] I suggest giving your child 200 mg of vitamin C and 200 mg of bioflavonoids three times each day at the first sign of an attack. If your child regularly suffers from cold sores, regular doses of vitamin C may help keep these at bay. I suggest 250 mg of vitamin C per day for a 40 kg child.

Selenium
Another nutrient that might help to reduce cold sore attacks is the mineral selenium. Selenium has the ability to inhibit several viruses, including the herpes virus. Taking a multivitamin and mineral preparation that contains selenium each day may also help prevent cold sores in the longer term.

Topical treatments
Vitamin E oil
For topical relief I recommend vitamin E oil from a soft gelatine capsule. The contents of a vitamin E capsule can be used to soak a small piece of tissue and this can be applied to the cold sore. If this is done for 15 minutes, twice a day, the cold sore will often resolve in a day or two.[80–81]
Vitamin C cream
Vitamin C applied topically to a cold sore may help healing.[82] Vitamin C creams are available in health food stores and may be applied to the cold sores three or four times a day.

Colds and flu

Colds and flu are caused by viruses, which means that they do not respond to antibiotics (which treat bacteria). One key to helping a child who is prone to such infections is to take steps to ensure their immune system is in good working order.

Diet
Sugar and dairy products
The strength of the immune system is intimately related to lifestyle factors, including what we eat. An important

dietary component in this respect is sugar. There is evidence that sugar has the capacity to disable the immune system.[83–4] Sugar should therefore be limited in your child's diet, particularly at the first sign of an infection.

Many children who are prone to colds may also tend to make mucus in and around the nose. These children tend to do quite well on a diet that contains less in the way of dairy products (dairy products tend to increase mucus secretion). For more information about food sensitivity and alternative foods, see pages 211–22.

Supplements
Vitamin C
Several natural agents have been found to be effective in treating the common cold, probably the best known of which is vitamin C. Vitamin C has several immune strengthening and anti-viral actions in the body. Most studies suggest that 1.5–4 g of vitamin C (in adults) taken in divided doses during the day at the first sign of a cold reduce the number of ill days by about a third.[85] However, in accordance with the work of the late Linus Pauling, an ardent proponent of vitamin C, larger doses tend to be more effective. For a 40 kg child, give 250–500 mg of vitamin C (either in tablet or capsule form, or as a powder dissolved in water or juice) every hour or two. This large dose of vitamin C can sometimes cause some loosening of the bowels, though this side-effect resolves once the dose is reduced.

Zinc
Another useful nutrient for combating the common cold is zinc. Zinc inhibits the virus responsible for the cold infections (rhinovirus). Sucking a zinc lozenge every two waking hours has been shown to reduce the average duration of colds by seven days compared to placebo.[86] There's also some evidence that regular intake of zinc can help to prevent colds and, like vitamin C, ensure that they are shorter and less severe when they do strike.[87] The precise form of the zinc in the lozenge is important – it should be zinc gluconate. Other forms of zinc may not actually liberate sufficient quantities of zinc to exert a significant effect. The lozenge should not contain citric acid, tartaric acid, mannitol or sorbitol either, as these can inactivate the zinc. Many children may find the taste unpalatable, but there are some good vanilla and lemon flavoured brands on the market. I recommend giving a zinc lozenge four to six times a day for five to ten days (for a 40 kg child).

Echinacea
The herb echinacea has gained quite a reputation over the last few years as a potent infection fighter. Echinacea has proven immune stimulating activity and a review concluded that there was good evidence to support its use in the treatment of the common cold.[88] One study showed that taking echinacea during a cold can reduce the duration from an average of nine days to six.[89] There are two main species of echinacea used therapeutically; purpurea and angustifolia. Purpurea is the type most commonly used, though angustifolia

certainly has merit and contains anti-viral agents called echinacosides, which are not found in the purpurea plant. Because of this, it is probably best to use a combination of both types of echinacea during a viral infection. Give 15–20 drops of tincture (alcoholic extract), every two to three hours on the first day of the illness, followed by three to four times a day for the next 10–14 days.

Sambucol

Another useful agent in the treatment of viral infections is sambucol. This product contains a blend of black elderberries (*Sambucus nigra*) and raspberries (*Rubus idaeus*), which have the ability to inhibit the flu virus. One study found that if sambucol was started within 24 hours of the onset of symptoms, 90 per cent of subjects became symptom-free in two to three days.[90] A sambucol supplement specifically designed for kids is available in health food stores. Give to your child as directed on the label.

Colic

Colic is a common problem in infants that usually causes sharp, gripey abdominal pains, abdominal bloating, drawing up of the legs and crying. It tends not to last longer than about three months, but it can be very distressing for parents, who may find it difficult to console a baby who is clearly in some pain. There is good evidence to suggest that colic is related to a reaction to cow's milk-based infant formulas.[91–2] In fact, one study showed that sensitivity to cow's milk is implicated in about 25 per cent of cases.[93] While breast-feeding might reduce the risk of colic, it does not make a child immune to it. Studies show that milk in the mother's diet may cause colic in breast-fed infants too. Breast-fed infants with colic often improve when cow's milk is eliminated from the mother's diet. Rice and oat milk make good alternatives. While cow's milk is commonly implicated in colic, it's not the only offender. One study showed that other foods in the mother's diet that commonly upset breast-fed children include cabbage, broccoli, cauliflower, onion and chocolate.[94] Breast-feeding mothers with colicky babies might consider eliminating these foods from their diet too.

Smoking during pregnancy and after the birth appears to double the risk of colic.[95] Avoiding exposing your child to cigarette smoke might help to keep colic at bay and may reduce the risk of other health issues, including asthma, too.

What to do

Change formulas

Some babies are simply unable to digest the large protein molecules in milk and this is often at the root of the bowel symptoms typical of colic. Switching a baby to a formula based on goat's milk or cow's milk specially treated to break down the protein molecules within it (known as 'hydrolysates') can often be very effective in reducing the symptoms of colic. More details on formula-feeding can be found on pages 277–80.

Feeding on demand

Another useful strategy in combating colic is feeding on demand. There is a theory that if too long is left between a child's feeds, discomfort may result.

This problem may be related to drops in the child's blood sugar level. One study showed that demand-based feeding dramatically reduced the incidence of colic.[96]

Probiotics

A breast-feeding mother may be able to ease the symptoms of colic by taking a probiotic supplement. This will help provide the baby's bowel with friendly bacteria, which may help ease digestion and help to resolve colic. A suitable supplement is INT B1, which contains the gut bacteria thought to be of particular importance in infants and small children (*Bifidobacterium infantis*). Give a quarter of a teaspoon in one feed each day. (For more details, see Useful contacts and information – under BioCare.)

Chamomile tea

Some breast-feeding mothers find that drinking a cup of chamomile tea or fennel tea, two or three times a day, helps to ease colic in their babies.

Other options

Carrying your baby and cuddling him or her can make a profound difference to the way he or she feels. One study found that crying babies respond dramatically to being carried .[97] At the time of peak crying (six weeks of age), infants who were carried more cried and fussed 43 per cent less overall, and 51 per cent less at the end of the day (4pm to midnight). Similar but smaller decreases occurred at four, eight and 12 weeks of age.

Flower essences

• Rescue Remedy is great to have on hand, both to soothe your baby and to take yourself! Many parents feel inadequate, frustrated and distressed by seemingly endless crying, and this remedy can help to take the edge off things.

Concentration – poor

See 'Attention deficit hyperactivity disorder', 'Autism' and pages 229–32 (DDAT and omega-3 fatty acids)

Conjunctivitis

Sometimes known as 'pinkeye', conjunctivitis is an inflammation of the white of the eye (the conjunctiva), which is a transparent membrane that lines the eyeball. In the early stages of conjunctivitis your child might experience burning or itching, and may complain that it feels like something is on the surface of the eyeball itself. There may also be some swelling of the eyelid and a yellowish discharge – normally evident in the morning.

There are many causes of this condition, including viral or bacterial infection, an injury to the eye, or a reaction to smoke, pollution or another irritant. Allergic conjunctivitis is normally caused by pollen and tends to be seasonal. There is also some evidence that slight vitamin A deficiency makes this condition more likely.[98] Babies less than a week old may experience conjunctivitis as a result of a blocked tear duct. This condition is fairly common and normally resolves itself by the time your baby reaches six months. It can, however, cause the fluid to back up and accumulate, creating a perfect setting for infection. In older children, the most common cause is viral infection, which is normally contagious.

Most cases of conjunctivitis last for about a week. If you are treating your child at home and there is no improvement after four or five days, seek medical advice.

Topical treatments
Warm water compresses
Simple compresses with warm water are generally effective because many of the micro-organisms that cause conjunctivitis are sensitive to heat. Cotton wool balls make good compresses, and they should be applied for about ten minutes, every two hours, throughout the day. The heat of the compress will also loosen the debris and increase the blood flow to the area, which will help healing. Avoid re-using the compresses as they can spread the infection. Also, take care to wash your hands before and after use.

Supplements
Oregon grape
A natural remedy that may well help in cases of conjunctivitis is the herb Oregon grape (*Mahonia aquifolium*). This plant extract is traditionally used to treat eye disorders, including blepharitis and conjunctivitis.[99–100] Oregon grape contains a substance called berberine, which has anti-microbial action and can therefore help to combat the infection that is often at the root of conjunctivitis.

Oregon grape should be applied to the outside of the eyes and taken internally for best effect. To make a soothing eyewash, simmer 10 g of the herb in 600 ml of water for 20 minutes. The resulting fluid should be strained and allowed to cool. This mixture can then be applied via an eye bath or cotton wool balls. The eyes can be bathed for 10 minutes, twice a day, wiping gently from the corner of the eye to the outside.

Constipation
Children's bowel habits are often slightly erratic as their bowels tend to be more sensitive to changes in diet than adults. However, if your child's daily habits change, significantly decreasing in the number or consistency of the bowel movements, or if there is pain or difficulty passing stools, you can be sure he is suffering from constipation. It's worth noting that breast-fed babies tend to have fewer bowel movements than bottle-fed babies. This might be, at least in part, because breast milk tends to be efficiently used and there is less waste to get rid of. Babies under the age of four months may go as long as two or three days without a bowel movement. As long as they are comfortable and eating normally, there is unlikely to be anything amiss.

There are a few different causes of constipation, the most common of which is too little fibre in the diet along with insufficient fluid intake. Without enough fluid and bulk, the faeces can become hard and rough. On passing, these rock-like entities can cause quite a lot of pain and may even cause small tears in and around the anus known as fissures. Children who find passing a stool is painful may tend to resist the call of nature, which in the long term can set up a vicious cycle that can be quite a challenge to crack. However, a nutritional approach – and a degree of patience – will usually solve the problem.

Diet
Fibre
Start by increasing the amount of fibre in your child's diet, in the form of brown rice, oats, beans, pulses, fruits and vegetables. A lot of parents opt for high-bran breakfast cereals in an effort to add fibre to their child's diet. Wholemeal bread is another favoured food for constipation. However, despite their healthy reputation, wheat-based products such as wholemeal bread and bran-based cereals are common instigators of undesirable digestive symptoms such as bloating, discomfort and constipation. Oat-based cereals and whole rye bread seem to be easier on the gut and are generally better options.
Dairy products
There is some evidence that dairy products can cause constipation in children.[101–2] For more details about how to identify problem foods in your child's diet, see pages 211–22.
Magnesium-rich foods
Foods high in magnesium are generally helpful for a constipated child. Magnesium is important to help keep the muscles in the lining of the gut working normally. Eating green leafy vegetables, along with pulses, nuts and seeds, will help keep magnesium intake up, but supplementation (150–250 mg per day for a 40 kg child) may help.
Bulking agents
Another way to get a bit more roughage into the diet is with bulking agents such as psyllium seeds, linseeds or guar gum (*see also* below). These generally soften the stool, making it easier to pass.
Water
Along with increased fibre, however, it's important that your child has plenty to drink.[103] For more advice on the recommended amount of water for children, see pages 181–3.
Prune juice
For children over the age of four years, try giving a cup of prune juice mixed with 1 tbsp of lemon juice. Taken before bedtime, this normally has the desired effect the next morning.

Exercise
Ensure that your child gets plenty of activity and exercise as this seems to help ensure bowel regularity, as well have having a host of other benefits too.

Supplements
Probiotics
Probiotics (supplements of healthy gut bacteria) seem to help resolve constipation as well as improve the general health of the gut.[104] For more information about probiotics, see page 16.

Flower essences
• The Australian Bush essences Bluebell, Bottlebrush and Boronia are recommended.
• Dr Bach's Crab Apple remedy tends to work well for children who believe that opening their bowels makes them **dirty or unclean**.

Coughs

Coughs are often a sign of an underlying health problem and it's generally best to treat this rather than just the cough. There are many causes of coughs, including bacterial or viral infections of the airways, e.g. bronchitis, laryngitis, pneumonia, croup or bronchiolitis. Sometimes, coughs are caused by inhaling irritating substances such as dust, cigarette smoke and pollen.

Diet

Food allergies

Both upper and lower respiratory tracts can be affected by food allergies. One study found, for example, that one of the classic signs of food allergy was chronic coughing and wheezing.[105] The authors of the study recommended that food allergy should be considered when there is a history of prior intolerance to a food in childhood or of symptoms beginning soon after a particular food was introduced into the diet. On this basis, it might be worth looking at the possibility of food sensitivity in your child (see pages 211–22).

Supplements

Vitamin C, zinc and echinacea

If a child seems to be coughing as the result of an infection, then supporting their immune system may help. A combination of vitamin C, zinc and the herb echinacea is usually quite effective in getting on top of an infection (see 'Colds and flu').

Thyme

A commonly used herb for a cough is thyme (*Thymus vulgaris*). This herb has a long history of use in Europe for dry cough. It also seems to help clear mucus. Add 1–2 g of thyme to boiling water to make a tea. This should be drunk several times a day. Your child may be more inclined to drink this if you add a little honey. Honey has been shown to help control organisms in the throat that might be a factor in coughing.

Flower essences

• The Australian Bush essences Illawarra Flame Tree, Dagger Hakea and Red Helmet are all indicated for coughs.
• Vervain (a Bach flower essence) will generally help **ease the stress** of a cough.
• Olive (a Bach flower essence) may help a child who is **worn out** by coughing.

Cracks at the corners of the mouth

See 'Angular stomatitis'

Cradle cap

Cradle cap is an infantile form of skin condition known as 'seborrhoeic dermatitis'. It is characterised by the presence of thick yellow scales on the skin of the scalp. Other sites for this condition include the face, neck and the nappy region. The condition is not related to poor hygiene or lack of cleanliness and is harmless.

Supplements
Biotin

There is some evidence that cradle cap is related to a deficiency in the nutrient biotin, which is one of the B-group vitamins.[106] Biotin supplementation may help to control the condition. If you are breast-feeding your child, take 500–1000 mcg of biotin per day. If you are bottle-feeding, put 50–100 mcg of biotin in your baby's feed each day.

Topical treatments
Starflower oil

The application of starflower oil (also known as borage oil) to children's seborrhoeic dermatitis in the nappy region often leads to considerable improvement in their condition. This approach is also certainly worth trying in cradle cap too. Rub 10 drops of starflower oil into the affected region, twice a day for two weeks. This can be repeated as necessary.

Cramp

Cramp is a painful spasm in a muscle caused by excessive or prolonged contraction of muscle fibres, often in the calves, feet or back of the thighs. Cramps usually last for a few moments, but can quite commonly occur at night, which may disrupt your child's sleep.

Diet
Calcium and magnesium

Cramps are quite often related to nutritional deficiency, often in the minerals calcium, magnesium or potassium. Sesame seeds, tahini (sesame seed paste) and tinned fish are good sources of calcium. Magnesium can be found in nuts, seafood, whole grains and green leafy vegetables, while bananas and other fruits are rich in potassium. Encouraging your child to eat more of these foods can sometimes be all it takes to stop recurrent cramp attacks.

Supplements
Magnesium

Taking magnesium in supplement form often puts a stop to cramp attacks within a few days or weeks. For a 40 kg child, give 150–250 mg per day. Supplementing with magnesium is often very effective in relieving cramp in pregnancy too. In one study, magnesium was found to reduce the severity of the cramps by more than 70 per cent.[107] If you are suffering from cramps in pregnancy, take 300–500 mg of magnesium each day.

Flower essences
• Rescue Remedy can be offered in the throes of a cramp, to relax and reduce pain.
• The Bush flower essences Grey Spider Flower and Bottlebrush also seem to work well for all types of muscular cramps.

Crohn's disease

Crohn's disease is caused by inflammation in the wall of the bowel and is characterised by bouts of pain and diarrhoea, which can be bloody. The condition can affect any part of the gut, but classically causes inflammation in the last part of the small intestine.

There are two approaches to Crohn's disease that tend to be quite effective in many individuals. One of these is to eliminate refined carbohydrates, and in particular, sugars known as 'disaccharides' (e.g. sucrose and fructose). The concept here is that these foods feed organisms within the gut, which might trigger or worsen Crohn's disease. More details about the specifics of this diet can be found in Elaine Gotschall's book entitled *Breaking the Vicious Cycle* (Kirkton Press, Kirkton, Ontario, Canada). There is at least some experimental evidence that suggests that a low carbohydrate diet can be effective in controlling Crohn's disease. In one study, a low-sugar, high-fibre diet led to a 70 per cent reduction in hospitalisations compared to individuals who did not change their diet.[108]

The other major approach that tends to be effective for Crohn's disease centres around the identification and treatment of food sensitivities. There is some evidence that food intolerance can be a factor in Crohn's disease. In one study, the most common food triggers were found to be cereals, dairy and yeast.[109] Identification and elimination of problem foodstuffs does seem to help a substantial proportion of Crohn's sufferers. For more information about food sensitivity, see pages 211–22.

Supplements

Multivitamins and minerals

Crohn's sufferers can have multiple nutritional deficiencies because they tend not to absorb nutrients very effectively. It is a good idea for sufferers to take a potent, high quality multivitamin and mineral preparation every day. Nutrients that might be of particular importance are zinc, vitamin B12 and folic acid, as they can help in the repair of the cells that line the intestinal tract. More details about suitable supplements for children can be found on page 14.

Fish oils

Fish oils such as eicosapentaenoic acid (EPA) and docosahexaenoic acid (DHA) might also help to control Crohn's and this may be related to their anti-inflammatory effect. One two-year study showed that a high fish diet substantially reduced the relapse rate in sufferers.[110] The fish richest in EPA and DHA are the 'oily' fish such as salmon, trout, mackerel, herring and sardine. In addition, it may help to take 2–3 g of concentrated fish oils each day.

Croup

Croup is an infection of the upper respiratory tract that results in swelling and inflammation of the area below the vocal cords. The condition is almost always caused by a virus, which may also affect the membranes above and below the larynx (voice box). Croup is most common in children aged three months to three years. Before the onset of the infection, a child may have a cold, sinus infection or sore throat. When the condition sets in, however, it gives rise to a characteristic barking cough as well as a harsh, low-pitched wheezing sound heard with each intake of breath. While the condition is not life threatening, it can cause a child to be breathless, which can be quite distressing. The infection will not last for more than three days. If your child does not seem to be getting better, or if you are worried for whatever reason, seek medical attention.

Supplements
Vitamin C and echinacea
A child with croup may be helped by taking steps to boost his immune system. Liquids containing vitamin C powder and/or the herb echinacea may help with this. See 'Colds and flu' for details.

Cuts and scrapes
Few children will make it through childhood without a few cuts and scrapes. Although the majority of such injuries are not serious, it is worth remembering that any break in the skin can open up the body to infection, so it's important that you treat even minor grazes as soon as possible. Serious injuries will obviously require medical care immediately.

Cleaning the wound
Wash and dry the cut or scrape gently with clean warm water. Adding a drop or two of tea tree oil to the water may help keep infection at bay. Tea tree is well known for its potent antimicrobial properties. One study found that tea tree was even effective against bacteria resistant to all known antibiotics.[111] It can be applied neat to scrapes or cuts, though it tends to sting.

Supplements
Vitamin C, zinc and echinacea
To boost the immune system and to help healing, make sure your child gets plenty of vitamin C and zinc. If your child is not taking one already, then a good multivitamin and mineral might help. The herb echinacea may also help to enhance immune function and reduce the risk of infection (see 'Colds and flu').

Topical treatments
Calendula cream
Apply calendula cream to the wound after cleaning. *Calendula officinalis* (marigold) is traditionally used for the treatment of skin disorders and is believed to have bacteria-killing, antiseptic and anti-inflammatory properties. Apply once or twice a day.
Honey
Many studies have demonstrated that honey has antibacterial activity, and a small number of clinical case studies have shown that application of honey to severely infected wounds is capable of clearing infection from the wound and improving tissue healing. It is also known that particular honeys from Australia and New Zealand have enhanced antibacterial activity, and these honeys have been approved for marketing as therapeutic honeys.[112–13] Manuka honey seems to be the best bet for wound healing. Brands to look out for in the UK are MediBee and Comvita. Apply twice a day.

Flower essences

• Rescue Remedy should be offered as soon as the injury occurs, which will help calm your child.
• The Bush flower essences Spinifex and Sturt Desert Rose are recommended for cuts and scrapes.

Cystitis

See 'Urinary tract infection'

Depression

Depressive disorders can have far reaching effects on the mental state and functioning of young people. Among both children and adolescents, depressive disorders increase the risk of illness and interpersonal difficulties and these may even persist long after the depressive episode has resolved. Depression is a diagnosis that seems to be commonly missed in adults, and the same is almost certainly true for younger individuals too. Often, signs of depressive disorders in young people are viewed as normal mood changes associated with transitions such as puberty or a change in schools. Also, there may be reluctance on the part of health professionals to 'label' someone as a depressive. However, it does seem sensible at least to be mindful of the fact that even young children can be depressed, so that they may be offered appropriate support if need be. In childhood, boys and girls appear to be at equal risk of depression. During adolescence, however, girls are twice as likely as boys to develop depression.

Sometimes, a child's depression is related to a specific situation in life. A child, for instance, may be depressed because of bullying at school or academic pressures. In general, it helps if a child is encouraged to talk about the problem. Open communication, followed by the appropriate support and action, may do much to allay the emotional distress that may be connected to life's circumstances.

Quite often, children may not be able to put their finger on what is troubling them. In these situations, depression may well be related to nutritional factors. Depression can have specific physiological and/or biochemical triggers. Common problems that I encounter in practice include anaemia and/or iron deficiency (see page 29), seasonal affective disorder (see page 133), food sensitivity (see pages 211–22), and blood sugar imbalance (see page 204). It can often help to eliminate certain foodstuffs that tend to upset brain chemistry. The major offenders here are generally sugar, caffeine and artificial sweeteners. In older children, alcohol or recreational drugs may be factors too. Getting these elements out of the diet often leads to a significant improvement in mood.

Diet

Omega-3 deficiency

There is increasing evidence that depression may be associated with a deficiency in the omega-3 fats found in oily fish such as salmon, trout, mackerel, herring and sardine. Omega-3 fats do seem to be very important for the normal function of the brain, and increasing the intake of these seems to help many conditions believed to be rooted in the brain such as dyslexia, hyperactivity and schizophrenia. One study showed that depression is far less common in people with a high consumption of fish and that fish eaters are more likely to report better mental health.[114] One study found that treatment with omega-3 fish oils (eicosapentaenoic acid) brought about significant relief from depression in a group of individuals who had not responded well to conventional antidepressants.

Children with mood disturbance should be encouraged to consume two or three servings of oily fish each week.

Supplements
Fish oils
It may help to supplement a child with omega-3 fats. For a 40 kg child, supplement 2–3 g of concentrated fish oils each day. Alternatives to fish oil supplements are discussed on page 246.
St John's wort
The herb St John's wort (*Hypericum perforatum*) has been shown to be effective in the treatment of depression. In one study, two-thirds of individuals with mild to moderate depression improved on St John's wort, compared to only about a quarter of individuals who were taking a placebo.[115] There is some evidence that the overall effect of St John's wort is to increase the levels of 'feel-good' brain chemicals such as serotonin, noradrenaline and dopamine.[116] The normal recommended dose for a 40 kg child is 150–200 mg of

herb extract, taken three times a day. St John's wort should not be mixed with other antidepressant medication.
Multivitamins and minerals
A range of nutrients seems to have an important influence on maintaining normal brain function and mood. These include vitamin B1 (thiamine). One study found that low B1 levels were associated with low feelings of composure and confidence and an increased tendency to depression in young women. Supplementation with vitamin B1 improved mood in the long term.[117] Another study, this time in young men, found that vitamin B1 deficiency was associated with inactivity, introversion, fatigue, decreased self-confidence and poorer mood. This study found that just two months of B1 supplementation led to an improvement in these men.[118]

Other nutrients that seem to play some role in the prevention and treatment of depression include folic acid[119] and selenium.[120] The taking of a good quality multivitamin and mineral supplement on a regular basis reduces the risk of deficiency in key nutrients and may help prevent or even treat depression in the long term. More details about suitable supplements can be found on page 14.

Flower essences
Flower essences were originally devised with emotional problems in mind, so it comes as no surprise that they have enormous potential value in the treatment of depression. A full list of the indications for specific flower essences can be found on pages 20–1.

However, of particular use may be:
- Agrimony for **deeply held emotional tensions** that are hidden from others.
- Gorse for **feelings of hopelessness.**
- Gentian for **mild depression** and despondency.
- Mustard for **black depression** and little or no feeling of joy.

See pages 19–24 for more details about flower essences and how to use them.

Diabetes mellitus

Diabetes is a condition characterised by abnormally high levels of sugar in the bloodstream. In the long term, diabetes can lead to a variety of health problems, including eye disease and blindness, kidney disease, heart disease, leg ulcers, gangrene and impotence. There are essentially two forms of diabetes; Type I and Type II. Type I diabetes (also known as 'juvenile onset' or 'insulin-dependent' diabetes) generally comes on early in life and is caused by a failure of the pancreas to secrete insulin. Sufferers of this form of diabetes must take insulin by injection to keep blood sugar levels from rising uncontrollably. There is some evidence to suggest that Type I diabetes is related to the consumption of cow's milk.[121–3] Some scientists have suggested that certain proteins in milk might trigger an immune reaction, which also leads to the destruction of cells in the pancreas responsible for making insulin.

Symptoms of Type I diabetes include increased frequency of urination, increased and often extreme thirst, weight loss and irritability and fatigue.

Bedwetting may be a feature too. If your child is exhibiting these symptoms, then it is important that you seek medical attention. Undiagnosed and untreated Type I diabetes can lead to coma, which may be life threatening.

In Type II diabetes (also known 'non-insulin dependent' diabetes) the problem is generally not that there is insufficient insulin, but that the body is resistant to its effects. Type II diabetes is very often related to excess weight and inactivity. Fortunately, sufferers of this form of diabetes may be able to control their diabetes through changing their diet and taking more exercise. If this fails, oral medication may be prescribed. A proportion of Type II diabetics may need insulin to control their condition. Until recently, Type II diabetes was found almost exclusively in middle and old age and, for this reason, was sometimes referred to as 'mature-onset' diabetes. However, in many industrialised countries the condition is being diagnosed in children as young as ten years old, which is why the term 'mature-onset' is generally no longer used.

Diet
Sugar and the glycaemic index
Diabetics are normally advised to limit their consumption of sweet, sugary foods, and to keep their diet based around starchy carbohydrates such as bread, potatoes, rice and pasta. The basis for this is that unlike sugar, starches need to be digested before they can be absorbed, slowing their release into the bloodstream. However, in contrast to conventional wisdom, many starchy foods can upset blood

sugar control because they actually release sugar quickly into the bloodstream (known as high glycaemic index foods). Foods that fall into this category include diabetic staples such as potatoes, white bread, white rice and pasta. As a result, individuals who eat a conventional diet for diabetes very often have continuing problems with their blood sugar levels. Basing the diet around low glycaemic index (slow sugar-releasing) foods is of paramount importance to individuals suffering from diabetes. Regular eating, preferably moderate amounts of food taken frequently, also helps to regularise blood sugar levels. More information about this and a list of the common carbohydrate foods and their glycaemic indices can be found on pages 206–8.

Prevention: Type I diabetes

Because of the link between Type I diabetes and cow's milk protein, it makes sense not to over-emphasise dairy products in a child's diet. Varying the diet and using alternative food products such as rice milk, goat's milk, sheep's yoghurt and goat's and sheep's milk is likely to reduce the risk of your child mounting the immune reaction that might cause some cases of Type I diabetes. More details about food sensitivity can be found on pages 211–22.

Vitamin D

There is good evidence that vitamin D can help protect against Type I diabetes.[124–5] Some scientists have suggested that vitamin D may have beneficial effects on the immune response and reduce the risk of unwanted reactions.

Taking a good quality multivitamin and mineral (containing vitamin D) during pregnancy and breast-feeding and having your child take a suitable supplement during childhood may help to provide some protection from Type I diabetes.

Prevention: Type II diabetes

Basing the diet around low glycaemic index foods and a regular pattern of eating will help prevent blood sugar imbalance. This, in turn, will reduce the risk of the high levels of insulin that are a common feature on the road to Type II diabetes. Apart from diet, studies have found that the other lifestyle factor that has an important bearing on the risk of diabetes is exercise. Ensuring that your child gets regular activity and exercise should also help provide protection from diabetes in the long term.

Supplements

Multivitamins and minerals

The basic dietary principles of a diabetic diet are covered above. However, certain nutrients and/or herbs may also assist in healthy blood sugar control. Some of the more important nutrients in this respect are chromium, vitamin B3 and magnesium. Taking a good quality multivitamin and mineral (that contains these nutrients) may help long-term blood sugar control.

Gymnema sylvestre

The herb *Gymnema sylvestre* can also help balance blood sugar levels. A 40 kg child should take 200 mg of *Gymnema sylvestre* per day.

Flower essences

• The Bush flower essences Paw Paw and Peach-flowered Tea-tree are recommended for problems relating to blood sugar.

Diarrhoea

See also 'Food poisoning and Gastroenteritis'

Short-term (acute) diarrhoea has a number of causes – normally viral (as in gastroenteritis), bacterial (salmonella, for example) or non-specific (in the case of eating a new, rich food, for example). Long-standing (chronic) diarrhoea can quite easily lead to dehydration. In children, common causes of loose bowels can also include food sensitivity (see pages 211–22) and excess yeast in the gut (see page 223). Working with and resolving these factors, if they seem to be present, often leads to an improvement in symptoms.

Fluid intake

Keeping your child well hydrated is extremely important. Offer small sips of water – larger quantities may make your child feel sick and increase the risk of vomiting. Diluted, freshly squeezed fruit juice can also help supply your child with some energy.

Diet

Keep foods light and easy to digest, such as ripe bananas, cooked vegetables, light soups and broths. It is a good idea to avoid too much in the way of wheat or other whole grains as they can irritate the lining of the gut and make the condition worse. Food containing added sugar should also be avoided as this tends to feed the organisms that may be causing the problem.

Supplements

Probiotics

If there is one 'cure-all' for diarrhoea, probiotics (supplements of healthy gut bacteria) are it, in my opinion. Probiotics may work in a number of ways to restore health to the gut. In particular, they seem to have the ability to 'crowd out' unhealthy organisms and perhaps even have an antimicrobial action of their own. Probiotics do not just help resolve diarrhoea, but also reduce the risk of a problem with an imbalance in the gut organisms in the long term. One study found that the use of probiotics was associated with a significantly reduced risk of diarrhoea lasting more than three days.[126] Probiotics also significantly reduced the duration of diarrhoea. Another study confirmed that taken regularly, probiotics reduce the risk of diarrhoea significantly in young children.[127]

For more information on suitable probiotic supplements, see page 16.

Zinc

There's also evidence that zinc can reduce the duration of a bout of diarrhoea and the risk of acquiring diarrhoea by about half.[128] Adding a multivitamin and mineral that contains zinc to your child's regime may help bring a problem with diarrhoea under control.

Flower essences
• The Australian Bush essence Paw Paw is specifically indicated for diarrhoea.

Down's syndrome
Almost all cells in the body contain genetic information in the form of structures called chromosomes. Normally the cells contain 46 chromosomes each (23 pairs of chromosomes). However, in Down's syndrome, individuals have one extra chromosome. Instead of there being two copies of chromosome number 21, there are three. This extra chromosome has been shown to increase the work-rate of certain enzymes that increase free radical production and enhance what is known as 'oxidative stress' on the body. What this essentially means is that the body ages more quickly, and is more likely to run into problems with degenerative conditions earlier in life.

Certain nutrients known as 'antioxidants' have the capacity to combat oxidative stress in the body. Nutri-Chem Pharmacies in Canada has formulated a multivitamin and mineral preparation specifically for individuals with Down's syndrome. (For more details, see Useful contacts and information.)

Dry eyes
The surface of the eye is kept moist by tears secreted by what are known as the 'lachrymal glands'. 'Sicca syndrome' is a condition characterised by dry eyes caused by insufficient tear production and is usually associated with a dry mouth.

Diet
Salt
On a dietary level, it is important to avoid salt. Salt in the body tends to draw moisture out of the surface of the eye and can therefore worsen a dry eye condition.
Essential fatty acids
Dry eyes are often a sign of a deficiency in healthy fats known as essential fatty acids (EFAs). Other symptoms of EFA deficiency include dry skin, abnormal thirst and behavioural or learning difficulties. More details about the role of EFAs in health can be found on pages 154–7. A child with dry eyes may benefit from eating more foods rich in EFAs, including extra virgin olive oil, avocado, oily fish and nuts and seeds.

Supplements
Hemp seed oil
It can also help to take an EFA supplement. Hemp seed oil is a good all-round supplement as it contains essential fats of both the omega-3 and omega-6 type (see pages 156–7). I recommend 10–15 ml (2 –3 tsp) a day for a 40 kg child. Children may be reluctant to take this oil off a spoon, so it may be best to put it in a soup, stew, sauce or casserole.

Dry skin
In general, dry skin is usually associated with a deficiency of healthy fats known as essential fatty acids (EFAs). In this respect, the condition has a similar cause to dry eyes and these two symptoms very often coincide. Increasing consumption of EFA-rich foods (see 'Dry eyes') is often effective in moistening the skin.

Supplements

Hemp seed oil

As with dry eyes, I recommend hemp seed oil as a good all-round supplement for children with dry skin as it contains essential fats of both the omega-3 and omega-6 type (see page 156). I recommend 10 ml (2 tsp) a day for a 40 kg child. Children may be reluctant to take this oil off a spoon, so it may be best to put it in a soup, stew, sauce or casserole.

Dyslexia and dyspraxia

Dyslexia is a condition that can manifest as problems in a range of areas, including reading, writing, spelling, mathematical ability, memory and concentration. Because dyslexics may have difficulties learning information in the way that it is commonly presented, they may be labelled as learning disabled or just 'slow'. However, many dyslexics are bright and often have many creative, artistic and practical skills. It has been estimated that about 10 per cent of the population is dyslexic.

Dyspraxia is a condition often characterised by problems with bodily co-ordination. Children with dyspraxia have difficulty learning new and unfamiliar tasks. With effort, a dyspraxic child may learn things that non-dyspraxic children appear to master more quickly. As a result, the phrases 'he could do it if he tried' and 'more effort required' is often applied to affected children.

Children with dyspraxia are also often described as being clumsy or awkward. They also may seem to have to think carefully about their movements and plan these to avoid making mistakes. Poor handwriting is quite common too. It has been estimated that at least 10 per cent of the population are affected by dyspraxia, and 70 per cent of dyspraxics are male.

Dyslexia and dyspraxia often coincide and it is quite likely that the two conditions have similar if not identical causes. Two prominent theories about what underlies these conditions relate to a deficiency of 'healthy' essential fatty acids in the diet, and abnormal function in a part of the brain called the cerebellum (cerebellar developmental delay). These issues, and their management, are discussed below.

Diagnosis

While the diagnoses of dyslexia and dyspraxia are generally in the domain of educational psychologists, there are tell-tale signs for you to look out for. These include:

Pre-school signs of dyslexia
• Family history of dyslexia
• Later than expected ability to speak clearly
• Jumbling of phrases, e.g. 'cobbler's club' for 'toddler's club', 'teddy-dare' for 'teddy-bear'
• Impulsiveness and quick thinking
• Mislabelling of objects, e.g. lampshade for lamppost
• Lisping
• Inability to remember the label for known objects, e.g. colours
• Confused directional words, e.g. using 'up' for 'down' or 'in' for 'out'

• Enhanced creativity, e.g. drawing skills and a good sense of colour
• 'Good' and 'bad' days for no apparent reason
• Aptitude for constructional or technical toys, e.g. bricks, puzzles, Lego blocks
• Enjoys being read to but exhibiting little interest in letters or words
• Has difficulty learning nursery rhymes
• Prefers or preferred to 'bottom shuffle' rather than crawl

Children of nine years or under
• Particular difficulty learning to read and write
• Persistent and continued reversing of numbers and letters, e.g. '15' for '51', 'b' for 'd'
• Difficulty telling left from right
• Difficulty learning the alphabet and multiplication tables, and remembering sequences such as the days of the week and months of the year
• Continued difficulty with tasks such as the tying of shoelaces, ball catching and skipping
• Inattention and poor concentration
• Frustration, possibly leading to behavioural problems

Children of nine to twelve years
• Continued mistakes in reading and/or problems with reading comprehension
• Strange spelling, perhaps with letters missed out or in the wrong order
• Taking an above average time over written work
• Disorganisation at home and at school
• Difficulty copying accurately from blackboard or textbook
• Difficulty taking down oral instructions

• Growing lack of self-confidence and increasing frustration

Children of 12 years and over
• Tendency to read inaccurately or without comprehension
• Inconsistent spelling
• Difficulty with planning and written essays
• Tendency to confuse verbal instructions and telephone numbers
• Severe difficulty with learning a foreign language
• Low self-esteem
• Difficulty with perception of language, e.g. following instructions, listening

Symptoms suggestive of dyspraxia
• Clumsiness
• Poor posture, poor body awareness and awkward movement
• Confusion over handedness
• Sensitive to touch and find some clothes uncomfortable
• Poor short-term memory, can forget tasks learned that day
• Writing/reading difficulties, holding of pens can be awkward
• Poor sense of direction
• Physical activities are problematic, cannot catch, run, skip, ride a bike or use equipment easily
• Phobias, obsessive or immature behaviour
• Difficulty with tasks requiring a sequence such as maths
• Problems with awareness of time
• Energy drain (dyspraxic children appear to tire easily and need longer periods of rest and sleep)
• Lack of awareness of potential danger, especially important in practical and science subjects

What causes dyslexia and dyspraxia?

It is not known for sure what causes dyslexia and dyspraxia. However, it is clear from the nature of the symptoms of these conditions that they are both likely to be related to problems with the normal functioning of the brain. An emerging theory about the precise nature of the neurological glitches in dyslexia and dyspraxia concerns a part of the brain called the cerebellum.[129] The potential role of the cerebellum in dyslexia and dyspraxia has led some scientists to explore the idea of improving cerebellar function in individuals affected by these conditions. Some doctors believe that it is possible to 're-train' the cerebellum with daily movements and exercises specifically designed to stimulate this area of the brain.

In a recent study, children with dyslexia were split into two groups. Children in one group were asked to perform specific exercises designed to improve cerebellar function each day for six months. Compared to children who did not go through the programme, those performing the exercises were found to enjoy significant improvements in a great number of areas, including posture, dexterity, reading and verbal fluency. These children were also found to perform significantly better on standardised tests of reading, writing and comprehension.[130]

DDAT, a UK-based company, has a number of centres that offer a comprehensive service for children with dyslexia and dyspraxia. At an initial three-hour consultation, children have their cerebellar function assessed. Then they are advised on the specific exercises that may help their cerebellar function. Follow-up appointments are usually at six-weekly intervals, with complete treatment normally in several months. There is some evidence that the benefits of these exercises remain even after a child stops doing them. (For more details, see Useful contacts and information.)

Diet

Essential fatty acids

Healthy fats known as essential fatty acids (EFAs) appear to have an important role in the normal and healthy functioning of the brain. A deficiency of these healthy fats in the body may possibly lead to problems with mood and behaviour. One study found that dyslexic adults were much more likely to show symptoms of EFA deficiency than non-dyslexics, and the more deficient they seemed to be, the worse the dyslexia.[131] Another small study has found that EFA supplementation brought benefits for both dyslexics and dyspraxics.[132] The omega-3 fats found in oily fish such as salmon, trout, mackerel, herring and sardine seem to be particularly important in the treatment of dyslexia and dyspraxia. Symptoms suggestive of EFA deficiency to look out for in your child include:

- Excessive thirst
- Frequent urination
- Dry skin
- Dry hair
- Soft or brittle nails
- Dandruff
- Follicular keratosis (a skin condition characterised by what look like permanent goosebumps, usually at the back of the upper arms)

For more details about EFA deficiency and how to correct it, see page 156. For children exhibiting some or all of these symptoms, EFA supplementation is likely to be of benefit. In cases of dyslexia and dyspraxia, I generally suggest an aggressive approach that includes decent amounts of all the major essential fats. For a 40 kg child, I recommend giving 10–15 ml (2–3 tsp) of hemp seed oil along with 2–3 g of concentrated fish oils each day.

Dysmenorrhoea
See 'Menstrual cramps'

Ear infections

Ear infections (also called 'otitis media' by the medical profession) are common in childhood and a frequent cause of earache. Such infections are quite often related to colds. Here the viral infection may lead to the build-up of fluid and congestion, which then makes infection with a bacterial agent more likely. Bacterial infections are usually treated with antibiotics.

Diet
Food sensitivity

In natural medicine it is often found that recurrent ear infections in children are related to food sensitivity. In one study in children with recurrent ear infection, 78 per cent tested positive for food sensitivity. Elimination of offending foods led to a significant improvement in 86 per cent of children.[133] Some foods are renowned for their ability to stimulate mucus formation in and around the ears, with dairy products being by far the most common culprits. It is usually beneficial to remove cow's milk and dairy products made from cow's milk, such as cheese and yoghurt, from a child's diet. These can be substituted with rice and soya milk (available from good health food stores), and cheeses made from goat's and sheep's milk.

If a child does not improve on this regime, it might be worth eliminating other commonly implicated foods, such as wheat, eggs and chocolate. More information on how to identify food sensitivities and appropriate substitute foods can be found in pages 211–22. Sugar should also be avoided as this suppresses the function of the immune system, which can make ear infection more likely.

Supplements

Multivitamins and minerals

Certain nutrients may help to maintain healthy immune function. For this reason, it is a good idea for children who are prone to ear infections to take a multivitamin and mineral supplement each day.

Probiotics

Another useful approach is for the child to take a course of probiotics (healthy gut bacteria) for a month or two. Children who have had ear infection will normally have been given antibiotics. While these may help fight bacterial infection in the ear itself, they can also kill many of the beneficial bacteria in the gut leading to imbalance in the organisms here. This can lead to problems with irritable bowel syndrome, yeast overgrowth and food sensitivity in the long term. Such supplements can be found in powder form or as capsules, which can be opened into water and drunk. If antibiotics have been given, a probiotic should be given for two to four weeks. More details about suitable supplements can be found on pages 16–17.

Eczema

Eczema is an inflammatory skin disorder characterised by patches of red, flaking skin. The condition can affect any part of the body, but is most common on the face, neck and the bends of the elbows and areas behind the knees. There is some evidence that food sensitivity is often at the root of eczema. One study found that up to 63 per cent of children with eczema showed reactions to certain foods.[134] In practice, the identification and elimination of problem foods is usually very effective in helping a child with this condition. Milk and other dairy products seem to be a particular problem, though any food might be at fault.[135] More information about food sensitivity and what to do about it can be found on pages 211–22.

Supplements

Essential fatty acids

Of particular importance here seem to be EFAs of the omega-6 class, including a fat known as linoleic acid.[136] One study suggests that research dating from the 1930s through to the 1950s has established that a deficit of omega-6 EFAs can lead to inflammatory skin conditions in both animals and humans. Also, eczema sufferers have been noted to have a tendency to be low in EFAs, and that supplementation with evening primrose oil (rich in omega-6 EFAs) could bring a significant benefit to eczema sufferers.[137] Evening primrose oil treatment has been found to reduce the severity of eczema and may also lead to a substantial reduction in the amount of steroid cream used by sufferers.

Linoleic acid

Supplements of linoleic acid have also been found to be of great benefit in the treatment of eczema. One study found that three months of treatment with 3 g of linoleic acid led to a reduction in eczema symptoms of between 80 and 90 per cent. In the UK, concentrated linoleic acid is available under the brand name Linatox. (For more details, see

Useful contacts and information – under Cedar.) This product is particularly suitable for children as it contains natural strawberry flavouring, which makes it more palatable than a lot of other oil products. The dose for children aged five to twelve years is 3 ml a day. Children older than this should take 6 ml a day.

Fish oils

Fish oils (which contain what are known as omega-3 fats) have also been shown to benefit eczema sufferers. One study found that symptoms were reduced by some 75 per cent in patients taking fish oils, compared to only 5 per cent in those who took a placebo.[138] For a 40 kg child, give 2 g of concentrated fish oils a day.

Hemp seed oil

Hemp seed oil is a good all-round supplement as it contains essential fats of both the omega-3 and omega-6 type. I recommend 10 ml (2 tsp) a day for a 40 kg child. Children may be reluctant to take this oil off a spoon, so it may be best to put it in a soup, stew, sauce or casserole.

Vitamins and minerals

A variety of nutrients, including zinc, magnesium and the vitamins B6, B3 and C, are needed to aid the conversion of EFAs into molecules that are critical to the health-giving effects of these fats. Lack of one or more of these nutrients can cause this conversion to stall, which means a child may not get all the benefits of whatever healthy fats it consumes via the diet or supplements. In addition to supplementing with EFAs, it can help a child to take a good quality multivitamin and mineral supplement each day (see pages 14–15).

Probiotics

Healthy gut bacteria seem to play some role in the prevention and treatment of eczema. It is believed that these have an important part to play in maintaining health in the gut, which in turn reduces the risk of food sensitivity problems. One study found that giving probiotics during pregnancy to the mother and then after the birth to the child substantially reduced the incidence of eczema in those children at the age of two.[139] Another study found the same thing, and showed that taking probiotics while breast-feeding also helps protect a baby from eczema in the first two years of life. Further research found that probiotics brought significant benefits to infants who developed eczema during breast-feeding.[140]

For the best protection from eczema and other allergic conditions, it is advisable for women to take a probiotic supplement during pregnancy and breast-feeding. In addition, children with eczema are likely to be helped by probiotic supplementation. Up to the age of two, this is best done with a product called INT B1 which contains the gut bacteria thought to be of particular importance in infants and small children (*Bifidobacterium infantis*). Give a quarter of a teaspoon in one feed each day. (For more details, see Useful contacts and information – under BioCare.) After this time, it is better to give a supplement containing the dominant organisms found in the digestive tracts of older children. More details about suitable supplements can be found on pages 16–17.

Topical treatments

Hemp seed oil cream

Hemp seed oil cream provides a good all-round cream for combating dry skin and inflammatory skin conditions such as eczema. It can be obtained by mail order from Fitzsimmons Herbals. (For more details, see Useful contacts and information.)

Allergenics

Allergenics is a range of skin products designed for eczema. They contain extracts of soya (soy sterols) and liquorice (glycyrrhetinic acid), which can calm inflammation in the skin but do not weaken it. The cream also contains other plant-based substances known to help soothe and heal irritated skin, including aloe vera and vitamin E. Allergenics products represent a natural alternative to steroid-based products, and are available in good health food stores. (For more details, see Useful contacts and information – under Optima Healthcare.)

Flower essences

• Bach flower essence Impatiens is useful for **itching and irritability**.
• The Australian Bush essences Dagger Hakea and Billy Goat Plum are recommended for eczema.

Endometriosis

During each menstrual cycle, the lining of the womb builds up and then is shed if pregnancy does not take place. In endometriosis, womb tissue is found outside the womb itself. Common sites for the endometrial tissue include the ovaries, fallopian tubes and ligaments that support the uterus, and the area between the vagina and rectum. This misplaced tissue develops into growths or lesions, which respond to the menstrual cycle in the same way that the womb lining does, and this can cause considerable pain and discomfort. Some of the most common symptoms of endometriosis include menstrual pain, pain during sex and painful urination and/or bowel movements during periods. The condition is also associated with some cases of infertility.

It is not clear what causes endometriosis. One theory is that it is related to exposure to environmental toxins called 'dioxins'. One study in rhesus monkeys found a clear correlation between dioxin exposure and endometriosis.[141] Many sanitary towels and tampons contain dioxins and it might be worthwhile avoiding products treated with these chemicals. Organic sanitary wear that is not contaminated with suspect chemicals is widely available in health food stores.

Epilepsy

Epilepsy, characterised by fitting, can be a serious condition, which may not respond to medication. Even when it does, however, the side effects of the medication can be persistent and troublesome. Not unusually, though, epilepsy responds to a natural and/or nutritional approach. It should be borne in mind, however, that epilepsy is a potentially serious condition and it is therefore advisable to work with a practitioner experienced in its management. In particular, it is sensible not to make changes to a child's conventional medication without first consulting your doctor.

Diet
Sugar
One potentially effective strategy is to ensure that the level of sugar in the bloodstream is maintained. Low blood sugar (hypoglycaemia) seems to be a common trigger factor in epilepsy. Frequent meals and snacks based on foods that release sugar slowly into the bloodstream should be taken. Also, certain nutrient supplements can also help stabilise blood sugar levels, including chromium, magnesium and vitamin B3. More about the regulation of blood sugar can be found on pages 204–10.

Food sensitivity
Food sensitivity may be a common factor in epilepsy in children anyway. One study found that 80 per cent of epileptic children who also had other symptoms of food sensitivity (e.g. migraine, hyperactivity, abdominal symptoms) improved on a diet that excluded the food to which individuals tend to be sensitive.[142] In this study, more than half of the children who excluded foods became completely seizure-free. More information about the diagnosis and treatment of food sensitivity can be found on pages 211–22.

Supplements
Vitamins B6 and E
There is some evidence that epilepsy might be related to nutritional deficiencies. One study showed that more than half of epileptic patients had a deficiency of vitamin B6, and that about half of these responded to vitamin B6 therapy at a dose of 160 mg per day.[143] In another study, vitamin E was found to help a significant proportion of epileptic children. Ten out of twelve children (83 per cent) who were resistant to drug therapy had a reduction in seizure frequency of at least 60 per cent when given vitamin E at a dose of 400 IU per day.[144] It may be that giving additional quantities of vitamin E and B6 (and perhaps other nutrients) may help to reduce a tendency to epileptic seizures. A good quality multivitamin and mineral each day is a good starting point, though more specialised management is best done under the supervision of a practitioner.

Fatigue
An unusually tired child can have one or more of a range of imbalances going on in the body. However, certain imbalances crop up commonly in children with fatigue, and identifying and correcting these factors can often really help to pick up a child's energy and sense of wellbeing.

Common causes of fatigue
Nutrient deficiency
To a degree, the body needs certain nutrients to run properly. A poor diet, low in nutrients and perhaps loaded with additives, simply does not make the best fuel for the body. Advice on what constitutes a healthy diet for children and some practical advice

about how to go about revamping a child's diet can be found on pages 187–91. One nutrient that is commonly deficient in children with fatigue is iron. For more details, see pages 165–6.

Blood sugar imbalance

Children prone to episodes of low blood sugar can find themselves unusually tired at certain times of the day. Mid-afternoon fatigue (and maybe some crankiness) is also common in children whose blood sugar levels are a bit unstable. Cravings for sweet foods or drinks is another common feature in this imbalance. If this sounds like your child, you can learn more about this problem and what to do about it on pages 204–10.

Food sensitivity

Food sensitivities very often cause fatigue. Some children may feel tired an hour or two after certain foods and this is worth looking out for. If a child is prone to conditions such as tonsillitis, ear infections, glue ear, a runny nose, eczema or asthma, then food sensitivity is very likely. If this sounds like your child, then I recommend you have a look at the section on food sensitivity on pages 211–22.

Yeast overgrowth

Overgrowth of yeast in the body, which generally occurs in children who have been treated with antibiotics, is a common cause of fatigue. If your child tends to be on the windy side and get fungal infections such as athlete's foot, then a yeast problem is likely. See pages 223–8 for more details about this.

Adrenal weakness

Weakness in the adrenal glands appears to be becoming more common,

even in children. If your child seems to be especially worn out after exercise, tends towards low blood pressure (and is perhaps prone to dizziness and fainting), needs to eat regularly and is slender in stature, then adrenal weakness is a likely problem.

What to do

A basic healthy diet (see pages 187–91) is a good place to start, whatever the cause of your child's fatigue. Adequate sleep is also important, and if there's any hint of insomnia, you might find the information on pages 101–3 useful.

Supplements

B-complex

B vitamins have a variety of roles to play in the body, one of which is to help in the reactions that convert food into energy. Deficiencies of B vitamins seem often to be a factor in childhood fatigue, which is not surprising when you consider that some of the foods richest in these nutrients (whole grains, vegetables, nuts and seeds) tend to be in short supply in many children's diets. For a 40 kg child, give a B-complex supplement that contains about 25 mg of the major B vitamins B1, B2, B3, B5 and B6.

Vitamin C

Deficiency of vitamin C may cause fatigue and depression, which usually responds to a bit of additional supplementation.[145] Plenty of fresh fruit and vegetables will help prevent this, though some additional supplementation as part of a multivitamin and mineral formulation makes good sense too. For a 40 kg child, give 500–1000 mg of vitamin C per day.

Iron
Iron deficiency is surprisingly common in children (see page 29). A diet that includes some meat, eggs, dark leafy green vegetables and even a bit of dark chocolate should help here. Including a multivitamin and mineral with some added iron is also a good idea. However, large doses of iron should not be given to a child unless blood tests reveal that they have a proven iron deficiency. The best test for this seems to be a blood test called 'serum ferritin' (see page 30).

Magnesium
Magnesium is a key nutrient for the production of energy in the body, but tends to be in short supply in the average child's diet. This problem may be worsened by stress and anxiety, which can reduce the amount of magnesium in the body.[146] It often helps children to take a supplement of magnesium, at a dose of 150–250 mg per day for a 40 kg child.

Liquorice
Liquorice is generally a good remedy for children who seem to have weakness in the adrenal glands (see above). For a 40 kg child, give 1–2 g per day of liquorice root. While high doses of liquorice should not be used in the long term, the lower doses recommended here are known to be safe.

Other tips for beating fatigue *Sleep*
Adequate sleep is key to banishing fatigue. As with adults, a child's sleep requirements are quite individual. Most parents have a good sense for if a child is getting enough sleep. If your child is having difficulties getting to sleep, or is waking in the night, see 'Insomnia'.

Exercise
Exercise and activity generally boost energy and wellbeing in children. One of the reasons for this may be that active children tend to sleep better, perhaps because exercise helps to burn-up 'stress' hormones that may disrupt sleep. Exercise also may help to lift mood and motivation.

Flower essences
• The best essence for **overwhelming fatigue** is the Bach flower remedy Olive.
• Gentian is good if your child feels **discouraged, despondent and pessimistic**.
• Hornbeam is ideal if your child tends to feel **stuck in a rut** and perpetually tired.

More details about the flower essences and how to use them can be found on pages 19–24.

Fainting
Fainting is sudden and temporary loss of consciousness that is the result of a lack of oxygen and/or nutrients getting through to the brain. Low blood pressure is often a feature in children prone to fainting. This is often made worse in the heat when blood vessels expand, which tends to lower blood pressure further. Individuals are more likely to faint when standing, as this can cause blood to pool

in the legs, increasing the possibility that not enough of it will get to the brain.

Fainting is made more likely by dips in blood sugar levels. Symptoms that are suggestive of this include fatigue in the afternoon, mood swings and cravings for sweet foods. If this sounds like your child, it may help to take steps to maintain blood sugar levels. This is dealt with in depth on pages 204–10. Fainting that can occur after exercise seems to be particularly related to episodes of low blood sugar (hypoglycaemia). One study found that some children experience hypoglycaemia 15–50 minutes after exercise, even of moderate intensity.[147] If this sounds like your child, then taking steps to ensure stable blood sugar levels is of prime importance.

Children who are anaemic and/or low in iron may also be prone to fainting. More information about these specific issues, and how to correct them, can be found on pages 29–3.

What to do

When a child faints, the priority is to increase blood flow to the brain. The child should be laid flat on his or her back, preferably on a slope with the feet higher than the head. This will help get blood back to the brain. Because low blood sugar is quite a common factor in fainting, it may help to give a child some diluted fruit juice as he or she comes round. If a child seems to have hurt him- or herself, or if you are concerned for any reason, seek medical advice.

Flower essences
• Offer Rescue Remedy or Emergency Essence immediately, to soothe

your child.
• In the longer term for a child with a tendency to low blood pressure, try the Australian Bush flower essences Southern Cross, Kapok Bush and Five Corners.

Fever

The normal human body temperature generally lies between 36 and 37°C (96.8 and 98.6°F). Temperatures over 37.8°C (100°F) are generally regarded as fever. A fever is a symptom of an illness, rather than a health condition in its own right. If a child has a fever, it's usually a sign that he or she has some sort of infection, and treating that infection is the key to overcoming the fever. Some of the most common symptoms associated with fever, and the infections they may be a sign of, are given in the box below.

What to do

In conventional medicine, parents are often encouraged to reach for the paracetamol in an effort to bring a fever down. However, this is not always the best course of action. Part of the function of a fever in the body is to stimulate the immune system, which helps the body fight whatever organism is infecting it. Unless your child is very uncomfortable or seems very unwell, it's probably best to avoid bringing their temperature down with medication.

To help your child feel more comfortable, sponge him or her with tepid water. A flannel soaked in cold water applied to the forehead will often help too. Fever provokes sweating, increasing the risk of dehydration.

This can add to feelings of general malaise and may impair the healing response too. For these reasons, it's important that your child drinks plenty of fluid during a fever. Water is the best fluid, though diluted fruit juice is another option. Your child should have enough fluid to ensure he or she passes water every hour or two during the waking day.

Symptoms associated with fever	Illness that these symptoms may be a sign of
Runny nose, sneezing, coughing	Cold (see pages 61–3)
Runny nose, sneezing, coughing and aches and pain	Flu (see pages 61–3)
Sore throat	Viral throat infection or tonsillitis (see pages 136–7)
Ear ache or a young child pulling on ear	Ear infection (see pages 80–1)
Catarrh and cough	Bronchitis (see pages 51–3)
Catarrh, cough and difficulty breathing	Bronchiolitis (see pages 50–1) or pneumonia (see pages 122–3)
Swollen glands in the neck, sore throat and fatigue	Glandular fever (see pages 93–4)
Itchy red spots	Chickenpox (see page 56)
Swollen face and difficulty swallowing	Mumps (see page 116)
Frequent urination, low abdominal pain and or pain or burning on passing water	Urinary tract infection (see pages 141–3)
Headache, stiff neck and discomfort from being in bright light	Meningitis (see page 107)
Nausea, vomiting and/or diarrhoea	Gastroenteritis (see pages 89–90)

Supplements

Whatever the precise nature of an infection in a child, it generally helps to supplement them with natural agents that can boost the immune function. Some of the most commonly used immune-boosters for combating fever are vitamin C and the herb echinacea.

Vitamin C

For a 40 kg child, give 250–500 mg of vitamin C (either in tablet or capsule form, or as a powder dissolved in water or juice) every hour or two. This large dose of vitamin C can sometimes cause some loosening of the bowels, though this side-effect resolves once the dose is reduced.

Echinacea

Echinacea has immune stimulating activity and this herb can therefore be useful in the treatment of a wide range of infections. There are two main species of echinacea used therapeutically: purpurea and angustifolia. Purpurea is the most commonly used form, though angustifolia certainly has merit and contains anti-viral agents called echinacosides, which are not found in the purpurea plant. Because of this, it is probably best to use a combination of both types of echinacea during a viral infection. Give 15–20 drops of tincture every two to three hours on the first day of the illness, followed by this dose three to four times a day for the next 10–14 days.

When to call a doctor

In certain circumstances, it can be useful to seek medical advice for a child with a fever. Such situations include:

- If your child is less than six months old
- If your child is between six months and three years of age and has a temperature of 38.9°C (102°F) or more
- If your child is four years or more and has a temperature of 40°C (104°F) or more
- If your child is showing signs of bronchiolitis, pneumonia, urinary tract infection or meningitis (see opposite)
- If your child is unusually listless, sleepy or irritable, seems distressed or just doesn't seem right to you

Occasionally, children with fever may suffer from a seizure – known as a febrile fit or febrile convulsion. Medical attention should be sought if this happens.

Flower essences

- Rescue Remedy can be offered at the first signs of a fever and throughout the recovery period.
- Following the illness, offer Olive to help **restore energy**.

Fifth disease

Fifth disease is a common viral (parvovirus) infection in children and is also known as slapped cheek disease. It starts as raised, rose-red spots on the cheeks, which then enlarge and converge. Within a few days, the rash usually spreads to form a lacy pattern over the limbs that may affect the trunk too. The condition can also cause fever. The rash usually clears after about ten days, but may recur.

What to do

The natural management of Fifth disease is the same as for other viral infections. For more information, see 'Colds and Flu' and 'Fever'.

Food allergy, sensitivity or intolerance

See pages 211–22.

Food poisoning and gastroenteritis

Food poisoning usually occurs as the result of eating food contaminated with a bacterium (such as Salmonella or Campylobacter) or virus. Gastroenteritis (inflammation in the gut) is also often caused by an infection. Usually, the infecting agent is a type of virus known as the rotavirus. These types of infection are particularly common in children under the age of two years, and are more common in the winter.

Food poisoning and gastroenteritis may cause abdominal pain, discomfort, nausea and vomiting and diarrhoea (which may be bloody). There may also be fever (see pages 87–9). The condition usually settles down of its own accord over a few days. However, if the condition does not appear to be resolving, or if you are concerned for any reason, do not hesitate to seek medical advice.

Diet
Fluid
Most children with food poisoning will generally feel too unwell to eat. However, fluid is essential to keep your child from becoming dehydrated. Water and diluted freshly squeezed fruit juice will help prevent dehydration and also provide some fuel. Encourage your child to take small volumes of fluid quite frequently. Large volumes may make nausea and vomiting more likely.

Supplements
Vitamin C
Because vitamin C has immune stimulating properties, it may help to take this during the illness. A convenient way of giving this is as a powder dissolved in some water or juice. For a 40 kg child, give 500 mg, three or four times a day.
Probiotics
Probiotics (healthy gut bacteria) are very useful for treating gut infections.

The organisms can help 'crowd out' the infecting bug and may also help to reduce the risk of longer-term imbalance in the gut. For children under the age of two years, I recommend a product called INT B1, which contains the gut bacteria thought to be of particular importance in infants and small children (*Bifidobacterium infantis*). Give a quarter of a teaspoon in one feed each day for two to four weeks. (For more details, see Useful contacts and information – under BioCare.) Older children are better off taking supplements designed for the more mature gut. More advice about suitable supplements can be found on pages 14–17.

German measles
German measles (also known as rubella) is a viral infection accompanied by a rash that starts as pink or light red spots, about 2–3 mm in diameter. The illness usually starts with a day or two of mild fever 37.2–37.8°C (99–100°F) and swollen glands that are usually found either in the neck or behind the ears. Typically, a rash appears on the second or third day and begins at the hairline and spreads downward onto the rest of the body. The spots may merge together to form patches of affected skin. As the rash spreads downwards on the body, it usually clears on the face. The rash generally will not itch and tends to last for between two and five days. As the rash passes, the affected skin may be shed in flakes.

Other symptoms of rubella may include: mild conjunctivitis

(inflammation of the lining of the eyelids and eyeballs), stuffy or runny nose, swollen lymph glands in other regions of the body, pain and swelling in the joints (especially in young women), and pain in the testicles in boys. An episode of German measles is a relatively harmless affair for most children. However, it can cause considerable problems if it affects a woman in pregnancy. Children infected with rubella before birth (a condition known as congenital rubella) are at risk of a range of abnormalities including: growth retardation; abnormalities of the heart, eyes, or brain; deafness; and problems affecting the liver, spleen and bone marrow. German measles is a rare infection these days, partly as a result of widespread immunisation with the MMR (measles, mumps, rubella) vaccine.

The German measles virus is spread by airborne droplets. The virus normally incubates for 14–21 days before any signs of illness appear. A child with German measles is contagious from approximately seven days before to five days after the rash appears – so if your child comes down with German measles, you should contact anyone who has been exposed to your child over the previous week. This is important because of the potential dangers to pregnant women.

What to do

Call your child's doctor if your child develops a fever over 38.9°C (102°F) or if his or her symptoms seem significantly worse than those described above. Otherwise, the condition should pass with little or no need for conventional intervention. Offer plenty of fluids in the form of water and diluted fruit juices.

Supplements
Vitamin C, zinc and echinacea
Give your child natural agents to help boost the immune system and help healing and speed recovery. A combination of vitamin C, zinc and the herb echinacea is usually very effective for this. For more details, see the section entitled 'Colds and flu'. Give at the recommended dose for 10–14 days, starting as soon as possible.

Topical treatments
Calendula cream
If the rash is itchy you may use Calendula cream as this encourages healing and will help to ease any discomfort caused by flaking skin.

Flower essences
• The Australian Bush flower essences Paw Paw, Jacaranda and Black-eyed Susan are generally recommended for viral infections.
• Also, you may offer Rescue Remedy during the illness to help encourage healing.

Gilbert's disease

Each red cell in the blood lives for about 120 days. When it dies, its chief ingredient, haemoglobin, is broken down in the liver. The main breakdown product of this process is a substance called 'bilirubin'. Most of the bilirubin formed by the liver passes into the gut in the bile and goes on to be excreted from the body in the stool. In Gilbert's disease, the ability of the liver to process bilirubin is faulty, causing bilirubin levels in the blood to rise.

Once thought to be very rare, Gilbert's disease is now thought to affect as much as 5 per cent of the population. Usually, the condition does not give rise to symptoms, though a proportion of sufferers may experience problems with loss of appetite, general malaise and fatigue.

Diet
As balanced as possible
Nutritionally, it is a good idea for sufferers of Gilbert's disease to avoid anything that tends to put stress on the liver. Following the guidelines for what constitutes a healthy diet for children and adolescents (pages 187–9) will go a long way to helping ensure your child does not tax the liver too much.

Supplements
Milk thistle
One natural substance that may help to protect the liver and minimise the effect of Gilbert's disease is the herb milk thistle (*Silybum marianum*). Milk thistle contains a substance called silymarin, which enhances liver function and helps in the regeneration of liver cells. For a 40 kg child, give 140 mg of silymarin (the main active ingredient in milk thistle) per day.

Gingivitis

Gingivitis is a condition characterised by red, swollen, often tender gums that tend to bleed easily. The condition can be caused by a bacterial infection where the gum and tooth meet and is often related to the build-up of plaque in this area. The condition is often uncomfortable and is a major cause of tooth loss.

The inflammation typical of gingivitis can be difficult to treat and sufferers often have persistent problems related to this condition. Certain nutrients, including vitamin C and substances known as bioflavonoids, are essential for gum health. A child with gingivitis may be helped by eating plenty of fruit and vegetables as these are generally rich in vitamin C and bioflavonoids.

Supplements
Vitamin C and bioflavonoids
Supplementation with vitamin C and bioflavonoids will generally provide additional benefits. One study showed that in combination (300 mg of each per day) these nutrients improved the health of the gum tissue.[148] A 40 kg child should be given 150–200 mg of both vitamin C and bioflavonoids per day.

Coenzyme Q10
Another nutrient that has been shown to help resolve gingivitis is coenzyme Q10 (CoQ10). This vitamin-like substance participates in the processes that generate energy within the body's cells and has also been shown to improve the health and condition of the gums.[149] A 40 kg child should be given 25 mg of CoQ10 each day. Piercing an oil-filled CoQ10 capsule and rubbing its contents into the gums from time to time might also help restore health to the area.

> **Toothpaste and gingivitis**
> A good natural toothpaste for children suffering from gingivitis is Aloe Dent. This contains aloe vera and an extract from horse chestnut

called aescin (both soothing and healing to the gums), tea tree oil (a natural antiseptic) along with CoQ10. You will find this product in independent health food stores.

Glandular fever

Glandular fever – also known as infectious mononucleosis – is an infection of the throat and lymph nodes caused by something known as the Epstein-Barr virus. Mononucleosis refers to the characteristic rise in the number of specific immune cells (known as mononuclear cells) seen in the condition. The virus is transmitted by saliva (which is the reason why it's sometimes called the 'kissing disease'), but it is also spread by coughing and sneezing. Common symptoms of glandular fever include fever, sore throat, swollen lymph glands and a red rash. Symptoms tend to be more dramatic in teenagers than in younger children, in whom the condition may be mild and even go unnoticed. The condition is normally diagnosed on the basis of the sufferer's symptoms, along with a blood test, which shows raised levels of mononuclear cells.

During the infection itself, a child will tend to feel unwell and is usually tired and listless. This phase of the illness generally lasts two to four weeks. However, a significant number of individuals seem to have lasting problems after a bout of glandular fever and may feel tired and mildly unwell for some months, and even years, after the original infection.

Diet
Sugar
Refined sugar has been found to suppress the immune system (see pages 149–51) and should be avoided as much as possible. The diet should be based on whole, unrefined foods. Fruits and vegetables are particularly important as these tend to be rich in nutrients that support the immune system, such as vitamin C and beta-carotene. Plenty of water is important, too, to help prevent dehydration and help with healing and recovery.

Supplements
Vitamin C, zinc and echinacea
A combination of vitamin C, the mineral zinc and the herb echinacea can really help to boost the immune system function and resolve the illness more quickly. For details about dosing, see 'Colds and flu'. Start supplementation as soon as possible and keep them going for two weeks. After this, I would continue with vitamin C until a month after the symptoms appear to have abated.

Long-term problems
Natural approaches can also be effective for individuals who feel they have long-term problems with energy that seemed to start after a bout of glandular fever. General measures to support the immune system, such as a healthy diet and supplementation with vitamin C and a good quality multivitamin and mineral can help. However, two specific approaches seem to be of particular help in individuals suffering from long-term problems after an infection with glandular fever.

Magnesium

Supplementation with magnesium often seems to pull individuals out of a problem with long-term fatigue. Magnesium is found naturally in foods such as green leafy vegetables, fish, meat, beans, pulses and nuts and seeds. Ensuring your child is getting enough of these foods will help ensure they get a decent amount of magnesium. However, it is almost always worthwhile supplementing with this nutrient at a dose of 150–250 mg of magnesium each day (for a 40 kg child) for several months. After this, it is a good idea to supplement with a good quality multivitamin and mineral preparation. More details about suitable supplements can be found on pages 14–17.

Liquorice for adrenal weakness

Individuals with long-term fatigue after glandular fever very often show signs of weakness in the adrenal glands (the chief glands in the body responsible for dealing with stress), including low blood pressure, easy tiring on exertion and the need to eat very regularly. Slender stature is another common feature. Liquorice is generally a good remedy for children who seem to have weakness in the adrenal glands (see above). For a 40 kg child, give 1–2 g per day of liquorice root. While high doses of liquorice should not be used in the long term, the lower doses recommended here are known to be safe.

Flower essences

• **Olive** is a good remedy for fatigue.

Glue ear

Glue ear is a condition caused by the accumulation of fluid within the ear. Many children with this condition are recommended to have grommets (small plastic tubes) inserted into the eardrum. Grommets allow air into the ear cavity, which can help fluid drain from this area. Interestingly, studies suggest that glue ear does not impair intellectual development and it is possible that the insertion of grommets may lead to some degree of hearing loss for several years after the procedure.

It is not uncommon for children with glue ear to have problems with their adenoids – glands (similar to tonsils) situated at the back of the nose. In some children, the adenoids enlarge, restricting breathing through the nose (sufferers often have a characteristic nasal voice), snoring and an increased risk of glue ear and ear infections. The usual medical management of enlarged adenoids is something called 'adenoidectomy', where the glands are removed surgically.

Diet

Food sensitivity

In practice, glue ear is often caused by food sensitivity. By far the most common food triggers of these problems are cow's milk, ice cream and cheese, with yoghurt often being a problem too. Other symptoms of dairy sensitivity include frequent colds and a blocked and/or runny nose. Often, children crave the foods that they are most sensitive to. If a child is especially keen on one or more dairy product, then this strongly suggests that he or she has a problem with this type of food. While dairy product sensitivity is quite likely to be a factor in glue ear, other foods may contribute to the problem too. For more details about food sensitivity, see pages 211–22. Experience shows that identification and elimination of problem foods from a child's diet usually put an end to problems with glue ear.

Growing pains

Growing pains are aches and pains that occur in the limbs of children. The pains usually occur at night and generally affect the calves, shins, thighs or knees of children between six and twelve years of age. Despite its name, it seems this condition is not necessarily related to the growth of a child. Occasionally, joint pains may be related to juvenile arthritis. For this reason, children who have joint pain and swelling should be seen by a doctor.

Diet
Food sensitivity
A common and frequently overlooked cause of growing pains is food sensitivity. Identification and elimination of problem foods usually bring considerable relief from growing pains. Advice about identifying culprit foods can be found on pages 211–22.

Supplements
Magnesium and vitamin E
Magnesium, which is essential for muscle health, can often help relieve growing pains, especially when combined with vitamin E, which improves blood flow to muscle tissues.

A daily dose of 150–250 mg of magnesium and 200 IU of vitamin E (for a 40 kg child) is often effective.

Gum disease
See 'Gingivitis'

Halitosis
See 'Bad breath'

Hand, foot and mouth disease

Hand, foot and mouth disease is a common viral infectious disease in children (especially toddlers), caused by what is known as the coxsackievirus. It is characterised by many small blisters (vesicles) in the mouth and on the palms of the hands and the soles of the feet. These may also appear on other parts of the body. There may be some difficulty in swallowing, a slight fever and vomiting. The disease is generally mild and normally lasts for only a few days. For the natural management of hand, foot and mouth disease, see 'Colds and Flu'.

Hay fever
Hay fever is caused by an allergic reaction to pollen, causing the release of a substance called histamine around the nose and eyes. Symptoms normally include red, itchy eyes and a runny or congested nose. The conventional medical approach to hay fever generally consists of three types of medication: antihistamines, which block the release

of histamine that is responsible for swelling and congestion; steroid-based nasal sprays; and decongestants such as ephedrine. However, dietary changes and natural supplements may significantly reduce or even eliminate the need for conventional medication.

Diet
Food sensitivity
Individuals with hay fever may have food sensitivities too. There is some thought that reactions to food 'sensitise' the tissues in the eye and/or nose, making it more likely that pollen will trigger and allergic reaction there. Any food may cause a problem here, but dairy products (particularly milk, cheese and yoghurt) are frequent underlying problems in hay fever. Identifying culprit foods and eliminating them from the diet very often brings tremendous long-term relief from hay fever. For more details about this, see pages 211–22.

Supplements
Vitamin C
Vitamin C has natural antihistamine activity in the body and there is some evidence that it can help control hay fever symptoms.[150–2] A 40 kg child should be given 250 mg of vitamin C, three or four times a day while symptoms persist.
Quercetin
Another useful natural agent for the treatment of hay fever is quercetin. This 'bioflavonoid' compound appears to reduce the release of histamine from immune system cells known as 'mast cells'.[153] In practice, quercetin does seem to help a proportion of hay fever

sufferers, although it seems to work best as a preventative rather than a treatment. A suitable dose for a 40 kg child would be 500 mg of quercetin per day.
Nettle
Nettle (*Urtica dioica*) has a long history of use in herbal medicine in the treatment of allergic conditions, including hay fever. For a 40 kg child, give 200–400 mg of nettle every four hours.
Antibiotics and probiotics
Antibiotic use in children in their first two years of life has been associated with a two-to three-fold increased risk of hay fever.[154] One major problem with antibiotics is that they tend to kill healthy bacteria in the gut and this may increase the likelihood of food sensitivity and maybe cause malfunctioning of the immune system. As a long-term strategy for the prevention and perhaps even treatment of hay fever, it is a good idea for any child who has had antibiotics to be given a supplement of healthy gut bacteria (probiotics). More details about this can be found on page 16.

Flower essences
• Rescue Remedy may help during a bad hay fever attack.
• The Bush flower essences Fringed Violet and Dagger Hakea are generally good for allergic conditions such as hay fever.

Headache
See also 'Migraine'
Headaches can have a variety of causes, most of which are harmless. However, sometimes headache can be a sign of a

potentially serious medical condition. If your child has developed a headache and is also shying away from the light, then meningitis (see page 107) is a possibility and medical attention should be sought. Very rarely, a headache can be a sign of a brain tumour. If your child seems to have other neurological symptoms (such as visual problems or muscle weakness), has nausea or vomiting or has had a seizure, then it is important to seek a medical opinion. In the grand scheme of things, meningitis and brain tumours are rare, but it is just worth bearing them in mind if your child seems very unwell.

Diet
Dehydration
Dehydration is a very common cause of headache in kids but it's often overlooked. The tissues that surround the brain are mostly composed of water. When these tissues lose fluid, they shrink, and this can cause pain and irritation. Low levels of fluid in the body may also encourage the accumulation of toxins, which have been implicated in headaches. Drinking more water is one of the simplest and most effective remedies for headaches. More information on the benefits of water, and how to gauge the right amount for your child, can be found on page 158–9.
Caffeine
Another dietary factor that is often related to headaches is caffeine. It is often between times of caffeine consumption (caffeine withdrawal) that the headache tends to strike. Regular caffeine takers normally find that stopping caffeine cold-turkey leads to

substantial headaches for a day or two, after which headaches tend to be much reduced or stop altogether. For the best results, all forms of caffeine-containing foodstuffs, including caffeinated soft drinks (e.g. cola), coffee and tea, should be eliminated from your child's diet. Naturally caffeine-free beverages such as herb and fruit teas and diluted fruit juices are the best alternatives. Carbonated soft drinks, in whatever form they come, are likely to impair your child's health in the long term and should be avoided as much as possible.
Food sensitivity
Food sensitivity seems to be a common cause of headaches in children. In practice, wheat is a frequent offender here. For more details about how to identify problem foods, see pages (211–22.).

Supplements
Magnesium
The mineral magnesium often seems to relieve headaches and some practitioners believe that headache is actually a symptom of magnesium deficiency. In fact, the statistics show that magnesium is one nutrient that children and adolescents often do not get in adequate amounts in their diets. Symptoms (other than headache) that may point to a problem with magnesium deficiency in your child include muscle twitching and/or cramping and general restlessness and/or hyperactivity. However, even in the absence of such symptoms, magnesium supplementation may help a child with frequent headaches. For a 40 kg child, give 150–250 mg of magnesium per day.

Flower essences

• At the first sign of a headache, offer Rescue Remedy, which should ease symptoms enormously, particularly if they are related to stress or heightened emotions.

• **Stress-related** headaches often respond to Vervain.

• Impatiens tends to soothe headaches caused by **irritability and tension**.

Head lice

Head lice are tiny insects that attach themselves to the scalp, where they lay eggs and multiply in seemingly impossible numbers and at great speed. Also known as 'nits', head lice are spread by direct contact. It's worth noting that poor hygiene is not a cause of head lice. In fact, if anything, they seem to prefer clean hair. Contracting nits tends to be the result of close proximity rather than anything else, hence the reason why they spread like wildfire through classrooms. It only takes one infestation to claim a whole classroom full of victims.

The lice appear as greyish round specks on the scalp and eggs may be evident on the shaft of the hair. Because female lice can lay up to five eggs a day, it helps to eradicate the infestation as soon as possible. Conventional treatments are based on what are known as organophosphate chemicals. Some scientists have suggested that organophosphates in the environment may pose considerable health risks for childen.[155] It therefore makes good sense to avoid these chemicals in favour of natural alternatives if you can.

What to do

Remember that nits spread easily from clothing, sheets, pillows, combs, brushes and anything else that has come into contact with them. Scrupulous domestic hygiene is important. Boil-wash linen and clothing, and soak combs and brushes in hot water with 1–2 drops of tea tree oil (see below).

Topical treatments
Tea tree oil

Tea tree oil has natural bug-killing potential, and can be added to water to make a good anti-lice treatment for your child's hair. Add 25 drops of tea tree oil to about 600 ml of warm water. Rub the mixture into your child's hair and scalp three times daily and comb your child's hair with a fine-toothed comb to remove lice and eggs from the hair shaft. Another good trick is to add 3–4 drops of tea tree oil to conditioner, apply it to the hair, leave it on overnight (with a towel on your child's pillow) and then comb it out the following day.

Polygonum

Polygonum is a herb that appears to have the ability to kill head lice. One study found that a preparation by the name of KINcare was effective in getting rid of nits in 90 per cent of cases. KINcare solution should be applied to a child's hair (as directed) on three consecutive days. (For more details, see Useful contacts and information.)

Hepatitis A

'Hepatitis' actually means inflammation of the liver. This condition can be caused by a number of factors, including drugs, chemicals and poisons. However, by far the most common cause of hepatitis is infection with the hepatitis virus. There are several strains of hepatitis virus, which are identified using letters of the alphabet. The most important strains are hepatitis A, B and C. Hepatitis A is passed through contact with infected water, food or faeces, while B and C are usually contracted through sex or via contact with infected blood.

Initial infection with the hepatitis virus often triggers a condition known as 'acute hepatitis'. This may start as a flu-like illness, after which jaundice (yellowing of the skin) may develop. In hepatitis A, the illness is usually self-limiting, though a proportion of sufferers may complain of vague symptoms for weeks or months after the original infection.

Diet

During the infection itself, the sufferer should avoid anything that tends to put stress on the liver, including fatty, processed and additive-laden foods. Plenty of water should be drunk (enough to ensure a child is passing water every hour or two) as this helps to reduce the toxic load on the body. In addition, certain natural substances may help.

Supplements
Milk thistle

The herb milk thistle (*Silybum marianum*) has been shown to have beneficial effects on liver function, and may help restore health to the liver. For a 40 kg child, give 140 mg of silymarin (the main active ingredient in milk thistle) per day for one to two months.

Vitamin C

Another nutrient that is likely to help is vitamin C. In addition to its immune stimulating and anti-viral properties, this nutrient is also well known to promote tissue healing and may therefore help to reduce the risk of damage to the liver in the longer term. For a 40 kg child, give 500–1000 mg of vitamin C, two or three times a day while symptoms persist, though this dose can be reduced as the condition resolves.

Selenium

There is also evidence that the mineral selenium inhibits the hepatitis virus. A 40 kg child should be given 300 mcg each day for one to two weeks.

Hives

Hives, also known as urticaria or nettle rash, is a condition characterised by red, raised itchy wheals on the skin surface. The rash usually affects the trunk or limbs, tends to come and go, and normally lasts for a few hours at a time. Urticaria is known to be triggered by a variety of factors, including prescription medication, extremes of temperature and sunlight. However, there is some evidence that many cases of urticaria are caused by reactions to food[156] or food additives, particularly colourings, flavourings (salicylates), aspartame and preservatives.[157–9] For more details about food additives and food sensitivity see pages 159–60 and 211–22 respectively.

Because urticaria seems to be related to the release of histamine, natural approaches that have antihistamine effect may help, including vitamin C, quercetin and the herb nettle. See the section 'Hay fever' for more details about these.

Hyperactivity

See 'Attention deficit hyperactivity disorder'

Impetigo

Impetigo is a contagious skin infection usually caused by a bacterium known as *Staphylococcus aureus*. This organism tends to make its way through a breach in the skin (such as a cold sore or patch of skin affected with eczema) to set up an infection. Characteristically, impetigo initially presents as red, fluid-filled blisters around the nose and/or mouth (though other areas of skin can be affected). The blisters eventually burst and dry out, leaving honey-coloured crusts. The condition is normally treated with antibiotics, administered orally and/or as an ointment. Treatment is normally successful within a few days.

What to do

Impetigo is generally very contagious, so try to keep your child away from other children. Ensure that your child washes his or her hands and face carefully in hot soapy water, both to prevent spreading the infection and also to prevent further infection by scratching. Clothing that has been in contact with the blisters can also spread the condition, so it's important to keep everything clean and dry and away from other members of the family. Pillowcases, towels and face cloths should not be shared and are best put in a good hot wash after use.

Supplements

Vitamin C, zinc and echinacea

The trick to getting on top of an impetigo problem naturally is to boost a child's immune system so that they have a decent chance of combating the organism that is at its root. In this respect, a combination of vitamin C, zinc and the herb echinacea is generally very effective. Zinc is especially important as it not only helps to support immune function, but is also important for skin healing. More details about dosing and how to administer these natural agents can be found in the section 'Colds and flu'.

Probiotics

If your child has had oral antibiotics, then it is a good idea to give him or her a course of probiotics (healthy gut bacteria) to replenish the good bacteria in the gut that might have gone by the wayside. For more details see pages 16–17.

Topical treatments

Tea tree oil

Tea tree oil has proven antibacterial power, including against Staphylococcus. However, neat tea tree oil is a bit potent, so should be diluted before use. Put about 10 drops of the oil in a cup of water and apply this to the lesions with cotton wool balls. Try to gently remove the crusts to allow the oil to reach the affected area beneath. Even diluted, tea tree oil may sting a bit. However, the results are usually worth a bit of discomfort.

Indigestion

Indigestion, the feeling of pain, discomfort or bloating after eating, is very often related to poor digestion. There are many potential reasons for this, but in children, the rapid eating that many partake in seems to be at fault. Hurried eating makes for poor chewing and generally sluggish digestion, and this can cause food to ferment in the stomach leading to bloating, belching and discomfort commonly referred to as 'stomach ache'. Thorough chewing is very important for digestion, mainly because it breaks up food into smaller particles, which dissolve more efficiently in the digestive juices in the gut. Ideally, your child should chew each mouthful to a cream before swallowing. Family meals are a good environment for children to learn the art of eating in an unhurried atmosphere. More details about the benefits of family meals can be found on page 195.

Some children tend to drink quite a lot of fluid with meals and believe that this can only help to 'wash food down'. Drinking with meals dilutes the acid and enzymes that do the digestive work, and can therefore cause problems with indigestion. Encourage your child to do the bulk of his or her drinking between meals, and not at meal time.

Helicobacter pylori

In some children, indigestion or abdominal discomfort can be related to infection with the organism *Helicobacter pylori*. This infection may respond to treatment with a natural substance known as mastic gum. This product is prepared from the resin of a tree that grows on an island in the Aegean Sea. Mastic gum has been found to kill *H. pylori* in the test-tube. Experimentally, mastic gum has been shown to reduce symptoms in 8 per cent of sufferers.[160] A 40 kg child should take 500 mg of mastic gum each day for two weeks.

Infectious mononucleosis

See 'Glandular fever'

Influenza

See 'Colds and flu'

Insomnia

Sleep disturbance can broadly be divided into two categories: difficulty in getting to sleep, and problems with waking in the night. Most parents find that one important approach to good sleep habits in children, particularly young children, is routine. Ensuring that a child goes to bed at about the same time each night, perhaps with a bedtime story, is a big part of helping a child establish a regular sleeping pattern. Children generally sleep better after an active day, so it's important to make sure your child is getting enough stimulation, physically and emotionally, during the day. In older children, certain situations may be causing undue stress, and these may need exploring. If something appears to be on your child's mind, then it can help to discuss this so that solutions can be sought.

Diet
Caffeine

Dietary factors also play an important part in determining our ability to get to sleep. For instance, one common cause of sleeplessness is caffeine, which has stimulant effects in the body. Studies have shown that caffeine consumers are more likely to suffer from sleep disruption. The effects of caffeine can linger for up to 20 hours,[161] so cutting out caffeine from your child's diet (caffeinated soft drinks are a common source in children) may do much to help regularise a child's sleep patterns. Camomile tea has mild sedative properties and, if drunk in the evening, may positively help to get a child off to sleep.

Supplements
Magnesium

Magnesium deficiency is common in kids, and this may manifest as sleeplessness and general restlessness. Other symptoms of magnesium deficiency include twitching and/or cramping in the muscles. Supplementation with magnesium often seems to help calm children and help their sleep in the longer term. A 40 kg child should be given 150–250 mg of magnesium each day.

Valerian

Valerian (*Valeriana officinalis*) has been widely used in folk medicine as a sedative. The root of the valerian plant contains a number of constituents, including essential oils, which have calming and sleep-inducing properties. Valerian, unlike many of the conventional sleeping medications, does not seem to be addictive. The normal recommended dose for a 40 kg child is 150–250 mg of root extract or 2.5 ml of tincture (alcoholic extract), taken one hour before bedtime.

Lavender oil

Putting a few drops of lavender oil in your child's bath water in the evening or on his pillow at night may help him or her get off to sleep.

Flower essences

• Olive is good for a child who seems not to sleep because he or she is **over-tired**.

• For children whose sleep seems to be affected by **concerns and worries**, try White Chestnut.

Waking in the night

Diet

While some children have difficulty dropping off in the evening, others tend to wake in the middle of the night. This problem is quite often related to a drop in the level of sugar in the bloodstream during the night. Normally, the body likes to keep an adequate and stable blood sugar level while we are asleep. Should the blood sugar level drop, the body secretes certain hormones, notably adrenaline, to correct this. Peak adrenaline secretion is often at around 3 or 4am, which is perhaps why this is a common time for waking in the night. If your child has other symptoms of blood sugar imbalance such as cravings for sweet foods, erratic mood and fatigue in the mid-late afternoon, then taking steps to stabilise blood sugar levels may reap enormous dividends in terms of better sleep through the night. One strategy that often works for this problem is to give a child something light to eat shortly before bedtime. A piece of fruit or some dried fruit can pick up blood sugar levels and reduce the risk that they will drop into the danger zone in the middle of the night. For more details about how to stabilise blood sugar levels, see pages 204–10.

Flower essences

If a child is waking in the night because of nightmares or night terrors, try the Bach flower essence Rock Rose.

Irritable bowel syndrome

Irritable bowel syndrome (IBS) is a common digestive problem, typical symptoms of which are bloating, excessive flatulence, abdominal discomfort and constipation and/or loose bowels. Very often, IBS can be effectively dealt with by considering one or both of two main underlying problems: food sensitivity and an imbalance in the organisms that normally inhabit the gut (especially yeast overgrowth).

In children with food sensitivity issues, wheat is a very common trigger of IBS-type symptoms, although dairy products are often at fault here too. For more information about how to identify specific food sensitivities, see pages 211–22.

If a child has been treated with antibiotics, there is a reasonable likelihood that he or she will have an imbalance in the organisms in the gut. This problem often manifests as excess wind, and the bowel motion can tend to be loose from time to time. Advice about re-balancing the ecosystem in the gut can be found on page 16. Of particular importance here is supplementation with healthy gut bacteria (probiotics). See page 16 for more details about this, too.

Juvenile arthritis

Juvenile arthritis (JA) is an inflammatory condition characterised by inflammation in the fingers, toes, wrists or other joints of the body. It most commonly starts at around two to four years of age or at puberty. It is more common in girls than boys. JA is what is known as an 'auto-immune' disease. Here, the immune system mounts an immune response against the body's own tissues causing inflammation.

Diet

Food sensitivity

It is not known what causes JA, but the condition is quite similar to the adult condition rheumatoid arthritis (RA). There is some evidence that it can be triggered by food. In one study of 22 RA sufferers, 20 improved on elimination of certain foods from the diet.[162] The worst offending foods in this study were grains, milk, nuts, beef and egg. If your child has JA, it is certainly worthwhile exploring potential food sensitivity problems. More information about the identification of individual food sensitivities can be found on pages 211–22.

Essential fatty acids

RA sufferers may benefit from eating plenty of foods rich in healthy essential fatty acids (EFAs), such as oily fish (mackerel, salmon and trout), extra virgin olive oil and pumpkin, sunflower and sesame seeds. There is some evidence that both omega-6 fatty acids in the form of borage oil,[163–4] blackcurrant seed oil,[165] evening primrose oil[166–7] and omega-3 fatty acids in the form of fish oil[168–73] can be effective in controlling the symptoms of RA. Emphasising a diet rich in EFA (e.g. oily fish, olive oil, nuts and seeds and avocado) may help reduce a tendency to inflammation.

Supplements

Fish oils

Fish oils (especially rich in omega-3 fats) are also generally useful for children with JA. I recommend 2–3 g of concentrated fish oils each day.

Flaxseed oil

Flaxseed oil is also rich in omega-3 fats (alpha-linolenic acid) and is a useful supplement for vegetarian children. Give 10–15 ml (2–3 tsp) a day.

Green-lipped mussel extract

Green-lipped mussel extract has developed a reputation as a useful agent in the treatment of arthritis. Research has identified a compound called eicosatetraenoic acid (ETA), which was found to have anti-inflammatory actions more potent than that of commonly prescribed painkillers. One study found that treatment with green-lipped mussel extract (1050 mg per day of dried powder or 210 mg per day of a special extract) brought significant improvements in 68 per cent of RA sufferers.[174] Half this dose is appropriate for a 40 kg child. Green-lipped mussel extract is widely available in health food stores.

Lactose intolerance

Milk contains a sugar called lactose, which is made up of two other sugars – glucose and galactose. Lactose is normally broken down into its constituents prior to absorption. However, some individuals lack the enzyme in the gut that is responsible for digesting lactose, a problem that can give rise to diarrhoea, bloating and wind. This condition is called lactose intolerance, and is especially common in individuals of Asian, African and Middle Eastern descent.

Supplements

Acidophilus

In the gut, certain bacterial species have the ability to metabolise lactose. One of the most important in this respect is *Lactobacillus acidophilus*. Taking a good quality acidophilus supplement for two to three months, perhaps followed by a maintenance dose of this organism, seems to enhance lactose-digesting ability.[175]

Lactase

Another option is to treat milk with the enzyme responsible for digesting lactose called 'lactase'. Lactase can often be found in liquid form, which can be added to milk 24 hours before it is consumed. Lactase may also be available in tablet form, to be taken when consuming milk or milk products such as ice cream. However, another approach is to avoid lactose-containing products and to give your child naturally lactose-free foods such as soya milk-based products (e.g. soya milk and yoghurt) and oat and rice milk. More details about alternatives to conventional dairy products can be found on page 179.

Lice

See 'Head lice'

Measles

Measles is a potentially serious and extremely contagious viral infection. Immunisation for measles (as part of the MMR vaccine) saw a decline in the incidence of measles. However, concerns about the safety of the MMR vaccine have led some parents to shun immunisation. There have been reports of an upsurge of measles cases in some parts of the country.

Once contracted, the disease will incubate for between nine days and two weeks, after which symptoms such as fever, fatigue, nausea, coughing, a runny nose and conjunctivitis will generally begin to appear. These symptoms tend to worsen over a few days, after which a rash (brownish or purplish red) will appear on the face and neck. The rash is normally slightly itchy, and generally spreads to the torso, arms, hands, legs and feet within a few days. Another sign of measles is what are known as 'Koplik's spots' – red spots with a blueish/white centre that tend to appear 12 hours before the rash starts.

Children with measles are contagious for at least seven days after the beginning of the illness. The average duration of measles is about ten days. Near the end of the illness, the rash fades and gradually disappears, a sign that the infection is no longer contagious.

Measles is generally a pretty harmless affair. However, complications such as ear infections are quite common. More serious, however, are potential problems with pneumonia and encephalitis (inflammation of the brain). Encephalitis occurs in about one in every 1000 cases of measles and, in extreme circumstances, may lead to seizures, coma and even death. These problems are rare, but it is wise to look out for early warning signs of problems, which include headache, drowsiness and vomiting, starting seven to ten days after the rash first appears.

What to do

The fever that accompanies measles will rev-up the immune response, but it does need keeping an eye on. Information about the management of fever can be found on page 87.

Plenty of fluids, in the form of water and diluted fruit juices, will help keep your child hydrated. Some children aren't particularly keen on drinking when they are ill, as they feel so unwell. Persistence is important here, because a well-hydrated child will tend to feel better and recover more quickly.

Supplements
Vitamin A

Vitamin A is a useful natural remedy in the treatment of measles. It is believed that vitamin A deficiency increases the risk of a child succumbing to a measles infection (and its complications). While vitamin A deficiency is generally thought of as a condition that occurs in developing countries, there is evidence that it can occur in industrialised countries too. One study in California in the USA among supposedly well-nourished children found that 50 per cent of children with measles were vitamin A deficient.[176] Vitamin A appears to be a useful nutrient in children who have measles. In one

review, vitamin A supplementation in young children with measles was described as one of the best-proven, safest and most cost-effective interventions in international public health.[177] The World Health Organisation (WHO) recommend an oral dose of 200,000 IU per day for two days to children over the age of two (100,000 IU to infants) with measles where vitamin A deficiency may be present. At this dose there is evidence of a reduced risk of complications and mortality.[178]

Vitamin C and zinc

Other nutrients that might help in the treatment of measles include vitamin C and zinc, both of which have immune-stimulating and anti-viral properties. Zinc supplementation may also help to correct low levels of this nutrient that are caused by the diarrhoea that can sometimes come during and after measles infection.[179] In laboratory studies, vitamin C has been shown to help boost the activity of certain infection-fighting white blood cells that are often suppressed during measles infection.[180] Give 500–1000 mg of vitamin C in three or four divided doses during the day. Also, 10–15 mg of zinc can be given once or twice a day. Both of these nutrients can be given safely for the duration of the illness for children aged two years or more.

Echinacea

Echinacea is a good herb for stimulating the immune system and helping to clear infections. There are two main species of echinacea used therapeutically – purpurea and angustifolia. Because each form of echinacea has slightly different properties, it is probably a good idea to combine them for maximum effect. Give 15–20 drops of tincture, every two to three hours on the first day of the illness, followed by this dose three to four times a day for the next 10–14 days.

Flower essences

• Olive can help with the **fatigue** that generally comes with a measles infection.

Meningitis

Meningitis is a term used by doctors to describe an inflammation of the membranes that surround the brain and/or spinal cord. The inflammation causing meningitis is normally the result of either a bacterial (bacterial meningitis) or viral (viral meningitis) infection. In general terms, viral meningitis is less serious than bacterial meningitis and is much less likely to lead to complications. The highest incidence of meningitis is between birth and two years, with greatest risk immediately following birth and at three to eight months.

The classic symptoms of meningitis are headache, neck stiffness (stiffness and discomfort on bringing the chin towards the chest) and photophobia (a dislike of being in the light, especially bright light). Two particular things to look out for are: if the knees are automatically brought up towards the body when the neck is bent forward (this is called Brudzinski sign), and a seeming inability to straighten a child's lower legs after they have been bent at the hips (this is called the Kernig sign and is a strong indication of meningitis).

Some of the most serious forms of meningitis are caused by the bacterium *Meningococcus*. This organism may cause a red rash that does not fade when a glass is pushed against it. This, along with other symptoms of meningitis, is a sign that urgent medical attention should be sought.

Other symptoms suggestive of meningitis

In infants

• Decreased liquid intake and vomiting
• Increased irritability
• Increased lethargy
• Fever
• Bulging fontanelle (soft spot on the top of the head)

In children older than one year

• Nausea and vomiting
• Headache
• Fever
• Altered mental status (such as confusion)
• Lethargy
• Seizure activity

Meningitis is a potentially life-threatening condition that can rapidly progress to brain damage and neurological problems. If you are at all suspicious that your child may have this condition, seek medical attention immediately.

Menorrhagia

Menorrhagia (pronounced men-orr-ay-jah) is the medical term for heavy periods. In some girls, menorrhagia can be a sign of low thyroid function. Other symptoms of this condition include sensitivity to cold, cold hands and feet and dry skin. If your daughter has symptoms suggestive of low thyroid function, it might be worthwhile consulting your doctor so that a blood test can be taken for this. However, it is worth bearing in mind that conventional blood tests for thyroid function are not foolproof. The reasons for this, and alternative methods of testing, are discussed in my book *Ultimate Health – 12 Keys to Abundant Health and Happiness*.

Supplements

Vitamin A

One nutrient that seems to be very effective in treating menorrhagia is vitamin A. One study showed that 25,000 IU of vitamin A taken twice a day for 15 days brought about a significant reduction of menstrual flow in more than 90 per cent of women.[181] This dose is certainly safe to use in the short term, even in younger girls.

Iron

Another useful nutrient in treating menorrhagia is the mineral iron. It is well known that iron deficiency is a common consequence of menorrhagia.[182] Adolescent girls with heavy periods are very often deficient in iron. In extreme cases they may be anaemic too. However, it's worth bearing in mind that iron deficiency can occur without anaemia and may still cause problems with fatigue and low mood. More

information about how to test for low iron and what to do about it can be found on page 29.

An added spin-off benefit of iron treatment is that it can actually reduce the amount of blood lost during a period. Iron is believed to help blood vessels to contract, which is important to stem blood flow from the womb.

Flower essences

• The Australian Bush flower essences Billy Goat Plum, She Oak and Sturt Desert Rose are all indicated for menstrual problems.

• If your child feels **drained** during her period, try the Bach Flower remedy Olive.

Menstrual cramps

Many girls and young women experience pain and cramping during their periods, known as dysmenorrhoea. The body of the womb is made up of muscular tissue. During a period this muscle contracts to help expel the womb's bloody lining. Sometimes, the contractions can be very strong, and this can lead to severe pain and cramping. Painful periods affect about half of menstruating women and a significant number of adolescent girls. In a small but significant proportion of these, the symptoms can be very severe and incapacitating, and may necessitate rest and the use of painkillers for the first day or two of the period. The pain normally lasts for between 12 and 16 hours, but in some girls it can last for the duration of the period.

Other symptoms of dysmenorrhoea include mild to severe cramping in the lower abdomen, backache and a pulling sensation on the inside of the thighs. Conventional treatments for dysmenorrhoea are based on painkilling medication (non-steroidal anti-inflammatory drugs) and the Pill.

Supplements
Omega-3 fatty acids
Period-related pain is caused, at least in part, by inflammatory substances known as prostaglandins. Omega-3 fats (found most abundantly in oily fish such as salmon, trout, mackerel and sardine) can help reduce the production of inflammatory prostaglandins and may enhance the production of substances that have natural anti-inflammatory and painkilling properties in the body. More details about this can be found on pages 156–7. Two or three portions of oily fish a week may help reduce symptoms of dysmenorrhoea in the long term. An alternative or adjunct to this is to supplement with 1–2 g of concentrated fish oil each day.

Magnesium
Magnesium is essential to muscle function and, in particular, helps prevent cramping and spasm. In practice, many girls respond to magnesium supplementation. A useful dose is 200–300 mg per day. When symptoms are at their worst, additional supplementation with 100–200 mg of magnesium every four hours does seem to help relieve symptoms.

Vitamin E
This vitamin also appears to have an effect on the severity of pain during menstruation. In one study, vitamin E supplementation at a dose of 500 IU per day helped a significant proportion of sufferers.[183] Give 400–600 IU of vitamin E, starting two days before the period and stopping three days after the period is finished.

Cramp bark
Another good natural agent to use during the period itself is cramp bark (*Viburnum opulus*). Take 1/2 tsp (about 25 drops) of tincture three times a day during symptoms.

Migraine
See also 'Headaches'

The classic feature of a migraine headache is pain on one side of the head. The condition is believed to start as constriction in the blood vessels around the brain. After this initial constriction, the blood vessels tend to open out, and the 'rush of blood to the head' is believed to be what causes migraine.

The most common form of migraine is appropriately termed 'common migraine' by the medical profession, and occurs in about 80–85 per cent of sufferers. The headache is usually very intense and throbbing in nature and may be accompanied by symptoms such as photophobia (a dislike of being in the light), phonophobia (a dislike of loud sounds) and also gut-related symptoms such as nausea, vomiting and diarrhoea.

The remaining 15–20 per cent of migraine cases are what are known as 'classic migraines'. This type of migraine usually starts with other symptoms such as visual disturbance (such as flashing lights, blind spots, tunnel vision and temporary blindness) or numbness or pins and needles in the legs or arms. These symptoms generally last for up to an hour, after which there is normally an interval of about an hour before the headache begins in earnest.

Diet
Food sensitivity

In practice, migraine is very often related to food sensitivity, and there is also some scientific evidence to back this up.[184] Any food can cause problems, but wheat is a very frequent offender. Other foods that are commonly associated with migraine include coffee and chocolate. For more details about how to identify the foods that might be at the root of your child's migraine, see pages 211–22.

Blood sugar levels

Low levels of sugar in the bloodstream seem to have the potential to trigger migraine attacks in some children. If your child seems more prone to a migraine if they skip a meal, then suspect this problem. Regular meals, perhaps with healthy snacks, such as fresh fruit and nuts, in between should help keep migraine at bay if low blood sugar is a problem. More information about stabilising blood sugar levels, and the range of benefits a child may get from this, can be found on pages 204–10.

MSG and aspartame

MSG (monosodium glutamate, E621) is a chemical added to a whole variety of different foods, including many fast foods, crisps, soups and Chinese foods. In practice, it seems to have the capacity to trigger migraine and other headaches, and there is some evidence to bear this out.[185] The same seems to be true for aspartame, an artificial sweetener that is found in a huge range of products, including diet drinks, low-sugar yoghurts and sugar-free chewing gum.[186] It might take some fairly rigorous label reading, but it is likely to help to keep MSG and aspartame out of your child's diet as much as possible.

Caffeine

Caffeine can cause constriction in blood vessels, increasing the likelihood of a migraine attack once the vessels dilate again. As a general rule, caffeine is therefore best avoided by children who are prone to migraine. Unfortunately, it is found in a large range of food products, including chocolate, energy drinks, cola drinks and even painkillers. If there is quite a lot of caffeine in your child's diet (for instance, if they drink a lot of coffee, tea or cola), then abrupt removal of caffeine is likely to trigger a thumping headache (this is part of a syndrome called caffeine withdrawal). It's probably better (and kinder) to reduce caffeine gradually over three to four weeks.

Supplements
Magnesium

Low levels of magnesium in the body have been associated with migraines.[187] While it is not known for sure how magnesium may help prevent migraine attacks, it is known to be a blood vessel relaxant. Plenty of magnesium in the body is believed to reduce the risk of blood vessel constriction, thereby reducing the risk of the dilation that is believed to be a potent factor in migraine. In addition to increasing your child's intake of magnesium-rich foods, supplementation is likely to bring additional benefits in terms of migraine control. A 40 kg child should take 150–250 mg of magnesium per day.

Feverfew

Feverfew (*Tanacetum parthenium*) has a long history of use in herbal medicine in the treatment of migraines and is a godsend for many migraine sufferers. In studies, Feverfew has been found to reduce the frequency, severity and duration of migraine attacks.[188–90]

The main active constituent in Feverfew is thought to be a substance called 'parthenolide'. For a 40 kg child, give the equivalent of 125 mg of parthenolide a day. You might need to be patient with this remedy, as benefits may take several weeks to become apparent. Feverfew is not suitable for children under two years of age.

Flower essences

• Try Rescue Remedy as soon as your child starts to feel unwell.

• If **over-excitability** is a trigger, offer Impatiens.

• **Stress-related** migraines may respond to Vervain, Impatiens and Beech.

Miscarriage

A miscarriage (the medical term for which is spontaneous abortion) is a pregnancy that ends by itself within 20 weeks of conception. The term stillbirth refers to babies lost after 20 weeks. These problems are very common: experts estimate that about half of all fertilised eggs die and are miscarried, often very early on before women even know they are pregnant. Of pregnancies that the mother knows about, approximately 20 per cent end in miscarriage.

What causes a miscarriage?

It is not always possible to know what has caused a miscarriage. However, there is evidence that 50–60 per cent of miscarriages have a genetic root. In theory, higher levels of nutrients should help to prevent the glitches in DNA that are at the root of genetic abnormalities. Interestingly, Swedish researchers have found that higher intakes of folic acid, for instance, may reduce the risk of miscarriage.[191] The levels of folate were assessed in women who had lost a child between six and twelve weeks of pregnancy. These levels were then compared with those found in women who were between six and twelve weeks pregnant. The results showed that compared to women with normal folate levels, those with low levels of folate in their bodies were almost 50 per cent more likely to suffer a miscarriage. In addition, women with the highest levels of folate were 26 per cent less likely to suffer from a miscarriage compared to those with normal levels.

Another nutrient that is associated with miscarriage is selenium. One study found significantly lower levels of selenium in the blood of women who miscarried.[192] It seems that adequate selenium intakes are especially important early on in pregnancy, so ensuring a good intake prior to conception may be important. Supplementation with a multivitamin and mineral that contains folic acid and selenium may help to guard against miscarriage, especially if started pre-conceptually.

Homocysteine

Homocysteine (pronounced homo-sis-teen) is a breakdown product of a substance called methionine, itself derived from protein in the diet. Homocysteine helps to build and maintain tissues in the body, but in excess, has the capacity to injure the lining of the arteries in the body. Many scientists believe that such damage in the vessel wall is the first step in the process that ultimately leads to conditions such as heart disease and stroke. In addition, homocysteine can also thicken the blood, an effect that is likely to increase the risk of these conditions as well as blood clots in the leg known as deep vein thromboses (DVTs).

There is also evidence that raised levels of homocysteine may be a factor in some miscarriages. This seems to be especially true of women who have suffered recurrent miscarriages.[193] One study found that high levels of homocysteine in the blood, along with a folic acid deficiency (folic acid can reduce homocysteine levels) is a likely factor in recurrent miscarriage.[194]

Women who have suffered one or more miscarriages might do well to have their homocysteine levels checked. Homocysteine levels in the bloodstream are generally measured in units known as micromols per litre (mol/l) of blood. It is not clear what values represent 'healthy' levels of homocysteine, though existing research suggests that less than 10 mol/l is desirable.

Vitamin B6, B12 and folic acid

Homocysteine can be converted in the body into a harmless substance known as cystanthionine, and this conversion is dependent on vitamins B6, B12 and folic acid. Individuals with raised homocysteine levels may help themselves by upping their intake of these nutrients. The recommended supplemental levels of these nutrients for quelling homocysteine levels are 10 mg of vitamin B6, 400 mcg of vitamin B12 and 800 mcg of folic acid each day.

Caffeine

Another dietary factor that might affect risk of miscarriage is caffeine. One study found that pregnant women who consumed more than 100 mg of caffeine (which is roughly equivalent to a cup of coffee or two small cups of tea) were more likely to miscarry between six and twelve weeks of pregnancy than those who consumed less than this.[195]

In another study, drinking four to seven cups of coffee a day was found to be associated with a 40 per cent increase in the risk of stillbirth.[196] In this study, drinking eight or more cups of coffee a day appeared to more than double the risk. However, while this research showed that quite a lot of coffee may increase the risk of stillbirth, a small amount appeared to have the opposite effect: women drinking one to three cups of coffee a day were actually 40 per cent *less* likely to suffer a stillbirth compared to women drinking no coffee at all. Overall, it is likely that one cup of coffee or tea each day is generally safe for expectant mums and their babies.

Painkillers

Evidence suggests that the taking of aspirin or painkillers known as non-steroidal anti-inflammatory drugs (NSAIDs), such as ibuprofen, around the time of conception increases risk of miscarriage by 80 per cent.[197] An increased risk was not found for paracetamol. Pregnant women and women planning pregnancy are best advised to use paracetamol if there is any need for painkilling medication.

Insulin and miscarriage

Insulin is the hormone responsible for reducing blood sugar levels and stimulates the conversion of sugar into glycogen (a form of starch) and fat. Some individuals, particularly those that eat an abundance of sugar and refined carbohydrate, tend to secrete an excess of insulin, which can have unwanted effects in the body. High levels of insulin can increase the level of male hormones known as androgens in the blood, and these are though to participate in some cases of infertility and recurrent miscarriage. One study found that treating women with a condition known as polycystic ovarian syndrome (in which insulin and androgen levels are generally elevated) with a drug that lowered blood insulin levels helped to reduce their risk of miscarriage.[198] More details about how to control blood sugar and insulin levels can be found on pages 204–10.

Molluscum contagiosum

Molluscum contagiosum is a viral infection that gives rise to the presence of shiny, white, wart-like lumps on the skin. *Molluscum contagiosum* can affect any part of the skin, but the face, genitals and inside of the thighs are commonly affected. *Molluscum contagiosum* is more common in children than in adults and usually clears up of its own accord within a year a so. However, in a small percentage of sufferers, problems can persist for longer.

Supplements

Selenium

One nutrient that seems to help clear *Molluscum contagiosum* infection is the mineral selenium. Doses of 100–200 mcg of selenium per day should be given for a month or two.

Myrrh

Extracts of myrrh (*Commiphora molmol*) have potent anti-viral action and have been used historically to treat a wide range of infections. Dissolve 10 drops of essential oil of myrrh in 100 ml of almond oil. This mixture should be rubbed into the affected area two or three times a day.

Mononucleosis

See 'Glandular fever'

Morning sickness

Morning sickness is the term used to describe the nausea, and sometimes vomiting, associated with pregnancy.

Many women will bear testament to the fact that morning sickness can actually last right through the day. The condition is thought to affect up to 90 per cent of all pregnant women. Typically, the symptoms appear four to six weeks into the pregnancy, peak at eight to twelve weeks, and are normally over by week 20.[199] However, for a few poor unfortunates, symptoms can progress right through their pregnancy.[200] About 1 per cent of women develop very severe symptoms due to a condition known as hyperemesis gravidarum. This may require hospitalisation so that fluid and nutrients can be given through a drip.

Morning sickness has been associated with poor quality diets and large and infrequent meals.[201] Other suggestions for the cause of nausea and vomiting include nutrient deficiency, specifically of vitamin B6, and lower than normal weight.

Diet
Regular meals
Nausea and vomiting appear to be worse on an empty stomach and symptoms are often helped by eating small, frequent meals. Low levels of blood sugar can be a factor in nausea, and regular eating can help combat this too. Eating slowly and chewing food thoroughly will help digestion, which may help to reduce a tendency to feel sick.

Supplements
Vitamin B6
Vitamin B6 supplementation has been shown to be beneficial in morning sickness.[202] A good dose is 20–40 mg of B6 a day.

Ginger
Another good natural remedy for morning sickness is ginger. In one study, ginger was found to bring significant relief from vomiting in 28 out of 32 women.[203] Like vitamin B6, this is safe to take in pregnancy at the recommended dosage. Take 250 mg of ginger in tablet or capsule form, up to four times a day.

Motion sickness
Balance in the body is governed by delicate organs in the inner ear. Travel sickness is thought to be related to the effect of movement and vibration here, but it is not known why some individuals seem to be more sensitive to this than others.

Diet
Fatty foods
Avoid fatty foods before travel, as this can make your child more susceptible to nausea. Light snacks, such as fruit, dried fruit and nuts, taken before travelling and en route can help to maintain blood sugar levels. This does seem to help ease symptoms.

Supplements
Ginger
Certain natural remedies may help reduce or even prevent the nausea and sickness that is characteristic of travel sickness. One substance that is often very effective in this respect is ginger. The ancient Chinese mariners would ward off seasickness by keeping a slice of fresh root ginger between their cheek and gum. These days, ginger is available

in capsule and tablet form. A 40 kg child should take 125 mg of ginger every three hours, or 5 drops of 1:2 tincture in some water, three times a day. An alternative is to give your child some crystallised ginger to munch on. A packet of this stuff is useful to have around when you're on the move.

Acupressure bracelets

Another option for travel sickness is a bracelet that stimulates the acupressure points on the wrist connected with nausea. In the UK, these are marketed under a variety of different names, such as Seabands.

Flower essences

• The Bush flower essences Dog Rose and Paw Paw are recommended for travel sickness.

Mouth ulcers

Mouth ulcers are small, swollen, painful ulcers that occur on the lips or in the mouth. They usually start as a small red dot on the lip or the inside of the mouth, which then enlarges and develops a white head. Eventually the head ruptures, leaving an open ulcer that can make eating (and even talking) uncomfortable.

Mouth ulcers can have a variety of causes. One common, and often overlooked, factor is an ingredient in toothpaste known as sodium lauryl sulphate (SLS). SLS is a foaming agent, but is also thought to cause erosion of a substance called 'mucin', which lines and protects the mouth. One study showed that individuals suffering from recurrent mouth ulcers found significant relief by avoiding SLS in toothpaste.[204] Natural, SLS-free toothpastes are often available in health food stores. Most organic toothpastes do not contain SLS.

Mouth ulcers may also be related to nutritional deficiencies, especially in iron and B vitamins.[205–7] Another study found that patients who suffered from recurrent mouth ulcers tended to have low levels of calcium and vitamin C as well.[208]

Supplements

Multivitamins and minerals

Taking a good quality multivitamin and mineral that contains the B-complex vitamin may help build a child's nutritional reserves in time, and this may help make them much less prone to mouth ulcers. More details about suitable supplements can be found on page 00.

Deglycyrrhizinated liquorice (DGL)

A natural supplement that often works well for mouth ulcers is deglycyrrhizinated liquorice (DGL). This substance has natural soothing properties and can reduce the healing time for mouth ulcers. DGL is thought to work by increasing mucin production in the mouth. One study showed that 15 out of 20 patients with mouth ulcers experienced 50–75 per cent improvement within one day followed by complete healing of the ulcers by the third day.[209] Half a DGL tablet should be chewed 20 minutes before each meal for a week.

Vitamin E

Vitamin E can help soothe mouth ulcers and may promote healing too. For topical relief, the contents from a soft gelatine vitamin E capsule can be applied directly onto the ulcer(s) as often as necessary.

Mumps

Mumps is a viral infection that affects the salivary glands, usually the parotid glands, which are located in front of and below the ears. The condition is most common in children between the ages of five and fifteen years. It is transmitted by saliva and is generally less contagious than infections such as measles and chickenpox. After infection, the condition can incubate for up to three weeks before any symptoms appear.

The illness usually begins with fever, headache, loss of appetite and aching muscles. About a day later, there may be pain in the ears and under the jaw. Over the ensuing few days, the salivary glands swell up (to form the characteristic chipmunk appearance) and become tender. Symptoms will normally settle over the next week. The condition is contagious from about six days before the onset of the illness, to nine days after the glands have been swollen.

Mumps can lead to an inflammation in the testes known as orchitis. This affects about a quarter of boys. It normally only affects one testis. In rare cases, orchitis can affect both testes, and this may lead to problems with fertility later in life.

Diet
Sugar
Refined sugar has been found to suppress the immune system and should really be avoided. The diet should be based on whole, unrefined foods. Fruits and vegetables are particularly important as these tend to be rich in nutrients that support the immune system, such as vitamin C and beta-carotene. Plenty of water is important too, as this helps with healing and recovery.

Supplements
Vitamin C, zinc and echinacea
As with most infections, it is a good idea to supplement with nutrients and herbs to boost the immune system and speed healing. A combination of vitamin C, zinc and the herb echinacea are generally very effective in this respect. More details about dosing for these natural agents can be found in the section 'Colds and flu'. Start supplementation as soon as possible and keep them going for one week after the symptoms have cleared.

Flower essences
• Rescue Remedy can be offered to ease distress and discomfort.
• In addition you may try the Australian Bush flower essences Sturt Desert Rose for pain and Mountain Devil for fever.

Nails, brittle or weak

Weak nails are almost exclusively a female phenomenon, and can be a sign of imbalances within the body. The strength of the nails is dependent on the supply of certain nutrients, especially minerals such as iron, magnesium, calcium, zinc and healthy fats known as essential fatty acids. Weak nails in a young girl are generally a sign that she's not getting all the nutrients she needs.

Supplements

Multivitamins and minerals

If your daughter suffers from weak or brittle nails, taking a good multivitamin and mineral formulation may help strengthen the nails over time. Some companies have produced formulations specifically for this purpose and these are almost certainly worth a try. One nutrient that seems to be of particular value in strengthening nails is biotin. Biotin is a member of the B vitamin family and can be taken on its own or as part of a good B-complex tablet. In one study, 35 individuals were treated with 2500 mcg (2.5 g) of biotin per day. Some 63 per cent reported an improvement in the condition of their nails, though it took an average of two months before improvement was seen.[210] In addition to a good multivitamin and mineral, it might also be worth giving 1 mg of biotin per day.

Essential fatty acids

Supplementation with essential fatty acids (EFAs) may also help weak nails. If symptoms such as dry skin and dry hair are also present, this is suggestive of a deficiency in EFAs. Hemp seed oil is a good all-round supplement as it contains essential fats of both the omega-3 and omega-6 type (see pages 156–7 for more details). I recommend 10 ml (2 tsp) a day for a 40 kg child. Children may be reluctant to take this oil off a spoon, so it may be best to put it in a soup, stew, sauce or casserole.

Flower essences

• The Bush flower essence Fringed Violet is often recommended for nail-related problems.

Nappy rash

Nappy rash is a general inflammation of the skin within the nappy region. Most babies and toddlers will experience it at some point, though it can be persistent in some. The condition is believed to be caused by a reaction in the skin to chemicals and enzymes in the urine and faeces. These chemicals are held against the skin by the nappy, leaving it sore and tender. As well as redness and irritation, the skin may be swollen and even ulcerated.

Sometimes what looks like nappy rash can be caused by a fungal infection. In this case, the skin tends to be smooth, shiny and bright red. The rash will tend to be well defined and there may be scattered spots in the groin area. Generally, it helps to ensure that your child is getting plenty of fresh water to drink. This helps to dilute the acids present in urine and faeces. Changing the nappy as soon as it becomes wet or soiled will help too.

Supplements

Probiotics

Probiotics (healthy gut bacteria) are worth considering for nappy rash, as these appear to help repel the bacteria and yeast organisms that may be involved.[211] If you are breast feeding, take Bio-Acidophilus, 1 capsule each day for a month or two. The benefits of taking this supplement should be passed to your baby in your breast milk. Otherwise, you can treat your child directly with a product known as INT B1. This supplement contains a strain of probiotic that is especially suitable for children under the age of two. Give 1/4 tsp each day in some water, for a month or two. (For more details, see Useful contacts and information – under BioCare.)

Topical treatments
Calendula cream
Calendula cream is excellent for encouraging healing, acting as a light barrier cream and easing inflammation. Use liberally on the affected areas between nappy changes. If possible, keep your baby's nappy off after applying the cream. A bit of air to the region will help to encourage the healing process and give the skin a chance to renew itself, away from any irritating substances or fabrics.

Flower essences
• Rescue Remedy and Rescue Cream can both be used to soothe and calm your baby, particularly if he or she is in pain or distress. Rub the cream directly into the affected area.

Nausea and vomiting
See 'Food poisoning and Gastroenteritis' and 'Motion sickness'

Nettle rash
See 'Hives'

Nosebleeds
Nosebleeds come from ruptures in the blood vessels that line the nose and are generally caused by a blow to the nose, blowing the nose too hard, inflammation from a cold or an allergy, or even some overzealous picking. In the first instance, lean your child forwards and pinch under the bridge of his or her nose. He or she should breathe through the mouth. After 10–15 minutes, you can release the pressure. Most nosebleeds will have stopped in this time. If it hasn't, reapply pressure under the nostrils. If the bleeding has not stopped after 25 minutes, seek medical attention.

Homeopathic treatments
Arnica
The homeopathic remedy Arnica is indicated for nosebleeds, particularly if they are the result of an injury. Offer Arnica at 30C dilution every ten minutes during an attack, and three times a day for ten days. If nosebleeds are recurrent, it can be taken once daily until the problem is in hand.

Supplements
Vitamin C and bioflavonoids
Vitamin C and nutrients known as bioflavonoids are important for the health of the walls of blood vessels. Increasing the levels of these in the body can strengthen blood vessels and make them less prone to rupture. Try to ensure your child gets plenty of fresh fruit and vegetables. In addition, you might like to supplement with 500 mg of vitamin C and 500 mg of bioflavonoids each day (for a 40 kg child).

> **Swallowing blood**
> Blood can be swallowed during
> a nosebleed, which may cause
> children to feel sick. They may even
> vomit. Children who have swallowed
> quite a lot of blood may also pass an
> unusually dark and offensive stool
> about a day later.
>
> If your child's nosebleeds
> seem unusually common or you
> find that it can be difficult to
> stop the bleeding, it may be
> worthwhile seeking your doctor's
> advice. It is important to make sure
> there is no underlying reason for
> the problem, such as an inability
> to make blood clots.

Flower essences

• Offer Emergency Essence or Rescue
Remedy during an attack, particularly if
your child is frightened or has suffered
an injury.

Obesity

See 'Overweight and obesity'

Osgood-Schlatter disease

The thigh muscles attach to the
shinbone (tibia) via a tendon that runs
underneath the kneecap (patella). This
tendon inserts into the shin at a point
called the tibial tuberosity. Osgood-
Schlatter disease is a characterised by
the painful enlargement of the tibial
tuberosity. The pain associated with
the condition is generally worse during
exercise and the area below the knee

is usually tender to the touch.
Osgood-Schlatter disease normally
affects boys between the ages of ten
and fourteen years, though it can affect
girls too. The condition is generally
worsened by exercise, which is why
doctors tend to recommend that
sufferers lay off sport while it heals.
The condition usually clears up of its
own accord over about six months or
a year, though it is usually advised
that a child avoids running-based
exercise during this time.

Supplements

Vitamin E and selenium
In practice, a combination of vitamin
E and selenium can be very effective
in treating Osgood-Schlatter disease.
A dose of 400 IU of vitamin E each day
along with 100 mcg of selenium, twice
a day is likely to give relief within six
weeks. After this, half the dose should
be given for a further six weeks to
reduce the risk of a recurrence. In the
long term, it can help a child to take a
good quality multivitamin and mineral
containing selenium and vitamin E as
a preventive.

Overweight and obesity

Children obviously come in all sorts
of shapes and sizes. While a lot of kids
may harbour a bit of puppy fat at some
stage during childhood and even
adolescence, more significant amounts
of excess weight may have important
implications to physical (as well as
emotional) wellbeing. The most
commonly used measurement of weight

is something known as the body mass index (BMI), which is calculated by dividing the weight of an individual in kilograms by the square of their height in metres. The resulting number indicates if you are underweight, normal weight or overweight.

weight in kg ÷ (height in m)^2

BMIs of 20–25 are considered normal. However, BMIs above this range are considered as 'overweight'. A BMI of more than 30 is officially classified as 'obese'. According to the Office for National Statistics, rates of the percentage of overweight children increased from 14.7 per cent to 23.6 per cent between 1989 and 1998 alone. In the same time frame, rates of obesity almost doubled (5.4 per cent to 9.2 per cent). Excess weight and obesity are linked with an increased risk of a range of conditions, including heart disease, diabetes and joint problems. Not surprisingly, research shows that overweight children are more likely (though not necessarily destined) to turn into overweight adults too. Also, the impact that excess weight may have on a child's emotional wellbeing is sometimes underestimated. Overweight children as young as five years can develop a negative self-image, [212] and obese adolescents have been found to show varying degrees of low self-esteem, along with other emotional and social issues, such as sadness, loneliness and nervousness.[213]

There is always the risk that focusing on a child's weight can make him or her even more self-conscious. Generally, it seems to help not to be putting too much attention on the weight issue *itself*, but on behaviours that help combat the problem. The two fundamental lifestyle factors that are critical to achieving or maintaining healthy weight are diet and exercise.

Dietary strategies for weight control

Concerns about a child's weight may encourage parents to restrict food. However, evidence suggests that this approach tends not to work and may actually drive a tendency to overeat, especially unhealthy food. See page 194 for more information about this. It seems that having rafts of rules and regulations about what can be eaten, when and in what amounts, is unlikely to help a child, and may actually compound the problem. The key to having a child eat better is to ensure a healthy food culture in and out of the home. Chapter 3 covers this in depth.

Generally speaking, children with excess weight to lose will do this successfully by simply eating a healthy diet, as outlined in Chapters 1 and 2. A specific 'diet' is generally unnecessary. I would, however, be cautious about taking standard nutritional advice and opting for a low-fat, high carbohydrate diet. As discussed in Chapter 1, there is actually not much evidence for the link between dietary fat and excess weight. Also, too much carbohydrate (particularly refined carbohydrates such as white bread, white rice and pasta) may lead to weight gain. This is also discussed in Chapter 1. The emphasis should be on a diet based on whole, natural and unprocessed foods. The healthier the diet, the more likely your child is to lose weight healthily.

In addition, it can help to be mindful of specific factors that may impact on weight, including soft drinks, fast foods, portion size, activity levels and television watching habits.

Soft drinks

One carbohydrate rich foodstuff the consumption of which seems to have particular influence on weight is the fizzy drink. Results of one study showed that the total energy intake of kids consuming soft drinks is about 10 per cent greater than in children who don't.[214] Another study found that each additional serving of soft drink was associated with a whopping 60 per cent increased risk of obesity.[215] Bearing in mind the fact that soft drinks are likely to have other adverse effects on health too, these are certainly something to consume with extreme caution. As discussed on page oo, the benefits of artificial sweeteners has not been proven to help weight loss, and not a single study has looked at their effect in children. Bearing in mind the considerable doubt about their safety, my advice is to avoid 'diet' drinks as well as full-sugar varieties.

Fast food

In many ways, fast foods such as burgers, chicken nuggets, chips, soft drinks and milk shakes bring together the very worst elements in the standard Western diet. Many of these foods release sugar quickly into the bloodstream and are often laced with quantities of trans fats. The fact that these foods may be low on nutrients and high on additives does not help matters

either. The ever-rising popularity of fast food in our culture is almost certainly a factor in obesity (as well as a raft of other health issues). Had from time to time as an occasional treat, fast food is unlikely to put too much of a dent in a generally healthy diet. However, while it probably won't help to forbid it entirely, it won't do any harm to remind older children why fast food is something to be had in as limited quantities as possible.

Does portion size matter?

In general terms, my experience in practice is that it's much more important to concentrate on the quality of the diet, rather than its quantity. However, it is true that some children may have difficulty controlling the amount of food they consume. One factor here may be the amount of food children are served. On page 286 I look at one study that found that serving children (average age of four years) large portions of food led to them eating more than if they were allowed to serve themselves.[216] Another study found that feeding larger portions led to increased food intake in five-year-olds, but not three-and-a-half-year-olds.[217] These findings suggest that as children grow older, they become less responsive to internal signals and perhaps more reactive to their external environment, in deciding how much they eat. I suggest serving smallish portions to your child – you can always give him or her more if asked for or it seems like he or she is still hungry.

Activity and exercise

Many parents I know malign the apparent reduction in childhood activity that has been witnessed over the last couple of decades at least. Many of us will remember growing up in a culture where outdoor activity, even unsupervised by our parents or other adults, was a regular occurrence. In recent times, increasing concern about the potential dangers in our environment mean that parents have generally been less keen to give their children free rein. Also, the rise and rise of computer games and the Internet mean that more and more children are inclined to spend their leisure time sitting down rather than running about. None of this is helped, of course, by the selling off of sports fields and the national curriculum seems to be putting more and more emphasis on the importance of academic achievement, at the expense of sport and exercise-related activities.

However, there is very good evidence that even 'unorganised' sports such as cycling, skipping and kicking a football around can help to reduce the risk of being overweight and obesity.[218] Not all children enjoy sport, competitive or otherwise, and therefore tend not to gravitate towards it. My personal view is that this need not be a concern. What is most important is that children are *active*, and this can manifest in a variety of forms that are not perceived as formal exercise or 'sport'. Walking is a good place to start and it may be possible to weave this into the day's daily regime. If not, then you might want to think about how you might be able to get that activity at other times, including the early evenings and weekends, possibly as a family. It doesn't matter so much what the activity is, but more that it's happening at all. Whether it's a ball game in the garden, a cycle-ride in the park, swimming on Saturday morning or a walk in the woods on Sunday, it all counts.

Television viewing and weight

One area that has been the subject of considerable research is the link between television viewing with activity levels and weight. It is obvious that the more time a child spends in front of the television, the less time they will tend to spend being active. In one study, obesity risk increased by 12 per cent for each hour per day of television viewing, but decreased by 10 per cent for each hour per day of moderate-to-vigorous physical activity.[219] Another study found that in children aged seven to eleven years, those watching three to five hours of television a day were 50 per cent more likely to be obese compared to children watching zero to two hours of television each day.[220]

It may not only be the inactivity of television that causes problems. There is also evidence that more time spent in front of the TV may increase the amount of food a child gets through in a day.[221-2] It can also encourage unhealthy snacking and a stimulation of appetite at times when your child is not normally hungry. Some of this may relate to the constant bombardment of children with adverts for less-than-healthy foods via television advertisements. British children are exposed to about ten food commercials per hour of television time (amounting to thousands per year for many children), mostly for fast food, soft drinks, sweets, and sugar-sweetened breakfast cereal.[223-6]

What this amounts to is that television viewing is a pretty toxic force for many kids. Almost everyone has television in their homes. However, putting one in a child's bedroom seems to be a particular problem.[227] If your child already has a TV in the bedroom, it may be difficult to excise. However, whether he or she watches TV in his own room or in some communal area, it is probably worthwhile setting clear and consistent parameters about when he or she can watch it, and for how long.

Periods - heavy
See 'Menorrhagia'

Periods - painful
See 'Menstrual cramps'

Pinworms
See 'Worms'

Pneumonia

This is the medical term for inflammation in the lungs caused by an infection. Most cases are caused by bacteria or viruses. Viral pneumonia often begins as an upper respiratory infection such as a cold or flu. As the infection takes hold in the lung it often gives rise to a fever, cough and generalised fatigue. Eventually, the cough may become 'productive' (which means that phlegm comes up with the coughing). Phlegm in viral pneumonia is usually white. Lungs affected by viral pneumonia are more likely to become infected by a bacterial organism.

In general terms, bacterial pneumonia is a more serious illness than the viral type. A child with bacterial pneumonia will generally look and feel very ill, is likely to have a high fever, and with a high fever, may have difficulty breathing too. Coughing is usually a feature of the illness, and this tends to bring up phlegm that is coloured green or yellow.

If your child has symptoms of bacterial pneumonia, get a doctor's opinion. The likelihood is that antibiotics will be recommended. This may indeed be the best thing for your child. However, once taken, it is a good idea to give your child a good probiotic supplement (see page 16) for a month or two, as this will help restore healthy bacteria in the gut, which are likely to have been killed by the antibiotics.

Diet
Sugar and dairy products
If you suspect your child may be brewing a chest infection, early action

may help keep it from developing into something nasty. Keep your child's intake of refined sugar to a minimum, as there is evidence that sugar can disable the immune system, which will do nothing to help clear the infection. Keeping away from dairy products may help too, as these tend to cause mucus production, which won't help matters either.

The diet should be based on whole, unrefined foods. Fruits and vegetables are particularly important as these tend to be rich in nutrients that support the immune system, such as vitamin C and beta-carotene. Encourage your child to drink plenty of fluids (in the form of water and diluted fruit juices), which will help to keep him or her hydrated and speed recovery.

Supplements
Vitamin C
Vitamin C has been found to be a useful natural agent in fighting lung infection. Children with high levels of vitamin C in their bodies are less likely to succumb to pneumonia and are much more likely to recover quickly if they take it while they are ill.[228] Three studies have recorded a reduction of at least 80 per cent in the incidence of pneumonia in the group of individuals given vitamin C. Give your child 500 mg of vitamin C, several times each day while he or she is ill. This may loosen the bowels somewhat. If this happens, reduce the dose.

Zinc and echinacea
In addition, it may help your child to be treated with zinc and the herb echinacea, both of which have immune-stimulating properties. For more details

about how to administer these, see pages 61–2 in the section 'Colds and flu'.

Polycystic ovarian syndrome

As its name suggests, polycystic ovarian syndrome (PCOS) is a condition associated with multiple cysts in one or both ovaries. Other common symptoms of this condition include breast pain, menstrual irregularities, acne and excess facial and/or body hair (hirsutism). Sufferers of this condition are usually found to have raised levels of 'male' hormones known as androgens (such as testosterone), and this is thought to be a major reason for the acne and hirsutism often seen in the condition. A mainstay conventional treatment for women with PCOS is the oral contraceptive pill based on the drug cyproterone acetate (Dianette). Cyproterone acetate works by blocking the effect of androgens in the body. Women with PCOS may fail to ovulate normally, which can give rise to problems with fertility.

There is some evidence that PCOS is related to a condition known as insulin resistance syndrome. Here, higher-than-normal levels of insulin in the bloodstream appear to increase the production of androgens from the ovaries, and also strengthen their action in the body.[229] Some doctors are using anti-diabetic drugs to treat PCOS. However, another way of getting better control over insulin levels is to adjust the diet. Of particular importance here is balancing blood sugar levels, which is dealt with in depth on pages 204–20. In the long term, eating a diet designed to normalise blood sugar and insulin levels in the body (essentially a diet lower in carbohydrate-based sugars and starches) can be very effective in controlling PCOS.

Supplements
Saw palmetto
The symptoms of PCOS can often be helped with an herbal approach. The main androgen is a hormone called testosterone. Testosterone in the body can be converted into a more active form of this hormone called dihydrotestosterone. The herb saw palmetto (*Serenoa repens*) slows down the conversion of testosterone into dihydrotestosterone and may therefore help to control symptoms due to high levels of testosterone such as acne and hirsutism. Saw palmetto can be found in health food stores. The standard dose is 320 mg of standardised extract per day. (For more details about PCOS, see Useful contacts and information.)

Pre-eclampsia
Pre-eclampsia is a disorder that occurs in about 5 per cent of pregnancies and can harm both mother and child. The condition is characterised by high blood pressure, swelling due to fluid retention (also known as oedema) and protein in the urine. In extreme circumstances, blood pressure can rise to a very high level and cause fitting. This is a medical emergency, which usually results in the delivery of the baby by Caesarian section.

Quite what causes pre-eclampsia is unknown, though weight-related factors have been implicated. Ensuring you maintain a healthy weight (BMI of 25) (see page 119–29) may reduce risk.

Diet
Free radicals
Pre-eclampsia also seems to be related to damaging molecules known as free radicals. Free radicals are formed as by-products of many biochemical reactions in the body and seem to have the capacity to affect the function of blood vessels in pregnant women and the placenta.[230] It is believed that free radicals can stimulate the release of chemicals that contribute to high blood pressure and the leakage of protein into the urine.[231]

There is some thought that one way to help prevent pre-eclampsia is to reduce the effects of free radicals in the body. What are known as antioxidant nutrients, such as vitamins A, C, E and the minerals zinc and selenium, may help here. One study found that supplementing women at risk of pre-eclampsia with 1000 mg of vitamin C and 400 IU of vitamin E per day significantly reduced the risk of this condition.[232] Other research has been less conclusive, but that may be because studies have generally looked at giving supplements late in pregnancy. It makes sense that, if supplementation is to work, the earlier it is commenced, the better. Selenium might also be helpful, as it has been shown to reduce the risk of high blood pressure in pregnancy.[233] Women who have had problems with pre-eclampsia in a previous pregnancy may help to protect themselves from further problems by supplementing with 1000 mg of vitamin C, 400 IU of vitamin E and 100 mcg of selenium each day throughout subsequent pregnancies.

Pre-menstrual syndrome

Pre-menstrual syndrome (PMS) is the presence of physical and/or psychological symptoms in the second half of the menstrual cycle, which are normally relieved quite soon after menstruation begins. It's called a 'syndrome' because it is made up of a complex combination of symptoms, including psychological symptoms, such as irritability, aggression, tension, anxiety and depression, and physical changes, such as fluid retention, breast tenderness, headache, feeling of bloating and weight increase. The severity of symptoms varies widely between individuals: while some girls may get mild symptoms for a day or two before their period, others may get quite debilitating problems for a week or more.

The precise cause of PMS has not been elucidated and it is likely that it can be related to a number of underlying causes. One major theory about the cause of many cases of PMS is that it is related to an imbalance in hormone levels during the run-up to a period. Two of the key hormones involved in the regulation of the female cycle are oestrogen and progesterone. These hormones are secreted by the ovaries, although this process is largely governed by the pituitary gland, which sits at the base of the brain. There is some thought that an excess of the

hormone oestrogen relative to progesterone is a common factor in PMS. This situation, sometimes referred to as 'oestrogen dominance', typically gives rise to problems with irritability, fluid retention and breast tenderness.

Diet

Blood sugar levels

Research suggests that women who suffer from PMS consume more sugar and refined carbohydrates (like white bread) and lower levels of fibre and nutrients than non-sufferers. A diet based on whole, unrefined foods may help. Getting good control over blood sugar levels is generally a good ploy (see pages 204–20), as this will help prevent fluctuations that can drive symptoms such as food cravings and mood swings. In practice, sugar and caffeine both seem to increase the risk of PMS. Caffeine has been clearly implicated in PMS, and should be avoided as much as possible.[234]

Exercise

Another lifestyle factor that is well known to affect PMS in the long term is exercise.[235] Half an hour's exercise such as jogging, aerobics, cycling or swimming on most days does seem to help control the symptoms of PMS.

Supplements

Agnus castus **(chaste tree)**

The medicinal herb *Agnus castus* is very often effective for the treatment of PMS. It seems to work for the vast majority of sufferers, often within one or two menstrual cycles. *Agnus castus* seems to help increase production of the hormone progesterone, which helps balance the excess of oestrogen, the seeming common underlying factor in PMS. One study found that offering this herb daily for three months caused a good reduction in symptoms in the women taking part, and found that when the treatment ceased, the symptoms returned.[236] Another study found Agnus castus is effective in treating breast pain associated with PMS.[237] Finally, a 2001 study found that improvements in irritability, mood alteration, anger, headache, breast fullness and other symptoms such as bloating were significantly greater in the group treated with Agnus castus than those given a placebo. Give 40 drops of Agnus castus tincture (alcoholic extract) once a day, or 20 mg of herb extract (in tablet or capsule form), twice a day. Results can normally be expected within two or three menstrual cycles.

Calcium

There is some evidence that calcium deficiency may be a cause of PMS in some girls. In one study, calcium supplementation reduced problems with low mood, pain, fluid retention and food cravings.[238] By the third month, the calcium effectively halved the severity of symptoms. Ensuring that your daughter gets a decent intake of calcium-rich foods (e.g. natural yoghurt, green leafy vegetables, pulses, nuts and sesame seeds) is important, as statistics show that the majority of adolescent girls do not get the recommended daily amount of calcium. In addition, it may help to supplement with about 500 mg of calcium a day.

Magnesium

Magnesium deficiency is also considered to be a factor in some cases of PMS.[239] Again, as with calcium, the vast majority of adolescent girls simply do not get the recommended amount of this mineral in their diets. Increasing intake of green leafy vegetables, beans and pulses, and nuts and seeds should help. Also, supplementation at a dose of 200–400 mg of magnesium per day, generally helps. In one study, supplementation with magnesium helped to correct mood problems common in PMS.[240]

Vitamin B6

Vitamin B6 does seem to be quite an effective treatment for PMS. It appears to be important for the production of mood-enhancing brain chemicals such as serotonin and dopamine. Adequate levels of B6 are important if magnesium is to do its job in the body, and these two nutrients do seem to work very well together in the treatment of PMS. Even on its own, however, vitamin B6 supplementation has been found to help relieve PMS in many sufferers.[241-2] I suggest 50 mg per day.

Flower essences

• The Bach flower essence Impatiens often helps with **irritability and tension**.
• Try Mustard for **depression**.
• Try Olive for **fatigue**.

Prickly heat

Prickly heat is a 'heat' rash that affects babies and small children. The condition is thought to be caused by blocked sweat glands. When the glands become blocked, the sweat does not reach the surface of the skin, where it is normally released. Instead, it becomes trapped, causing irritation and itching. It often causes a rash that is characterised by small blisters with bumps at the centre of each of these. It can affect the face, neck, shoulders or torso.

What to do

Cooling your child will help, as more sweat will not be produced to exacerbate the problem. Offer a lukewarm bath, and dress your child in as few clothes as possible. Your child should avoid any undue exertion that may lead to further sweating.

Topical treatments
Vitamin C

Studies suggest that vitamin C spray applied topically to the rash can help calm prickly heat.[243-4] You can make your own spray or lotion by mixing 2 table-spoons of vitamin C powder (available at good chemists or your local health food shop) with 125 ml of aloe vera gel (which itself has soothing properties). This can be sprayed or applied onto the rash two or three times a day.

Calendula cream

Calendula cream can also be applied to the affected area to ease discomfort and promote healing.

Flower essences

• Rescue Remedy will help ease discomfort and soothe your child.
• The Bush flower essences Red Grevillea or Black-eyed Susan may help reduce itching.

Psoriasis

Psoriasis is a chronic skin condition that normally gives rise to raised, red and scaly patches of skin, often on the knees, elbows, scalp and behind the ears. The condition seems to be linked to rapid growth in the outer layers of the skin. A percentage of psoriasis sufferers develop a form of arthritis known as psoriatic arthritis.

Although the precise cause of psoriasis is unknown, it does seem to be linked to certain factors. Psoriasis can tend to run in families suggesting that a predisposition for the condition may be inherited. The development of psoriasis may also be linked to our emotional state, with a significant number of sufferers reporting that the condition started after a time of particular stress. Other theories regarding the cause of psoriasis include the consumption of too much animal fat in the diet, a malfunctioning immune system and a build-up of toxins in the colon.

Diet
Food sensitivity

Some foods do seem to aggravate psoriasis, including citrus fruits, fried foods, refined foods and sugar. Meat and dairy products should be particularly avoided because they contain the substance arachidonic acid, which can make the psoriatic lesions turn red and swell. Two underlying factors that tend to crop up in some (though not all) cases of psoriasis are food sensitivity and yeast overgrowth. More information about how to diagnose and treat these problems can be found on pages 211–21 and 221–7.

Supplements

Essential fatty acids

Healthy fats known as essential fatty acids (EFAs) seem to have an important part to play in skin health and are often useful in the treatment of psoriasis. Some EFAs, particularly those of the omega-3 class such as alpha-linolenic acid, have an anti-inflammatory effect, which may help calm and soothe patches of psoriasis on the skin. In fact, there is some evidence that sufferers of psoriasis are deficient in alpha-linolenic acid.[245] Flaxseed oil is rich in alpha-linolenic acid and should be given at a dose of 15 ml (1 tbsp) per day.

Oregon grape

The herb Oregon grape (*Mahonia aquifolium*) proves useful in the treatment of psoriasis. There is some evidence that it helps to reduce the proliferation of skin cells that is typical of the condition.[246] Preparations of Oregon grape are available from health food stores and should be taken in accordance with the instructions on the label.

Milk thistle

The herb milk thistle (*Silybum marianum*) helps liver function, which is believed to help clear toxins in the body that might participate in the development of psoriasis. In practice, taking milk thistle seems to help a proportion of psoriasis sufferers after about eight weeks of treatment. Preparations of milk thistle are available from health food stores and should be taken in accordance with the instructions on the label.

Topical treatments

A number of natural substances applied topically to psoriasis may provide relief.

Aloe vera

One study found that application of aloe vera cream for 16 weeks cured 83 per cent of psoriasis sufferers (compared to only 7 per cent of those using an inactive cream).[247]

Fish oils

Topical application of fish oils has been found to help psoriasis sufferers.[248] The contents of fish oil capsules can be spread on the affected areas twice each day.

Flower essences

• If the condition has affected your child's **self esteem**, the Bach flower essence Larch may help.

• Crab Apple is cleansing, which can help with the detoxifying process, and also helps where a child **feels unclean** as a result of the condition.

Raynaud's disease

Raynaud's (pronounced ray-nodes) disease is characterised by poor circulation in the extremities. Here, constriction in the vessels that supply blood to the fingers and/or toes leads to problems with poor circulation. Typically, when first exposed to the cold, the affected digits turn white, then blue, and then finally red once they warm up again. As they warm, it is not uncommon for the digits to become painful for some minutes. Although there really is no conventional medical treatment for Raynaud's disease, certain natural approaches may help.

Diet

Caffeine

Caffeine tends to constrict blood vessels in the body and should therefore be avoided. Ginger, on the other hand, has a warming and circulation enhancing effect. To make ginger tea, simmer some grated or finely chopped root ginger in some water for about ten minutes.

Supplements

Magnesium

Magnesium may reduce spasm in the vessels of the fingers and toes and can often reduce the frequency and severity of attacks. A 40 kg child should take 150–250 mg per day.

Ginkgo biloba

The herb *Ginkgo biloba* is renowned for its ability to boost the circulation and is often effective in combating the symptoms of Raynaud's disease. A 40 kg child should take 60–120 mg of ginkgo extract each day.

Reye's syndrome

Reye's syndrome is a rare condition that can cause brain and liver damage (and even death) shortly after a viral infection such as cold, flu or chicken pox. The condition is almost entirely restricted to children under the age of 15 years. The symptoms of Reye's syndrome include uncontrollable vomiting, lethargy, memory loss, disorientation and delirium. In extreme cases, swelling in the brain may lead to seizures, heart rhythm irregularities and coma.

> **Emergency treatment**
> Reye's syndrome needs prompt medical care. If you are at all suspicious that your child may have it, seek medical attention immediately. Conventional treatment is based around fluids given into the vein and steroid drugs designed to reduce swelling in the brain.

Prevention

There seems to be a strong link between Reye's syndrome and the drug aspirin. One study found that of 56 children with Reye's syndrome, 82 per cent had been given aspirin.[249] Because of this association, parents are advised not to give their children aspirin, although paracetamol is permitted. Statistics show that this message appears to be getting through and there has been a steep decline in the incidence of Reye's syndrome as a result. The natural remedy White Willow (on which aspirin is based) should be avoided too.

Ringworm

Ringworm is not actually a worm but a fungal infection that thrives on the outer layers of the scalp, skin and nails. This fungus (called tinea) is the same one that causes athlete's foot and a red, itchy rash in the groin (almost always in boys). It is contagious and tends to spread between children via contaminated gyms, shower rooms and swimming pools.

Ringworm typically appears as a slightly scaly mark on the skin that starts as a small, round, itchy red spot. The infection heals from the inside of the lesion to the outer rim of the circle, which gives the appearance of a ring, hence the name. The spots can spread from one area of the body to another. Although not serious in itself, ringworm can be persistent if not treated, and may lead to considerable itching and discomfort.

Diet
Yeast

Yeast in the body feeds on sugar, and it is therefore a good idea to limit this in your child's diet. Some children with ringworm may have a more general problem with yeast overgrowth, often as a result of taking antibiotics. For more details about this, and how to tackle it, see pages 221–7.

Supplements
Probiotics

It generally helps to give probiotic supplement (healthy gut bacteria) to children with ringworm as this can help counteract any underlying problems with yeast overgrowth. See pages 221–7 for more details about this.

Topical treatments
Aloe vera, neem oil, oregano oil and grape seed extract

Certain natural substances have anti-fungal properties and may therefore be useful in the treatment of ringworm. Some of the most commonly used agents include aloe vera, neem oil, oregano oil and grape seed extract liquid. Apply one or more of these to the affected area, two or three times a day.

Rubella
See 'German measles'

Scalp – itchy

Itching in the scalp is almost always related to head lice or infection with yeast organisms (generally *Pityrosporum orbiculare*). If head lice is the problem, then this is usually obvious to the eye (see 'Head lice'). If yeast infection is the underlying feature, then the scalp is often flaky, and dandruff might be a feature too. In practice, children with yeast-related problems have overgrowth of yeast (usually candida) in the gut. This should be particularly suspected in children who have had antibiotic treatment. Making some dietary adjustments to correct this, along with the use of healthy gut bacterial supplements (probiotics), is usually key to getting lasting relief from an itchy scalp. More details about the general management of yeast overgrowth in the body can be found on pages 221–7.

Topical treatments
Tea tree oil

In addition to an internal approach to yeast, it may be useful to use natural topical agents too. A commonly used treatment for fungal (yeast) infections is tea tree oil, and this has proven yeast-killing ability.[250] Using shampoos and/or scalp treatments based on tea tree oil may help provide relief from itchy scalp. Another option is to add 3–4 drops of tea tree oil to a tablespoon of your child's regular shampoo and wash as normal. It is also generally helpful to choose shampoos for your children that are lower in chemical additives as this can help prevent irritation in the scalp. More 'natural' shampoos, some of which are specifically designed for children, can be found in most health food stores.

Flower essences
• Crab Apple is believed to help detoxification and can help a child who **feels 'dirty'** because of the condition.

Scalp – painful
Some children will experience quite severe pain when their hair is combed, brushed or pulled. Occasionally, the scalp may be tender to the touch too. In clinical practice, this problem is usually related to a deficiency in vitamin D. In its severe form, vitamin D deficiency can give rise to a condition called rickets, which is characterised by bone abnormalities such as bow legs and curvature of the spine. It is possible that even mild vitamin D deficiency may interfere with normal growth and development.

Diet
Vitamin D
Foods rich in vitamin D such as salmon, herring and mackerel should be emphasised in the diet. In addition, exposure to sunlight is important, as vitamin D is formed in the skin in response to sunlight.

Supplements
Vitamin D and multivitamin and mineral
Vitamin D may be added in supplement form. Give 200 IU per day for a month, followed by a multivitamin and mineral that contains vitamin D.

Scarring
See also 'Surgery - recovery from'. Scarring in the skin can be caused by a variety of things, including severe acne, burns, cuts or surgery. Whatever its precise cause, natural treatments can often be effective in improving a scar's appearance.

Topical treatments
Rosehip oil
A natural remedy for scarring does exist in the form of rosehip oil. Rosehip oil contains beneficial fats that are believed to help in the regeneration of the skin protein called collagen. Applied once or twice a day for some months, rosehip oil can often be quite effective in reducing all forms of scarring, including surgical scars, injuries and the type of scarring that may follow acne. One study found that it had beneficial effects in patients with a variety of skin-related scarring, including burns.[251]

Rosehip oil is available in the UK under the brand name Rosa Mosqueta from Rio Trading Company. (For more details, see Useful contacts and information.)

Vitamin E oil

Another natural remedy that seems to help reduce the appearance of scars is vitamin E oil. As with rosehip oil, this should be rubbed into the affected area once or twice a day for several months. It is sometimes possible to buy bottles of undiluted vitamin E oil. However, an alternative is to use the contents of soft gelatine capsules containing vitamin E oil.

Seasonal affective disorder

Seasonal affective disorder (SAD) is a condition that is characterised by depression related to reduced exposure to sunlight. Generally, the depression will start in the autumn or winter and disappear in the spring. The condition is common, with estimates of one in 20 people being affected to some degree. In countries where daylight is very much reduced during the winter, such as Scandinavian nations, SAD seems to be a particular problem, with rates of depression and suicide tending to rise significantly in the winter months. If your child suffers from low mood and/or depression, it is worthwhile seeing if this is in any way related to the seasons. If your child's symptoms are worse in the winter, then this suggests he or she might be suffering from SAD.

The conventional treatment for SAD is anti-depressant drugs. However, natural approaches are often an effective alternative and are less likely to give rise to unwanted side effects. Because SAD is essentially caused by lack of sunlight, it makes sense to get as much natural daylight as possible. Even on a dull day, the amount of natural light available outside is far higher than levels found in most indoor settings. Encouraging plenty of outdoor activity, especially in the winter, should help maintain mood. Exercise and activity have a natural anti-depressant effect, and this should help too.

It is also worthwhile considering purchasing a 'light box' for use at home or work. These devices, which give off light with the specific characteristics of the sun's rays, can often help to combat the symptoms of SAD. (For more details, see Useful contacts and information.)

Diet
Omega-3 fats

Dietary approaches to depression, including the role of omega-3 fats, can be found on the section on depression (pages 71–2).

Supplements
St John's wort

Many SAD sufferers find that taking a preparation based on the herb hypericum (St John's wort) helps relieve their symptoms. This finding has also been supported scientifically.[252-3] The usual adult dose of hypericum is 300 mg of standardised extract, taken three times a day, though this may be adjusted according to the weight of the child.

Seborrhoeic dermatitis

Seborrhoeic dermatitis is a skin condition characterised by a red, greasy, scaly rash that is usually found on the face, especially around the nose, forehead, chin and in the eyebrows. Other common sites include the armpit, groin and the skin over the breastbone (sternum) in the middle of the chest.

While the precise cause of seborrhoeic dermatitis is not known for sure, it often seems to be related to overgrowth of the yeast organism *Candida albicans* in the system. If the rash is itchy, then this is a bit of a clue that candida may be an underlying factor. More information about the diagnosis and treatment of yeast overgrowth can by found on pages 223–9.

Supplements
B-complex

Taking a B-complex supplement each day can sometimes benefit seborrhoeic dermatitis. For a 40 kg child, give a B-complex supplement that contains about 25 mg of each of the main B vitamins, B1, B2, B3, B5 and B6.

Topical treatments
Starflower oil and tea tree oil

The application of starflower oil (also known as borage oil) to seborrhoeic dermatitis often leads to considerable improvement in the condition. Rub 10 drops of starflower oil into the affected region, twice a day for two weeks. Two drops of tea tree oil added to this may also help, as tea tree has natural anti-fungal properties. This can be repeated as necessary.

Seizure
See 'Epilepsy'

Sicca syndrome
See 'Dry eyes'

Sickle cell anaemia

Blood contains red cells that transport oxygen around the body. The oxygen-carrying function of the red cells is actually performed by a substance called haemoglobin. In children with sickle cell disease, the haemoglobin is abnormal, which causes some red blood cells to become distorted and sickle-like in shape. The red blood cells affected in this way can become stuck in the body's smallest vessels (the capillaries), which in turn may lead to painful 'crises' requiring hospitalisation and treatment with painkillers and intravenous fluids. Sickle cell anaemia is an inherited condition, which occurs primarily in individuals of Afro-Caribbean origin.

Supplements
Vitamin B6, folic acid and vitamin B12

Vitamin B6 appears to have the ability to inhibit sickling of red blood cells and this nutrient has been shown to improve wellbeing and significantly reduce the number of painful attacks in sickle cell disease sufferers.[254–5]

Another study found that children with sickle cell anaemia responded to treatment combining folic acid, vitamin B12 and vitamin B6.[256] Give a B-complex supplement that contains 25 mg of vitamin B6 (for a 40 kg child) each day. In the UK, there has been much debate about the safety of vitamin B6. Studies show that doses of at least 200 mg per day are safe in adults.[257]

Vitamin E

Vitamin E has been shown to reduce the percentage of diseased cells in sickle cell anaemia sufferers.[258] Give 300 IU per day for a 40 kg child.

Garlic and vitamin C

Garlic appears also to have an effect on the abnormal cells that cause the painful crises and anaemia. One study found that aged garlic extract (available in health food stores) inhibited the formation of the abnormal cells when tested in a laboratory. The same study found that vitamins C and E could also do this.[259] Give 500 mg of aged garlic extract and 500 mg of vitamin C each day for a 40 kg child.

Flower essences

• The Bach flower essence Olive may help **restore energy** in children affected by sickle cell anaemia.

Sinusitis

The sinuses are air-filled cavities in the bones at the front of the head and face. The sinuses are lined with membranes similar to the lining of the nasal passages and their main role is to filter incoming air, moistening and warming it before it reaches the lungs. Occasionally, the membranes lining the nose become swollen, blocking the ducts that lead to the sinuses. This prevents them from draining properly, causing congestion and swelling, which can lead to infection in the sinuses – also known as sinusitis. When the sinuses are blocked,

congested, irritated and inflamed, secondary symptoms may include a headache, earache, toothache and facial pain with tenderness over the forehead and cheekbones. If your child finds gentle tapping over his or her cheekbone or forehead painful, then this suggests a problem with sinusitis.

Diet

Food sensitivity

In practice, many children who are prone sto sinus congestion and/or infection have an underlying problem with food sensitivity (see pages 211–21). While any food may be at fault, it seems as though dairy products are frequent offenders and are renowned for their mucus-forming and congestion-inducing potential.

Supplements

Vitamin C

One study found that there are reduced levels of antioxidant nutrients in the tissues of sinusitis suffers.[260] Another study found that supplementing antioxidants was effective in the treatment of acute sinusitis.[261] While many antioxidants may be of benefit, taking a simple approach with vitamin C may be effective, as this nutrient has healing, antioxidant and immune-stimulating properties. In an acute infection, give 250–500 mg of vitamin C, three or four times a day (for a 40 kg child).

Bromelain

A natural remedy that is often helpful in clearing an attack of sinusitis is bromelain.[262] This extract of pineapple has the ability to break down protein in the body, and may therefore help to loosen up and help clear the congestion characteristic of the condition. Give 250 mg of bromelain three or four times a day.

Vitamin C and bromelain should be continued for two weeks. However, if the infection does not seem to be clearing, or if you are concerned, then seek medical advice. Antibiotics are likely to be advised in this situation. If these are taken, it is a good idea to follow them with a course of healthy gut bacteria (probiotics) to help prevent any long-term imbalance in the organisms in the gut and elsewhere in the body. For more information about this, see pages 16–17.

Flower essences
• The Australian Bush essence Dagger Hakea is indicated for sinusitis.
• In acute situations where your child is in discomfort, try Rescue Remedy.

Slapped cheek disease
See 'Fifth disease'

Sleep problems
See 'Insomnia'

Sore throat and tonsillitis
There are many causes of sore throats, most of which are thought to be caused by viral organisms, for which antibiotics are ineffective. However, some cases of tonsillitis (a common cause of sore throats in kids) may be due to bacterial organisms, and antibiotics may therefore provide relief. Bacterial infection can cause a condition known as 'strep throat', named after the organism – streptococcus – that is the cause of the trouble. Streptococcal infections are also responsible for scarlet fever and may also give rise to rheumatic fever, which can have potentially serious consequences. Strep throat is usually treated with antibiotics. If these are deemed necessary, then it is a good idea to follow them with a course of healthy gut bacteria (probiotics) to help prevent any long-term imbalance in the organisms in the gut and elsewhere in the body. For more information about this, see pages 16–17.

In practice, infections such as tonsillitis and strep throat seem to be related to the ingestion of dairy products. Some practitioners have noticed that if children exclude dairy products from their diets, then sore throats caused by tonsillitis and streptococcal infection tend not to occur. Why this may be is not known for sure, but it is possible that an immune sensitivity to dairy products (this is quite common in children) diverts the immune system, making it more likely for infections to take hold in the body. Another theory is that the mucus dairy products tend to induce in the throat and ears makes an ideal medium for the growth of bacterial organisms such as streptococcus.

Supplements

Vitamin C, zinc and echinacea

All these natural agents have immune-stimulating properties and, when combined, tend to be very effective in clearing all sorts of sore throats and throat infections. Details about the administration of zinc lozenges can be found in 'Colds and flu'. This section also includes information on dosing for vitamin C and echinacea.

Tea tree oil

Tea tree oil has been proven in many studies to fight bacteria. One study found that it was even effective against bacteria that had become resistant to antibiotics.[263] Put 2–3 drops of tea tree oil in some warm water and have your child gargle with this if he or she is old enough. This mixture should be spat out, rather than swallowed, after gargling.

Honey

Honey has natural anti-microbial action, which may explain its presence in folk remedies for sore throats (e.g. honey and lemon).[264-5] One particular type of honey that seems to be effective in this respect is Manuka honey, which comes from Australia and New Zealand. Look for honeys that are labelled AMF 10 +. AMF stands for active manuka factor – the part of the honey believed to be responsible for its therapeutic properties. The particular brands to look out for are MediBee and Comvita.

Give your child 1/2–1 tsp, three times a day. This is probably best taken neat, directly from the spoon. However, it can be mixed into food or a warm drink if preferred.

Grapefruit seed extract

Grapefruit seed extract is another natural agent that may help to combat the organisms that are often behind sore throats.[266] Add 1–2 drops to about 100 ml of water and use as a gargle for older children. The solution can be swallowed after gargling. For small children, mix 1–2 drops into any palatable heavy syrup (such as Manuka honey), which will slow the product as it goes down the throat. The honey will also help conceal grapefruit seed extract's bitter edge.

Flower essences

• For any problems affecting the throat, try the Australian Bush essences Bush Fuchsia, Bush Iris and Flannel Flower.

Stomach ache

See 'Indigestion' and 'Nausea and vomiting'

Stye

A stye is an infection of the edge of the eyelid that occurs in one or more oil-secreting glands located near the root of an eyelash. Styes are normally the result of an infection with a bacterial organism known as staphylococcus. When they emerge, styes appear as a red and swollen area on the rim of the eyelid. After this, pus usually forms, giving rise to a raised lump that is yellow in the centre. A stye will often appear in your child's line of vision, which means that he or she may be tempted to rub or scratch it, which may cause more pain and irritation. Left to their own devices, styes normally burst of their own accord within two or three days and then heal over in a few more.

Topical treatments
Warm water
Make a compress by dipping cotton wool or cotton wool pads in some warm water. Apply this over the affected eye (with the eye closed) for about ten minutes, three or four times each day. This should help bring the stye 'to a head', helping to speed the healing process overall.

Flower essences
• Try the Australian Bush essences Black-eyed Susan, Mountain Devil and Dagger Hakea.

Sunburn
Sunburn is caused by exposure to UV radiation from the sun. Sunburn has a general ageing affect on the skin, and may also increase the risk of skin cancer. However, not all the effects of sunlight are negative. For one thing, ultraviolet radiation from the sun increases the formation of vitamin D in the skin and this nutrient is important to the health of the bones, muscles and the immune system. Perhaps even more importantly, vitamin D appears to have cancer-protective qualities too. There is evidence from test-tube and animal experiments that shows vitamin D has the ability to combat the development and spread of cancerous tumours.

Increasing evidence suggests that sunlight reduces the risk of several types of cancer and the smart money is on vitamin D as the critical factor. One study found sunlight exposure afforded significant protection from cancers of the breast, colon, ovary and prostate.[267]

Other cancers that showed this same association with sunlight, though to a lesser degree, included those affecting the bladder, womb, oesophagus (food-pipe), rectum and stomach. The message seems to be that exposure to sunlight is beneficial, but burning is to be avoided.

Prevention
One of the most effective ways of avoiding sunburn is to stay out of direct sunlight when it is at its hottest. Appropriate clothing is useful here, though sunscreens may be more comfortable and practical for children, especially when they are by water. If your kids are out in the sun a lot, then a high sun protection factor (SPF) such as 25 or 30 is probably wise. Children with darker skin, or kids who are only out for a little time each day, can probably get away with SPF 15. Babies and children under the age of five years should always use 25 SPF. Remember to reapply often, particularly if your child is swimming, and look for 'waterproof' and 'sweatproof' brands. Obviously, the more natural the sunscreen, the better. (For more details on sunscreens based on organic ingredients, see Useful contacts and information – under Green People.) The company Green People make a range of sunscreens based on predominantly organic ingredients and are available in good health food stores and some pharmacies. See www.greenpeople.org for more details.

Diet

Beta-carotene

The undesirable effects of sunlight on the skin are believed to be triggered by the production of damaging, destructive biochemical entities known as free radicals. Free radicals are quenched by substances known as antioxidants, many of which are available in the food we eat. One antioxidant that is believed to play a particular role in skin protection is beta-carotene. Carrots, spinach, apricots, cantaloupe melons and mangoes are all rich in beta-carotene and make good summer food for kids for this reason.

Supplements

Beta-carotene

Supplementation with beta-carotene may prove a convenient and economical way of getting maximum protection from this nutrient. Give 10–15 mg of beta-carotene each day for the duration of the summer. Other antioxidant nutrients that may also protect the skin from sunburn are vitamins C and E.

Treating sunburn

Sunburn is normally a first-degree burn, which means that it damages only the outermost layer of the skin (see 'Burns'). The sunburned skin will be hot, red and painful. If the skin blisters and swelling develops, this is a sign that the burn is second-degree. If your child seems unwell, or if you are worried, you should seek medical advice.

Topical treatments

Aloe vera and essential oil of lavender

In most instances, sunburn can be self-treated. One of the most effective natural remedies for superficial burns such as this is aloe vera.[268] Spread aloe vera gel over the affected area several times each day. It is a good idea to add a few drops of essential oil of lavender to the aloe vera. Lavender can help calm and soothe a child, but is also renowned to help in the healing of burns and other skin wounds.

Surgery – recovery from

The body's healing mechanisms are to a degree dependent on the supply of certain nutrients. For speedy healing, it is always a good idea to provide the body with an adequate supply of some of the most important nutrients. Generally, supplementation should be started about a month before surgery, finishing about six weeks later.

Supplements

Vitamin C, Vitamin B12, folic acid and zinc

One of the most important healing nutrients is vitamin C. This vitamin promotes the healing of the supporting tissues in the body. Take 1 g of vitamin C, twice a day. Other important nutrients for healing include zinc, vitamin B12 and folic acid. The main function of these nutrients is to stimulate new cell formation. For a 40 kg child, give 15 mg of zinc, 250–500 mcg of vitamin B12 and 250–500 mcg of folic acid each day.

Gotu kola

To this regime it often helps to add a supplement of the herb gotu kola (*Centella asiatica*). This natural agent has been found to reduce healing time and improve the strength of healing tissue.[269–70] Give 30 mg of standardised extract one to two times a day or 2–3 ml of tincture, three times a day.

Teething

Teething is the undoubtedly normal process by which an infant's first teeth erupt through the gums. It normally begins between six and eight months of age. Once your baby's first tooth arrives, it is usual for another new one to appear about every month or so. Eruptions continue until the child's complete set of 20 baby teeth has appeared, usually by the age of 30 months.

Signs of teething include sore, inflamed gums, a low-grade temperature, drooling, a fondness for biting on hard objects, irritability, difficulty sleeping and loss of appetite. The pain, discomfort and inflamed gums that a teething child experiences result from the pressure that is exerted against the gum tissue as the crown of a tooth breaks through the membranes.

Topical treatments
Apple rings

Children who are teething generally like to bite down on something. A good natural food that is perfect for this is dried apple. These are readily available in health food stores and some supermarkets.

Clove oil

Clove oil is a natural anaesthetic and often works to ease pain and soreness in the gums. It is best used diluted, as in its most concentrated form it can cause blistering. Blend 1 drop of clove oil with 2 tbsp of olive oil. Use a cotton bud (or a clean finger) to gently massage the mixture into your child's gums.

Homeopathic treatments
Chamomilla

Chamomilla is a commonly used homeopathic remedy for teething. Give the 6c dilution every hour as needed up to a total of six doses. This is a wonderful and effective treatment, which has been proven scientifically to reduce symptoms associated with teething.[271]

Flower essences

• Rescue Remedy or Emergency Essence will soothe your baby, and help to get him or her back to sleep if wakening in the night. The essence can also be rubbed directly into the gums and this may offer some relief.

Thirst – excessive

Excessive thirst is sometimes a sign of diabetes. If your child complains of fatigue, it is important for him or her to be checked by a doctor for this. However, in most cases, excessive thirst is not related to diabetes, but to a deficiency in healthy dietary fats known as the essential fatty acids (EFAs). Other symptoms suggestive of this include dry skin, dry hair and mood and/or behaviour disturbance. For more details about EFA deficiency and how to correct it see page 232.

Threadworms

See 'Worms'

Tongue – sore

Certain vitamin deficiencies can lead to problems with soreness and discomfort in the tongue and inside of the mouth. Perhaps the most important nutrients in terms of oral health are the B vitamins. Individuals lacking in folic acid tend to develop sore mouths and throats. Too little vitamin B3 (niacinamide) in the diet can cause soreness of the gums, mouth and tongue. If the discomfort in the mouth is like a 'burning' sensation, then B6 deficiency is likely. If the cracks at the corners of the mouth are sore, this generally indicates a lack of vitamin B2 (riboflavin). Sore lips have also been noted to be related to deficiencies of folic acid, vitamin B5 (pantothenic acid) and vitamin B6.

Supplements

B-complex

Taking a B-complex supplement that contains about 25 mg of the major B vitamins (B1, B2, B3, B5 and B6) along with B12 and folic acid will usually resolve a sore tongue in a few weeks.

Tonsillitis

See 'Sore throat and tonsillitis'

Tooth decay

The principal dietary approach to preventing dental caries is the avoidance of sugar in the diet. Sugar feeds the bacteria in the mouth that cause the acidity responsible for dental decay. Limiting foods and drinks rich in sugar is important, including fruit juices and fruit drinks. Regular brushing and flossing is obviously important. Fluoride is often touted to be important for the prevention of tooth decay. Its use in toothpastes and other oral health products is widespread. However, there is some concern over the toxic effects of fluoride, so it is important to educate your child to swallow as little fluoridated toothpaste or mouthwash as possible. The issue of water fluoridation is dealt with on page 183.

Travel sickness

See 'Motion sickness'

Urinary tract infection

Urinary tract infection (UTI) is the medical term for an infection in the bladder and/or kidneys. Bladder infection, also known as 'cystitis', is the most common type of UTI. A child with UTI may complain of a burning pain on urination, and may pass cloudy or even foul-smelling urine. Your child may also experience the urge to urinate frequently, but may only pass a small amount of urine each time. Additional symptoms include wetting the bed at night, stomach ache, back ache or fever. Very small children with UTI may suffer from fever, vomiting, diarrhoea, lethargy and irritability. In some children, recurrent UTI are related to the leaking of urine from the bladder back up to the kidneys (known as vesico-ureteric reflux). If this is suspected, special investigations may be necessary.

Because of the structure of the female urinary tract, UTIs are more common in girls than boys. This is generally thought to be because the pipe that takes urine from the bladder to the outside (the urethra) is shorter in girls. This makes it more likely that bacteria will make their way up the urethra into the bladder. The most common cause of UTI is a bacterium known as E. coli. This organism is often to be found on the skin in the genital area.

Prevention of UTI

A few basic approaches can often be effective in reducing the risk of this organism getting the opportunity to become established in the bladder. Encourage your child to drink plenty of fresh water throughout the day as this helps to flush out organisms in and around the urethra and bladder before they get a foothold. Personal hygiene is obviously important, and washing should be done on at least a daily basis using a mild, unscented soap. When you teach your children to use the lavatory (toilet training), encourage her to wipe from the front to the back, which reduces the risk of organisms being brought into the vicinity of the urethra. In boys, it's also good practice as it prevents the risk of contact with the end of the penis.

In some children, recurrent urinary tract infections are related to an imbalance in the organisms in the gut and around the genital area. This

---

is often the result of antibiotic therapy killing healthy bacteria that help keep unhealthy organisms at bay in the region of the urethra. While antibiotics may kill the bacteria responsible for a UTI, they may also encourage an imbalance, which makes UTIs more likely. More information about how to combat this problem can be found on page 16.

Supplements
Cranberry

Over the last decade there has been a lot of interest in the role of cranberry in the treatment and prevention of UTIs. Cranberry contains substances called 'proanthocyanidins', which help to prevent E. coli sticking to the bladder wall. In one study, women taking 400 mg per day of cranberry had a reduced risk of UTI compared to women taking a placebo over a three month period.[272] I recommend 200–400 mg of cranberry extract per day. Avoid cranberry juice, however, as this is rich in sugar and/or artificial sweetener.

Probiotics

A common folk remedy for the prevention of UTIs is 'live' yoghurt. Yoghurt contains organisms known as lactobacilli, which may help to 'crowd out' unhealthy organisms such as E. coli in and around the vagina, thereby helping to prevent infections. Lactobacilli also make the vagina more acidic, which helps to inhibit E. coli. Acidophilus pessaries are available under the name YeastGuard. (For more details, see Useful contacts and information – under BioCare.) For older girls, one pessary should be inserted each day for a week.

Taking a probiotic orally is also likely to help restore bacterial balance in the body generally, and may therefore help keep unhealthy bacteria at bay. I recommend giving a probiotic for two to three months. More details about probiotic supplements can be found on page 16.

Urticaria

See 'Hives'

Warts and Verrucas

Warts and verrucas are caused by infection with the human papilloma virus. Verruca is actually a term used to describe a wart on the sole of the foot. The management of warts and verrucas is the same. Conventionally, warts and verrucas are often frozen with liquid nitrogen – a treatment referred to as 'cryotherapy'.

Topical treatments
Duct tape and greater celandine
In one study, cryotherapy was pitted against a lower-tech and more economical remedy that involved treating warts by covering them with duct tape.[273] In this study, individuals receiving cryotherapy had treatments every two or three weeks for up to six treatments. Those using duct tape were instructed to apply the tape over the affected area for up to two months. The duct tape was changed every six days. Before renewing the tape, individuals

were asked to soak the warts in warm water and then rub them with a pumice stone or emery board. At the end of the study, 60 per cent of those having cryotherapy were cured of their warts, compared to 85 per cent of those using duct tape.

You might like to give this DIY remedy for warts a go. I suggest you also use a preparation of greater celandine (*Chelidonium majus*), a traditional topical remedy for the treatment of warts. Chelidonium contains substances that appear to inhibit the wart virus. Apply a tincture of this herb (available in health food stores) to the warts after you abrade them each time you change the duct tape.
Banana peel
Banana peel contains a substance that is believed to be effective for destroying warts. Place a small amount of peel (inside of peel against wart) against the wart and hold it in place with tape. Change the peel once or twice daily. Repeat for three weeks or until the wart is gone.

Whooping cough

Whooping cough is an infectious childhood disease that mainly affects children under the age of five years. It is caused by the bacterium *Bordatella pertussis*. The condition is rare, partly because of the immunisation programme for this disease that has been going on since the 1950s.

Whooping cough normally starts with a runny nose, dry cough and raised temperature. As the cold symptoms appear to improve, however, the coughing attacks worsen, and may be particularly noticeable at night. The child may have breathing difficulties and may make the characteristic 'whooping' sound as they gasp for air. The prolonged coughing may be accompanied by bouts of vomiting, particularly in young babies who tend not to whoop, but may go blue during a coughing fit. The disease is highly contagious (especially in its early stages) and affected children should be kept away from school or nursery.

The diagnosis of whooping cough is usually made on the basis of the symptoms and the conventional medical treatment is centred around antibiotics. After antibiotics, I recommend giving your child a course of probiotics (healthy gut bacteria). More details about this can be found on page 16. In about half of cases, hospitalisation is deemed necessary, where oxygen and intravenous fluids may be given.

Supplements
Vitamin C and echinacea
Whatever course the disease is taking, it helps to take steps to support your child's immune system. For specific recommendations about how to do this, see 'Colds and flu'. For additional supportive advice, see 'Fever'.

Worms
Threadworms, also known as pinworms, are small, thin white worms about 1–1.5 cm in length. These parasitic worms are extremely common in children, with about a fifth of all children in the UK

being affected at any one time. A child becomes infested when he or she eats the eggs of the worm. The eggs are normally transferred under the fingernails or by clothing, bedding, house dust and food. They are easily spread and if one member of the family is affected, it's likely that all will be. After being swallowed, the eggs hatch, and then the worms make their way to the large intestine. At night, adult female worms travel to the area around the anus, where they deposit eggs. This can be enormously itchy and irritating. Scratching will generally cause eggs to get under the fingernails, which may lead to re-infection and a repeat of the cycle.

What to do
To prevent spreading pinworms, or to prevent reinfestation, your doctor may suggest that all family members be examined and treated, especially in persistent cases. There are, however, a number of natural treatments that can help.

Generally preventative measures include keeping your child's nails short, and ensuring that their hands are kept as clean as possible. Washing hands on waking and getting a brush under those nails may especially help by getting rid of eggs that may have made their way under your child's nails in the night. Adding some tea tree oil to the water used to rinse hands might help eradicate the worms.

Supplements
Garlic
Garlic has natural anti-parasitic properties. I recommend giving a child

1000 mg of garlic extract, once or twice a day for two weeks.

Grapefruit seed extract

Grapefruit seed extract is believed to have strong anti-parasitic action. Give 5–10 drops of this in some water or diluted fruit juice, three times a day for a week.

Probiotics

After treatment with garlic and/or grapefruit seed extract, give a probiotic (healthy gut bacteria supplement) for a month (see page 16). This can help restock the gut with healthy bacteria, which makes it more likely that your child will repel any unwanted invaders such as worms or other parasitic infections.

Topical treatments

Calendula cream

Calendula cream, rubbed into the area around the anus, should help to ease inflammation and itching. If you're applying this to your child, make sure you wash your hands well too.

Flower essences

• Rescue Remedy can be taken before bedtime to help sleep and to reduce the sensation of itching.

• If your child feels **frightened** by the thought of worms, I suggest giving the Bach flower remedy Mimulus.

Wound Healing

See 'Surgery – recovery from' and 'Scarring'

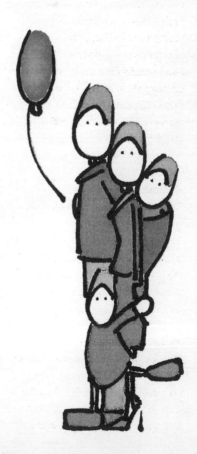

Part three

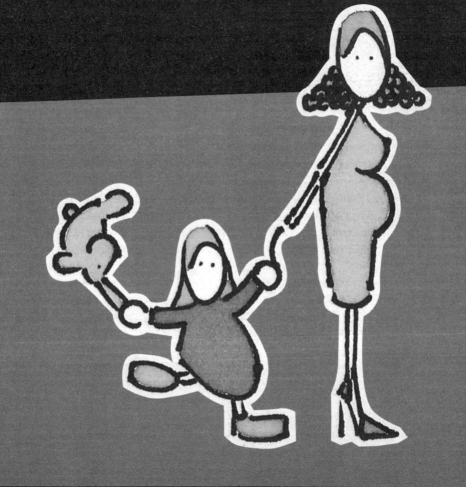

Chapter 1
Food
fundamentals

The growth and development that go on in the first few years of life are staggering. By the age of two years, a child will have usually tripled or even quadrupled his or her birth weight. At the same time, he or she will have probably transformed from a gurgling mass into a toddler capable of complex psychological and physical actions, such as walking and talking. After this time, most young children will grow about 5 cm (2 in) and gain about 2–3 kg (4–7 lb) each year. Between the ages of six and twelve, youngsters will add an average of 30–60 cm (1–2 ft) to their height and almost double in weight. Puberty and adolescence normally bring with them considerable accelerations in growth, and will metamorphose a child into an adult.

The essential ingredient in the growth and development of children and adolescents is food. What a child eats and drinks provides the raw materials to make new tissues such as bone, muscle and skin. Food also feeds the brain and contributes not just to the physical, but also the psychological wellbeing of a child. We really are what we eat. With this in mind, it is obvious that a child's diet has the potential to both help and hinder his or her development and health. There is little doubt that a child may gain much from eating a balanced, nutritious diet.

While few dispute the potential benefits offered by a healthy diet, unfortunately, there is no real consensus on what this actually means. There is a lot of nutritional information out there, but much of it seems to be inconsistent and sometimes downright contradictory. In an effort to cut through the confusion, this chapter looks at the major elements of the modern-day diet and explores their potential impact on the health and wellbeing of your child.

One critical theme that runs through the core nutritional information is the importance of eating as natural and unprocessed a diet a possible. Even more than that, the science shows that the best diet for all of us is one made up of the foods that we have been eating for large portions of our evolution, including meat, eggs (yes, *eggs*), fish, fruit, vegetables, nuts and seeds and water. These primal foods have always been in the human diet, and our physiology and biochemistry are therefore well-adapted to them. Despite the commonly held beliefs about the hazards of saturated fat (found, for instance, in red meat and eggs), a close look at the evidence reveals very little, if any, cause for concern.

On the other hand, newer foods, some of which we have been consuming for only a few decades, appear to be more of a worry. Despite the fact that we have been encouraged to emphasise carbohydrate-based foods, such as bread and pasta, in the diet, there is mounting evidence that this may be fuelling the rising rates of obesity and diabetes in children. While 'regulatory bodies' attempt to allay any concerns we may have about artificial additives and pesticide residues, there is actually good evidence that these can cause harm.

This chapter is designed to give you the basic facts about what's in our food. This core nutritional information is then used to make recommendations about specific foods (everything from fruit to fast food) in the next chapter.

Carbohydrates

Carbohydrates are compounds in the diet that are made of the elements carbon, hydrogen and oxygen. They come in two main forms, sugars and starches, and their main function is to provide fuel for the body.

Sugars

The basic building block of all carbohydrates is a single sugar molecule known as a monosaccharide (e.g. glucose, fructose). Sugars that contain two monosaccharides joined together are known as disaccharides (e.g. sucrose, which is made of a molecule each of glucose and fructose). Some sugars, such as those in fruit and vegetables, are found naturally in food. In general, sugars that are inherent in food have a place in a healthy balanced diet. This is not necessarily true, however, for sugars that are added to food.

Sugar is a common ingredient in many child-oriented foodstuffs such as soft drinks, chocolate, sweets, biscuits, ice cream, breakfast cereals and yoghurts. Most parents will be aware of the link between sugar-sweetened foodstuffs and dental decay. However, added sugar in the diet has plenty of other hazards besides. For instance:

- Sugar can suppress the immune system[1] and weaken the body's defences against bacterial infection.[2]
- Sugar can cause hyperactivity, anxiety, concentration difficulties and mood disturbance in children.[3]
- Sugar can cause drowsiness and decreased activity in children.[4]
- Sugar has been associated with lower academic achievement.[5]
- Sugar has been associated with an increased risk of short-sightedness (myopia).[6]

Excess sugar in the diet will tend to cause fluctuations in blood sugar levels, which in turn may increase the risk of conditions such as diabetes and excess weight. This important nutritional concept is dealt with in depth on pages 204–10.

Added sugar in food products is not always simply labelled as 'sugar'. Other pseudonyms to look out for (and be wary of) include:

- Sucrose
- Corn sweetener
- Corn syrup
- Fructose
- Fruit juice concentrate
- Glucose (dextrose)
- High-fructose corn syrup
- Invert sugar
- Lactose
- Maltose

Fructose

The sugar fructose is being used increasingly in processed and sweetened foods in the UK. Fructose is generally regarded as a healthier form of sugar compared to sucrose (table sugar), essentially on account of the fact that it is said not to cause blood sugar or insulin levels to rise. Because of this, fructose has traditionally been seen in a favourable light as an added sweetener, and has generally been recommended as the sugar of choice for diabetics (who tend to have raised levels of sugar and insulin in their bloodstreams). However, studies show that fructose can impair the body's ability to handle sugar and can reduce the effectiveness of insulin. What is more, animal experiments reveal that long-term consumption of fructose can indeed lead to elevated levels of both sugar and insulin. These effects strongly suggest that added fructose in the diet may increase the risk of weight gain and diabetes.[7]

Other studies show that fructose may push up blood levels of unhealthy blood fats called triglycerides and seems also to have the capacity to raise blood pressure. These effects would be expected to increase the risk of conditions such as heart disease and stroke. Generally, foods rich in fructose such as fruit juice and processed foods sweetened with fructose or 'high-fructose corn syrup' should be eaten in moderation.

Starch

Also referred to as complex carbohydrates, dietary starch is made of chains of sugar molecules. Examples of starch-based foods include vegetables, bread, pasta, rice, potato, beans, pulses and breakfast cereals.

Grains such as wheat, rice, corn and oats are made up of three main components: the endosperm (starchy part, which comprises about 80 per cent of the grain), the germ and bran. Unrefined (wholegrain) starches include all three parts of the grain. The germ and bran (the outer parts) are mainly lost when grains are refined, which substantially reduces the amount of fibre they contain. In addition, many nutrients can be lost too. Wholegrain products are important sources of nutrients, including vitamins E, B1, B5, B6 and minerals such as folate, iron, zinc, magnesium, copper and manganese.

For these reasons, unrefined starches, such as wholemeal bread, brown rice and wholewheat pasta, are generally regarded as nutritionally superior to their refined counterparts, such as white bread, white rice and regular pasta. Another advantage unrefined starches have over their refined forms is that they tend to give slower, more sustained release of sugar into the bloodstream. There is increasing evidence that eating slower-sugar-releasing foods can help combat a wide range of health issues, including excess weight and diabetes.[8–9] The importance of the speed at which foods release sugar into the bloodstream is dealt with in depth on pages 204–10.

GOOD SOURCES OF UNREFINED STARCH-BASED FOODS
- Wholemeal bread
- Whole rye bread
- Brown rice
- Wholewheat pasta
- Oats

Fibre

Fibre – also referred to as non-starch polysaccharide (NSP) – is indigestible plant material. It comes in two main forms: soluble and insoluble fibre. Soluble fibre dissolves in the gut to form a gel-like substance that slows down the release of some nutrients, particularly sugar, into the bloodstream. It appears to help control cholesterol levels in the bloodstream, which may reduce the risk of heart disease.

Insoluble fibre (sometimes referred to as 'roughage') does not dissolve in the digestive tract and adds bulk to the waste product in the gut (the faeces). Getting enough insoluble fibre in the diet is important because it helps ensure regular, healthy bowel motions. As a child progresses into adulthood, a diet rich in roughage may help to prevent conditions such as haemorrhoids (piles), diverticular disease (abnormal pockets on the lining of the large bowel that can become infected and cause bleeding or perforation of the gut wall) and cancer of the colon.

GOOD SOURCES OF FIBRE
Soluble fibre
- Fruit
- Vegetables
- Beans
- Oats
- Barley
- Rye

Insoluble fibre
- Whole (unrefined) cereals such as wholemeal bread, brown rice, wholewheat pasta and oats
- Beans
- Lentils
- Nuts
- Seeds
- Fibrous vegetables such as carrots, celery and cabbage

Protein

Within the body, proteins form the structural basis of many tissues, such as hair, skin, muscles, tendons and cartilage. Adequate protein in the diet is essential for normal growth and development. Other proteins include enzymes (which promote the biochemical reactions in the body), many hormones (such as growth hormones) and various proteins in the blood, such as haemoglobin and antibodies.

Protein is composed of molecules known as amino acids. Amino acids that come from protein in the diet are used as building blocks in the manufacture of many structures and tissues in the body, including bone, muscle, skin, nails and hair. Amino acids are also used in the manufacture of enzymes and DNA – substances that have key roles in maintaining healthy structure and function within the body.

There are 22 amino acids, most of which can be made in the body and therefore do not, strictly speaking, need to be provided in the diet. However, children are unable to make ten amino acids and their presence in the diet is therefore crucial to optimum health. These are referred to as the essential amino acids.

Some foods provide a good balance of essential amino acids and are generally regarded as superior sources of protein than those foods that may be lacking in one or more essential amino acids. In general, animal-derived proteins are regarded as more 'complete' in terms of their component amino acids than vegetable sources of protein. For this reason, those who do not eat animal foods generally do well to eat a broad range of protein-containing foods, including beans, pulses, nuts, seeds and perhaps soya-based products (e.g. soya milk and tofu) too.

GOOD SOURCES OF PROTEIN
- Meat
- Fish
- Eggs
- Dairy products such as milk, cheese and yoghurt
- Some non-animal foods, such as beans, lentils, peas, nuts and seeds

Fat

Fat in the diet provides the body with a source of energy and is also a component of the walls of the body's cells and certain hormones. The basic building blocks of fats in the diet are known as 'fatty acids'. These are essentially composed of chains of carbon atoms with hydrogen atoms attached. The three main forms of fats found naturally in the diet are saturated, monounsaturated and polyunsaturated fats.

Saturated fats

Saturated fats are found in animal products such as butter, cheese, whole milk, ice cream, cream and meat. They are also found in some vegetable oils, such as coconut and palm oils. Saturated fats, and particularly those that are found in animal products, have gained a reputation for having the ability to increase the risk of a variety of conditions, in particular heart disease and obesity.

However, there is good evidence that the saturated fat may not be the dietary spectre it is often made out to be. It is often said, for instance, that eating saturated fat can put up cholesterol levels (raised cholesterol levels are believed to be a risk factor for heart disease). However, there are several scientific studies that simply do not bear this out.[10–12] Some doctors and scientists believe that the role of saturated fat in heart disease has been over-stated, perhaps partly as a result of misquoting and misinterpretation of the studies in this area.[13] A number of studies show that in individuals with heart disease, the proportion of the diet made up from saturated fat is no higher than those without heart disease. Also, there is very little evidence that reducing fat in the diet has significant benefits for health. In one comprehensive review published in the *British Medical Journal* it was concluded that reducing fat intake had only a small effect on risk of cardiovascular disease, and had practically no effect on overall risk of death.[14] It appears that reduction of saturated fat is of very limited benefit in terms of overall health, which supports the notion that it is not as damaging to health as we have traditionally been led to believe.

The link between saturated fat and body weight is also tenuous. In the short term, it appears that reducing the proportion of fat in diet can lead to modest reductions in body weight. However, in the longer term, studies show that the amount of fat in the diet has little, if any, bearing on body fat. Also, government statistics show that over the last 20 years there has been a decline in the amount of fat (particularly saturated fat) in the diet. Despite this, rates of obesity have approximately trebled in both men and women over the same time period. A recent comprehensive review on this subject concluded that dietary fat is not a major determinant in body weight, and that eating less fat is unlikely to bring lasting weight loss.[15]

In balance, it appears that saturated fat is a more benign dietary component than it is often said to be and that including it in the diet in moderate amounts appears not to be harmful to health. While this notion may go against the grain of conventional dietetic thinking, it does make sense if we think about the diet we humans ate for much of our evolution. Saturated fat has been part of the human diet for at least hundreds of thousands of years and, because of this, it is something that the human body is likely to be very well adapted to. This theory, and an increasing amount of research, suggest moderate amounts of saturated fat in the diet in the form of meat, eggs, butter and other dairy products, are compatible with a healthy diet.

Monounsaturated fats

Monounsaturated fat is a form of fat that is believed to have benefits for the body. The inclusion of monounsaturated fats (see box, below) in the diet appears to lower blood levels of low-density lipoprotein (LDL) cholesterol – the type of cholesterol that is believed to increase the risk of heart disease. The consumption of monounsaturated fats may also raise the level of high-density lipoprotein (HDL) cholesterol – the 'healthy' form of cholesterol that is believed to protect against heart disease. A high intake of monounsaturated fats is believed to be one of the reasons certain populations such as the southern Italians and the Greeks have relatively low levels of heart disease.[16] The consumption of monounsaturated fat rich foods is to be encouraged in the diet.

GOOD SOURCES OF MONOUNSATURATED FATS
- Olives and olive oil
- Avocado
- Nuts
- Seeds

Polyunsaturated fats

Polyunsaturated fats are found in two main types in the diet: omega-3 fatty acids and omega-6 fatty acids. The major omega-6 fatty acid in the diet is known as linoleic acid, which is found most abundantly in plant oils. The major omega-3 fatty acids come in the form of alpha-linolenic acid (from plant sources such as flaxseed) and fats known as eicosapentaenoic acid (EPA) and docosahexaenoic acid (DHA) (see opposite). The omega-3 and omega-6 fats have important roles to play in maintaining the health of a variety of the body's systems and structures, including the brain, nervous system, immune system, cardiovascular system, eyes and skin.

The effects omega-3 and omega-6 fats have in the body come about as a result of their conversion into hormone-like substances known as eicosanoids (pronounced eye-coz-ah-noids). Eicosanoids made from omega-6 fats tend to be potent in nature and generally encourage processes such as inflammation, blood vessel constriction and clotting in the body. These eicosanoids are believed to increase the risk of conditions such as heart disease, stroke and inflammatory conditions such as arthritis.

Eicosanoids derived from omega-3 fats are quite different, however. In general, they are less likely to encourage inflammation, and some are positively anti-inflammatory in nature. Also, the eicosanoids derived from omega-3 fats tend to reduce the risk of clotting and help to relax blood vessels. As a result, omega-3 fats are believed to help reduce the risk of conditions such as heart disease, stroke and inflammatory conditions such as arthritis.

Because omega-3 and omega-6 fatty acids have roughly antagonistic actions in the body, it is important for them to be balanced in the body. Some scientists believe that the ideal ratio of omega-6:omega-3 fats in the diet is 1:1. However, a general decline in foods rich in omega-3 fats, coupled with an increase in our intake of omega-6 fats (for instance in the form of vegetable oils in margarine, processed food, fried and fatty fast foods) has led to an imbalance in omega-6:omega-3 ratio – with the most recent Government statistics showing that it now stands at 6:1 (MAFF 1997). This high omega-6: omega-3 ratio is believed to be an important factor in the development of many chronic diseases, including cardiovascular disease and some forms of cancer.

Constructing a diet that provides more in the way of omega-3 fats, and/or limiting omega-6 consumption, does seem to be a key strategy in promoting the physical and psychological wellbeing in children. Some telltale signs of an essential fat imbalance in the body include behavioural problems, hyperactivity, dry skin, dry hair and excessive thirst. More details of about this issue, and how to correct it, can be found on pages 229–33.

GOOD SOURCES OF POLYUNSATURATED FATS
Omega-6 fatty acids
• Plant oils, such as hemp, pumpkin, sunflower, safflower, sesame, corn, walnut, soya
Omega-3 fatty acids
• Oily varieties of fish, such as salmon, trout, mackerel, herring and sardine
• Some nut and seed oils including flaxseed (linseed) oil and walnut oil

---

Trans fatty acids

Trans fatty acids are a form of fat formed as a result of the processing of fat in food manufacturing. Many of the fats that are used in food processing (such as those from vegetable sources such as nuts, seeds and beans) are liquid at room temperature and unsuitable for addition to foods. However, these oils may be treated chemically to make them solid through a process known as 'hydrogenation'. During hydrogenation, fats are heated to a high temperature and hydrogen is added. This makes the fats more solid and also gives them a longer shelf life. However, hydrogenation damages fats and may lead to their conversion to unusually-shaped fats known as 'trans fatty acids', or 'trans fats' for short. Trans fats are found in a wide range of foods, including commercial baked goods (biscuits, cookies, cakes, doughnuts, etc.), chocolate confectionery, fast foods, processed foods and many types of margarine.

Trans fats have only been in the human diet in significant quantities for a few decades. With this in mind, it is highly unlikely that these man-made fats are likely to be better for us than more natural forms of fat in the diet. If anything, common sense dictates that because we are not adapted for their consumption, they are likely to have detrimental effects on health. With this in mind, it comes as no surprise that trans fats have been found to increase LDL (unhealthy) cholesterol and reduce HDL (healthy) cholesterol levels.[17] There is evidence that trans fatty acids may increase the risk of many chronic conditions, including heart disease and diabetes. While it may be difficult to avoid trans fats completely, there seems little doubt that the less of these our children consume, the better.

British labelling law does not require food manufacturers to state how much trans fat a food contains. To work this out for yourself, look up the total fat in a food, and take away from this the figures listed for saturated, monounsaturated and polyunsaturated fats. The figure you are left with gives a pretty good guide to the trans fat content of a food. For the best health, foods that contain any amount of trans fat should be avoided as much as possible.

SAMPLE LABEL TO DETERMINE TRANS FAT CONTENT
Nut cutlets Per cutlet: Fat 16.9 g
of which saturated 3.4 g
of which polyunsaturated 8.9 g
of which monounsaturated 0.9 g
Estimation of trans fat content of cutlet =
16.9 − (3.4 + 8.9 + 0.9) g = 3.7 g of trans fat.

Unfortunately, many food products do not list all the different types of fat they contain, making this calculation impossible. In this situation, look in the ingredients label for 'partially hydrogenated vegetable oil' or 'partially hydrogenated oil'. Foods containing this ingredient are best avoided.

Water

A full 70 per cent of the body is water, which means that this most basic of fluids plays some part in countless reactions and processes, including the circulation, detoxification, nerve transmission and muscular function. Even mild dehydration (e.g. 1 per cent dehydration or about 40 ml of fluid for a 40-kg child) can impair essential body processes, and cause symptoms such as headaches, loss of appetite, heat intolerance, fatigue, muscle weakness, light-headedness and dryness of the eyes and mouth.

Water is not just important for general wellbeing, but also seems to help reduce the risk of chronic disease. Research indicates, for instance, that low levels of fluid consumption are associated with increased risk of certain forms of cancer, including those of the kidney, bladder, prostate, testes and colon.[18-20]

There is also evidence that drinking water may reduce the risk of heart disease. One study found that women drinking five or more glasses of fluid each day were at 41 per cent reduced risk of dying from a heart attack compared to women drinking two or less glasses each day. In men, drinking more fluid appeared to reduce risk of heart attack by 54 per cent.[21] Ensuring a child gets adequate amounts of water each day is likely to have a very profound bearing on his or her health in both the short and long term. Information about the relative merits of tap and bottled water are covered on pages 181–3.

Food additives

The majority of processed and convenience foods that fill supermarket shelves contain a cocktail of additives such as flavourings, colourings and preservatives. While these may have been passed as fit to consume by the relevant authorities, it is important not to lose sight of the fact that most of these additives are chemical, alien-to-nature compounds. As recent additions to our diet, the chances are that they have the ability to affect health in undesirable ways.

Many parents complain, for instance, that their children's behaviour may worsen when they consume certain additives. Food manufacturers and Government bodies have tended to dismiss these claims as anecdotal and lacking in scientific evidence. However, there is good evidence that food additives can lead to behavioural problems in kids.

In a 2002 UK government-funded study conducted by the UK's Asthma and Allergy Research Centre, a group of 277 three-year-olds were assessed for one month. Each day for two weeks the children were given a measured quantity of fruit juice laced with four artificial colourings (tartrazine E102, sunset yellow E110, carmoisine E122, ponceau 4R E124) and a preservative (sodium benzoate E211). The other two weeks they were given a similar fruit juice, but without the additives. Neither the children nor their parents knew which fruit juice was being administered at any given time. Parents were asked to assess problem behaviours such as interrupting, fiddling with objects, behaviour that disturbed others, problems with getting to sleep, concentration difficulties and temper tantrums.

The results of this study showed that the artificial additives were a potent cause of behavioural problems in children. The researchers commented that significant changes in children's hyperactive behaviour could be produced by the removal of colourings and additives from their diet. They estimated that if the additives tested were removed from the UK diet, the number of children affected by hyperactivity should fall by two-thirds. For a full list of more than 200 hundred foods that contain one or more of the suspect additives, go to: http://www.foodcomm.org.uk/additive_2002.htm and click on the link under 'Further Information'.

The additives tested in the hyperactivity study are but a few of the many additives that may be found in processed foods. The box (below) is a guide to some of the other additives that may crop up in your child's diet.

Potential food additives you may encounter

- Chemical E numbers that are best avoided include: E102, E110, E122, E123, E124, E127, E129, E131, E133, E142, E150C, E151, E153, E154, E155, E210–E224, E226, E227, E228, E232, E249, E250, E251, E252, E284, £285, E320, E321, E512, E533B, E621, E942, E954, E1440

- E-numbers from E300–304 (Vitamin C) and E307–309 (Vitamin E) are not thought to have any adverse effects

- E310, E311, E312, E320 and E321 may be dangerous to asthmatics as well as individuals who tend to react adversely to aspirin. These additives are actually banned for use in baby foods

- E621 (monosodium glutamine – MSG) is used to enhance meaty or savoury flavours. In some children, MSG appears to have the ability to trigger symptoms such as headaches, giddiness, nausea, muscle pains and heart palpitations

- The sweeter, more brightly coloured or flavoured a food, the higher the number of additives

---

Artificial sweeteners

Artificial sweeteners such as saccharin and aspartame (e.g. NutraSweet, Equal) have assumed a growing presence in the diet over the last few decades. They are sold on the basis that although sweet, they do not contain the calories of sugar. The suggestion here is that artificial sweeteners help to prevent weight gain and may promote weight loss. Despite being a multi-billion dollar industry, no long-term, well-conducted studies have been published that have looked at the effect of artificial sweeteners on weight loss. In fact, some studies have found that artificial sweeteners such as aspartame may actually stimulate the appetite and may cause us to eat more, not less.[22–3] Also, despite its widespread use in the diet, there is not one single, well-conducted long-term study on the supposed weight loss effects of aspartame.

There is also some concern over the safety of aspartame – the most widely used of artificial sweeteners. Despite the fact that the regulatory authorities in over 100 countries have deemed aspartame to be fit to consume, evidence exists to the contrary. Animal experiments show that aspartame has the capacity to alter the brain's chemistry,[24] while other studies have suggested aspartame may be responsible for a range of neurological symptoms.[25] Aspartame has been linked with headaches[26–7] and depression.[28]

What is particularly concerning is the apparent disparity in the results obtained in industry-funded and non-industry-funded research. A review of the scientific literature on this subject found that while 100 per cent of industry-funded research concludes aspartame is safe, 92 per cent of independently-funded research suggests it is not. This review can be viewed on-line at www.dorway.com/peerrev.html. To my mind, this review casts considerable doubt on the validity of the largely industry-funded research used to pass aspartame as fit for human consumption. My advice is for artificial sweeteners to be avoided as much as possible.

Salt

Salt (sodium chloride) has a role to play in health, and seems to be particularly important in the regulation of blood pressure and in maintaining the circulation. However, as with everything, too much can be a bad thing. One major effect of excess salt in the diet is that it can cause blood pressure to rise, which is believed to increase the risk of other conditions, including heart disease and stroke.

> **Recommended daily amounts of salt for different ages**
>
> Babies: 1 g
>
> Children aged one to three years: 2 g
>
> Children aged four to six years: 3 g
>
> Children aged seven to ten years: 5 g
>
> Adults and children aged over
>
> ten years: 6 g

While reducing the amount of salt we add during cooking or at the table makes good sense, the fact is, for most children, the vast majority of the salt they get comes already added in processed and fast foods. Some products aimed at children contain more salt in one serving than the recommended intake for a whole day. Even a ham and cheese sandwich on brown bread provides more than three-quarters of the daily recommended intake of salt for a four-year-old.

Generally speaking, for children and adults alike, foods containing 0.5 g of salt or more per 100 g should be avoided. If you start looking at nutritional information labels on food, you may start noticing just how salty some foods are, despite the fact that they may not even taste very salty. For instance, cornflakes, weight for weight, are even saltier than seawater (which contains salt at a concentration of about 2.5 g per 100 g). There has been a recent vogue for food manufacturers to list salt content not as actual salt, but as sodium. Those not wise to this ploy can easily underestimate the amount of salt in a food. To convert the sodium level into the salt equivalent, multiply by 2.5.

Vitamins and minerals

The diet provides the body with a range of vitamins and minerals that have important roles to play in health and wellbeing. The major nutrients, along with their dietary sources, key benefits and recommended daily amounts (also known as the reference nutrient intakes) are summarised on pages 162–7. This information is provided mainly for reference. It may be useful to refer to this table from time to time when specific nutrients are recommended elsewhere in the book.

You may notice that the nutrient dosage recommended for a specific ailment is often far higher than the recommended amount. The reason for this is essentially because the amount of a nutrient needed to treat a medical condition is generally much greater than the amount needed to prevent an obvious deficiency of a nutrient. This concept is dealt with in more depth in the Introduction, which provides a guide to using supplements in children.

VITAMINS AND MINERALS: THEIR SOURCES AND EFFECTS

Nutrient	Main food sources	Key effects
Vitamin A	Milk, butter, egg yolk, liver, oily fish. As beta-carotene (a precursor of vitamin A), in carrots, tomatoes, dark green/yellow vegetables	• Believed to be cancer protective • Important for night vision • Important for growth and development of all cells • Important for the health of the skin
Vitamin B1 (thiamin)	Cereals, nuts, pulses, wholegrains, green vegetables	• Supplementation may enhance mood and mental alertness • Important for carbohydrate metabolism • Important for maintenance of the nervous system
Vitamin B2 (riboflavin)	Liver, milk, eggs, green vegetables, yeast extract	• Important for metabolism • Important for the growth and development of all cells
Vitamin B3 (niacin)	Liver, beef, pork, fish, fortified breakfast cereals, yeast extract	• Important for metabolism • Plays a key role in the formation of red blood cells • Important for the nervous and digestive systems
Vitamin B5 (pantothenic acid)	Animal products, cereals, legumes	• A constituent of coenzyme A – essential for metabolism • Coenzyme A is important for the immune system
Vitamin B6 (pyridoxine)	Meat, fish, eggs	• May be important in reducing the risk of heart disease (in combination with folate and vitamin B12) by lowering homocysteine levels • Is required for the efficient functioning of the immune and nervous systems • Supplementation may be beneficial in the treatment of pre-menstrual syndrome
Vitamin B12	Liver, meat, eggs, milk, yeast extract	• May be important in reducing the risk of heart disease (in combination with folate and vitamin B6) by lowering homocysteine levels • Is important for the production of red blood cells

Vitamin C	Fresh fruit, especially citrus fruit, blackcurrants, kiwi fruit, and green vegetables	• Supplementation has been associated with a reduced risk of heart disease (especially in combination with vitamin E) • Some evidence exists to suggest that vitamin C may be important in cancer prevention
Vitamin D	Oily fish, e.g. mackerel, egg yolk, fortified margarine	• Important for regulating calcium in body and for bone health • Evidence suggests that vitamin D supplementation may play a role in cancer prevention (especially cancers of the colon and breast) • Evidence suggests that vitamin D supplementation may help prevent heart disease
Vitamin E	Nuts, vegetable oils, vegetables, wholegrain cereals, oily fish	• Appears to enhance immune function • Supplementation is associated with a reduced risk of heart disease in some studies • Evidence suggests that supplementation reduces the risk of prostate cancer • Evidence suggests that supplementation may slow the progression of Alzheimer's disease • Evidence suggests that supplementation (particularly in combination with vitamin C) lowers the risk of developing Alzheimer's disease
Vitamin K	Dark green leafy vegetables, e.g. spinach	• Evidence suggests supplementation may prevent fractures
Folic acid	Liver, orange juice, green vegetables, nuts	• Proven to reduce the risk of neural tube defects such as spina bifida • Supplementation lowers plasma homocysteine levels – believed to reduce risk of heart disease • Supplementation may be important in cancer prevention (especially cancers of the colon and breast)
Calcium	Milk, canned fish, pulses, sesame seeds, nuts	• Necessary for the formation and maintenance of strong bones and teeth • Important for the proper functioning of nerves and muscles

Magnesium	Nuts, pulses, wholegrain cereals	• Important for normal nerve and muscle function • Supplementation may be useful in a wide variety of cardio-vascular disorders • Supplementation appears to reduce blood pressure • Supplementation may reduce the risk of stroke • Supplementation may be associated with better lung function • Supplementation may be useful in reducing the symptoms of PMS
Zinc	Meat, eggs, milk, fish, wholegrain cereals, pulses	• Important for immune system function • Supplementation may modulate testosterone levels in men (especially in men who are mildly deficient)
Selenium	Brazil nuts, fish, liver	• Appears to be cancer-protective • Supplementation may be protective against asthma • Supplementation may improve immunity • Supplementation may improve mood
Iron	Red meat, cereals, pulses	• Essential for the formation of red blood cells • May be important for the proper functioning of the immune system • Essential for brain function • Essential for the proper functioning of the thyroid
Iodine	Seafood, seaweed, eggs, milk	• Essential for the synthesis of thyroid hormones, which regulate metabolic activity
Copper	Meat, wholegrains, nuts, seeds	• Important for the immune system • Promotes the normal formation of red blood cells
Potassium	Widespread in food	• Needed for proper nerve function • Aids in the maintenance of blood pressure
Sodium	Widespread in food	• Important for nerve and muscle activity

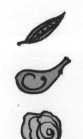

NUTRIENT INTAKES FOR VITAMINS IN CHILDREN UP TO 18 YEARS OLD

Age	B1 mg/d	B2 Mg/d	B3 mg/d	B6 mg/d	B12 g/d	Folate g/d	C mg/d	A g/d	D g/d
4–6 months	0.2	0.4	3	0.2	0.3	50	25	350	8.5
7–9 months	0.2	0.4	4	0.3	0.4	50	25	350	7
10–12 months	0.3	0.4	5	0.4	0.4	50	25	350	7
1–3 years	0.5	0.6	8	0.7	0.5	70	30	400	7
4–6 years	0.7	0.8	11	0.9	0.8	100	30	400	–
7–10 years	0.7	1.0	12	1.0	1.0	150	30	500	–
Males									
11–14 years	0.9	1.2	15	1.2	1.2	200	35	600	–
15–18 years	1.1	1.3	18	1.5	1.5	200	40	700	–
Females									
11–14 years	0.7	1.1	12	1.0	1.2	200	35	600	–
15–18 years	0.8	1.1	14	1.2	1.5	200	40	600	–

NUTRIENT INTAKES FOR MINERALS IN CHILDREN UP TO 18 YEARS OLD

Age	Cal mg/d	P m g/d	Mg mg/d	Na mg/d	K mg/d	Fe mg/d	Zn mg/d	Cu mg/d	Se g/d	I g/d
4–6 months	525	400	60	280	850	4.3	4.0	0.3	13	60
7–9 months	525	400	75	320	700	7.8	5.0	0.3	10	60
10–12 months	525	400	80	350	700	7.8	5.0	0.3	10	60
1–3 years	350	270	85	500	800	6.9	5.0	0.4	15	70
4–6 years	450	350	120	700	1100	6.1	6.5	0.6	20	100
7–10 years	550	450	200	1200	2000	8.7	7.0	0.7	30	110
Males										
11–14 years	1000	775	280	1600	3100	11.3	9.0	0.8	45	130
15–18 years	1000	775	300	1600	3500	11.3	9.5	1.0	70	140
Females										
11–14 years	800	625	280	1600	3100	14.8	9.0	0.8	45	130
15–18 years	800	625	300	1600	3500	14.8	7.0	1.0	60	140

Cal = calcium Mg = magnesium K = potassium Zn = zinc Se = selenium
P = phosphorus Na = sodium Fe = iron Cu = copper I = iodine

Key points

- Food provides the raw materials for children's growth and development.
- When used as a food additive, sugar appears to increase the risk of a wide variety of conditions, including dental decay, behavioural problems and immune system suppression.
- Unrefined starches (such as wholemeal bread and brown rice) are healthier than their refined versions because they release sugar more slowly into the bloodstream and are richer in fibre and nutrients.
- Protein is important for growth and development, and can be found most abundantly in the diet in meat, fish, eggs, nuts, seeds, beans and pulses.
- Saturated fat (found in foods such as red meat and dairy products) is a natural food constituent that science suggests can form part of a healthy diet.
- Monounsaturated fat (found in avocado, olive oil and nuts) is healthy fat and, among other things, appears to reduce the risk of heart disease.
- The omega-3 fatty acids (found in oily fish such as salmon, trout and mackerel and some nuts and seeds) appear to be particularly beneficial to general health and brain function.
- Trans fatty acids (found in many processed foods, fast foods and margarines) are unhealthy and should be avoided.
- Water is essential to general wellbeing but also appears to reduce the risk of major illness. Some of the constituents of tap water appear to pose health hazards, so it is best to filter tap water before drinking or use mineral water.
- Food additives may cause, among other things, behavioural problems in children.
- Artificial sweeteners such as aspartame have been linked to a wide variety of health issues, including headaches, depression and neurological symptoms.
- Salt, in excess, may increase the risk of high blood pressure and conditions such as heart disease and stroke in the long term.
- Vitamins and minerals in the diet have crucial roles to play in development, the maintenance of health and protection against illness.

Chapter 2
Specific foods

Knowing something of the main components of the diet and their effects on the body forms the foundation of constructing a healthy diet for your child. With these important fundamental principles in mind, we can now go on to look at the best foods that should form the bulk of a child's diet. Not all of the healthier foods may be immediately appealing to your child. However, don't panic – the next chapter contains lots of information and advice about how to upgrade your child's diet with the minimum of fuss.

In this chapter, I also touch on not-so-healthy foods, including fast and processed foods. It is unrealistic (if not impossible) to completely rid unhealthy fare from a child's diet. Besides, it's what a child eats most of the time, not some of it, that will ultimately shape his or her health and wellbeing. The information that follows is essentially a guide to which food to emphasise in a child's diet and which to use more sparingly. This is not about achieving some 'perfect' diet, but about *balance*.

I don't recommend attempting to make sweeping changes to your child's diet. As we shall see in the next chapter, gradual changes and encouraging a healthier food culture appear to work the best. Another thing to bear in mind is that children generally are quite resilient and tend to have enormous healing capacity. My experience in practice is that they generally snap back into shape pretty quickly, often even with relatively minor adjustments to the diet. Whatever improvements you make, however small, are quite likely to reap significant dividends in the long term.

The chapter ends with suggestions for healthy breakfasts and main meals, along with some ideas for healthy snacks and lunch-box items.

Fruit

Fruit is generally a nutritious and wholesome food for children of all ages. Being rich in high quality carbohydrate, fruit provides ready fuel for the body, but tends to give quite a sustained release of sugar into the bloodstream (a desirable quality that is covered in depth on pages 204–10). Fruit is also rich in fibre, which is not only important for healthy bowel function, but has also been linked with a reduced risk of several conditions, including gallstones, heart disease and cancer.

Many fruits are also rich in nutrients, such as vitamin C, beta-carotene and folic acid, which have health-promoting and disease-protective properties in the body. Fruit is also rich in health-giving substances called phytochemicals. Research suggests that these nutritionally active plant compounds have significant disease protective effects. Black grapes, for instance, have been found to contain the phytochemical resveratrol, which studies suggest may help protect against cancer and heart disease. Hesperidin, a phytochemical found in citrus fruits, is believed to stave off heart disease too. Strawberries and other berries are rich in ellagic acid, a compound that research is suggesting might have significant cancer-protective properties.

Bearing in mind the fact that fruit is packed full of nutrients, it comes as little surprise that eating more of it offers very real health benefits. Studies have found that the more fruit we eat, the lower our risk of cancer and heart disease. One study has even found that the benefits of fruit eating in childhood appear to extend into old age.[1] In this study of elderly individuals, those who had eaten the most fruit in childhood were found to be 40 per cent less likely to succumb to cancer compared to those who ate the least.

Fruit (and vegetable) consumption is also linked with strong and healthy bones.[2] One effect of fruit in the body is to make it less acidic, an effect that reduces the risk of calcium being lost from the bone.

Once children are eating solid food, it is generally safe for them to consume fruit. Recommendations for fruit are usually based on numbers of servings, where one serving is 80 g (which equates to a medium-sized apple, orange or banana, or two smaller fruits such as kiwi or plums). One serving of fruit each day is a good amount to aim for with toddlers. I suggest splitting this serving into two or more pieces to be given at different points in the day. For older children, two pieces a day is probably more appropriate. Teenagers should be encouraged to consume three or more servings of fruit each day.

Dried fruit

An alternative to fresh fruit is dried fruit. The drying of fruits does tend to make them intensely sugary, though many dried fruits still release their sugar quite slowly into the bloodstream. This is a desirable quality, the significance of which is discussed on pages 204–10. While dried fruit is almost certainly not as healthy as fresh, it is still a natural food that is a great deal better than foods rich in refined sugar, such as chocolate and confectionery.

Fruit juice

Fruit juices are often seen as healthy drinks that are roughly equivalent to whole fruit. However, in the juicing of a fruit, many nutritious elements, in particular its fibre and also a proportion of its nutrients, are left behind. Fruit juice also contains a hefty dose of the sugar fructose. While this sugar is traditionally thought of as quite healthy, there is evidence that it is really no better than other forms of sugar, such as sucrose (table sugar), and (in excessive quantities) may give rise to problems with weight gain, diabetes and heart disease. More details about the effects of fructose can be found on page 150.

Most commercially available juices are dehydrated and then reconstituted with water – processing that undoubtedly reduces their nutritional value too. The best fruit juices are those that are freshly squeezed. Home made is best, though diluting these with water (about half and half) is a good idea. It helps to temper their 'sugariness' by diluting the fructose in them. Commercially available 'freshly squeezed' juices are obviously not as 'fresh' as home prepared, and are also flash pasteurised (two factors that are likely to reflect on their nutrient content), but are generally a good second best to home-made stuff. Further down on the pecking order is the cartoned juices, which are made of concentrate (most of them) and are the worst of the lot.

Another option for fruit-based drinks is smoothies. These are generally better than juices as many of them contain whole fruit mashed up, rather than juiced fruit. Like freshly squeezed juices, these are pasteurised, but almost certainly retain many beneficial nutritional qualities. Look on the ingredients label – the best smoothies list fruit or fruit juice, and nothing else.

Fruit 'juice' vs fruit 'drink'
Do not be tempted to confuse fruit 'juice' with fruit 'drink'. Products labelled as 'fruit drink' need only to contain as little as 5 per cent fruit juice by law, and often contain a lot of unwanted additives besides. In particular, many contain artificial sweeteners. Fruit drinks are to be avoided, as is anything labelled 'fruit-flavoured': these do not need to contain any fruit at all.

Vegetables

Like fruit, vegetables also contain a range of health-giving nutrients, including fibre, vitamins, minerals and phytochemicals. Green vegetables are particularly rich in the mineral magnesium, a nutrient that tends to be deficient in the diet but is important for a number of processes within the body, including energy production. Green vegetables are also rich in folic acid, which appears to help reduce the risk of conditions such as heart disease and cancer. Vegetables such as broccoli, cauliflower, Brussels sprouts and cabbage are what are known as 'cruciferous' vegetables. These seem to be especially rich in phytochemicals, which are believed to have cancer-protective properties within the body. Also, along with fruit, vegetables seem to have an important part to play in ensuring healthy bones.

As with fruit, a standard portion of vegetables is 80 g, which equates to a medium-sized carrot or tomato, a couple of serving spoons of broccoli or peas, or a medium-sized bowl of salad. Studies show that frozen vegetables can be even more nutritious than fresh (the freezing process can 'lock in' nutrients soon after harvesting), so these definitely count. However, although canned vegetables count according to Government recommendations, these are not as good as fresh. The processing of canned vegetables almost certainly reduces their nutritional value, and may impart some unwanted sugar and salt too.

One specific vegetable that doesn't count towards a child's vegetable quota is the potato. Weight for weight, potato contains less fibre and nutrients that most other vegetables. It also tends to release sugar quite quickly into the bloodstream, which may have important implications for health, as explored on pages 204–10.

Fruit, vegetables and agrochemicals

While fruits and vegetables should assume a prominent place in a child's diet, there is always the potential that they will come laced with unwanted chemicals. A lot of fresh produce is quite liberally treated with agrochemicals such as pesticides and fungicides, which are designed to keep it free from attack by insects and moulds. Like a lot of things that appear in our diet these days, the agrochemicals may be deemed to be safe below a certain level, though common sense suggests that the less our children consume of these things, the better. There is also some evidence that links pesticide exposure to adverse health effects, including cancer, birth defects, reproductive problems, neurological damage and disruption of hormones in the body. More details about this can be found in a report entitled 'Our Children at Risk: The 5 Worst Environmental Threats to their Health', published by the Natural Resources Defence Council (NRDC). The report can be viewed on their website at www.nrdc.org. I recommend thorough washing of fruit and vegetable produce prior to consumption.

Is organic really better?

Organic fruit and vegetables are generally a better option than more intensively grown produce. Not only are they less likely to be contaminated with harmful chemicals (see left), but there is some evidence that they may contain higher levels of nutrients, including vitamin C, certain minerals and phytochemicals too. These findings, coupled with the concerns about the higher levels of chemical residues found in non-organic foods, means that opting for organic produce will almost certainly have benefits for health in the longer term. The benefits of organic produce are comprehensively dealt with in a 2001 report commissioned by the Soil Association (see www.soilassociation.org) entitled 'Organic Farming, Food Quality and Human Health'. The report is available to buy from the Soil Association website, though a summary of its findings can be had for free from their website too. While organic produce is the best choice for a number of reasons, its often premium-price can put it beyond the reach of many. Thorough washing of fresh produce will at least help to reduce the potential for pesticide problems in our kids.

It's difficult to overdo vegetables in the diet, so I generally suggest free rein with them. However, toddlers should be getting a serving or two each day if possible, increasing to about three or four portions a day by the time they are teenagers. Another major plus that comes from ensuring children get plenty of fruit and veg in their diet is that it makes it less likely that they will fill up on less healthy food.

Grains

As discussed earlier in this chapter, wholegrain foods such as wholemeal bread, brown rice, wholewheat pasta and rolled oats have a number of nutritional and health-related advantages over refined grain products such as white bread, white rice and regular pasta. As we will go on to discuss in the section on blood sugar balance on pages 204–10, there is growing evidence that the presence of copious quantities of sugar and refined grains in the modern-day diet is a major factor in the burgeoning rates of childhood obesity and diabetes. While I think grains do have a place in a balanced diet, it seems that too much emphasis has been placed on them generally. Also, if grains are to be consumed, then the more unrefined they are, the better.

Examples of wholegrain starches to emphasise in the diet include:

- Wholemeal wheat bread
- Whole rye bread
- Wholewheat pasta
- Brown rice
- Unsweetened, oat-based muesli
- Porridge oats
- Unrefined breakfast cereals, such as Shredded Wheat

Because refined starches are stripped of much of their nutritional content and also tend to liberate their sugar quite quickly into the bloodstream, they are best eaten in limited amounts.

Examples of refined starches include:

- White bread and rolls
- White rice
- Pasta (non-wholewheat)
- Crackers
- Most breakfast cereals
- Cakes and pastries
- Non-wholegrain noodles, such as egg noodles and rice noodles

One final point to bear in mind about grain-based foods is that they are quite a common instigator of problems connected with what is known as food sensitivity. Here, specific foods can initiate unwanted reactions, which may manifest in children in a variety of ways that include disordered behaviour, colic, earache, migraine and eczema. Of all the grains, wheat does seem to be the worst offender of all. More details about food sensitivity, and how to go about diagnosing it in your child, can be found on pages 211–21.

Beans and lentils

Beans (such as kidney beans and chickpeas) and lentils are known as pulses. They are the seeds of plants belonging to the family *leguminosae*, which gets its name from the characteristic pod – also known as a legume – that protects the seeds while they are forming and ripening. Pulses are a valuable source of protein and also tend to give sustained release of sugar into the bloodstream. Pulses are rich in fibre, too, as well as nutrients, such as many of the B vitamins and magnesium. All in all, pulses are a nutritious and wholesome food and certainly have a place in a healthy diet.

Pulses are often bought in their dried state. Most dried pulses need soaking for several hours before they can be cooked, though this does not apply to lentils, black-eye and mung beans. Soaking takes several hours (generally 4–12 hours) and the most convenient time to do this is generally overnight. The soaking water should be discarded and the pulses rinsed before cooking in unsalted water (salt tends to toughen the skins). An alternative to this lengthy preparation time is to buy canned pulses. However, before preparation, it is best to rinse them thoroughly as this will help to remove as much added salt and sugar as possible.

Pulses are ideal additions to, or bases for, salads and stews. Home-made hummus, the main ingredient of which is chickpeas, is another good option. Baked beans, on account of their high sugar and salt content, should be regarded as nutritionally inferior to less processed forms of pulses.

All beans and pulses can make children a little 'gassy'. This is because certain carbohydrate molecules within them tend to ferment in the gut. Proper soaking, cooking and rinsing of beans and pulses helps to keep this undesirable effect to a minimum. Another tip is to add some kombu seaweed (available in health food stores and some supermarkets) to the pot during cooking. Kombu contains glutanic acid, which improves the digestibility of beans and pulses and reduces their gas-forming potential.

Nuts and seeds

Because of the number of allergy scares, nuts have come off the menu in many households. But nutritionally, nuts most certainly have a place in a healthy diet. Nuts are rich in fat, though this mainly comes in the form of heart-healthy monounsaturated fat. Nuts are also rich in other nutrients believed to have disease protective properties, including magnesium and potassium. More than one study has found that those who include nuts in their diet tend to be at lower the risk of heart disease.[3–4] Seeds have a similar nutritional composition to nuts, and their health benefits are likely to be similar too.

Nuts and seeds make a healthy and nutritious snack (for the benefits of snacking, see page 196). For the very best health effects, they are probably best eaten in their raw (unroasted) and unsalted state. Adding nuts and/or seeds to breakfast cereals or salads is another way for children to get the benefits of these nutritious primal foods.

Fish and seafood

Fish and seafood (such as prawns, crab, mussels) are generally healthy foods that offer good quality protein, and may also supply other beneficial nutrients, including iodine, zinc and vitamin D. Of all the commonly available fish and seafood, probably the most nutritious of all are what are known as the 'oily fish', which include salmon, trout, mackerel, herring and sardine. These are especially rich in omega-3 fats, such as eicosapentaenoic acid (EPA) and docosahexaenoic acid (DHA). These fats are believed to be important for mental health and emotional balance (see page 229) as well as being protective for conditions such as heart disease, arthritis and certain forms of cancer.

Fish stocks in the sea are being depleted and fish farming is now increasingly being used to meet demand (and generally at a lower price too).

Fish farming often involves exposing fish to chemicals (such as antibiotics and colourings) that they do not come across in the wild. Generally, it is best to consume food in as natural and unadulterated a form as possible, so (in an ideal world) wild fish is better than farmed. However, fresh fish is generally very expensive and it's important to be at least mindful of those depleted stocks. It's also worth bearing in mind that eating farmed fish is almost certainly better than eating no fish at all.

Canned fish

Canned fish, though not as good as fresh from a nutritional perspective, probably represents a pretty decent alternative. The most popular canned fish in the UK is tuna. Tuna is often referred to as an 'oily' fish. However, while fresh tuna does contain some omega-3 (though not nearly as much as fish such as salmon and mackerel), much of this is removed before canning. Tuna is also one of the fish (along with marlin and swordfish) that tends to be contaminated with mercury – something that is believed to be toxic to the nervous system and is believed to have the capacity to interfere with normal neurological development. Better types of fish to have from a can are salmon, mackerel and sardine. These are richer in omega-3 fatty acids and tend not to be contaminated with mercury.

Meat

Compared to fish, meat does not have the healthiest of reputations. This is mainly on account of its saturated fat content, which is said to boost risk of conditions such as heart disease and obesity. However, as discussed in the previous chapter, saturated fat's effect on health seems to be quite benign. Remember also that meat is a food that evidence suggests we have been eating for a very long time indeed, and it is therefore something we are generally well-adapted to eating.

My reservations about meat come not from the food *per se*, but from the methods used to rear the animals that give up their meat and on any processing that may occur afterwards. Many commercially reared animals are intensively farmed and often exposed to drugs and chemicals that taint their meat, which may have undesirable effects when subsequently consumed by humans (especially children). One of the worst meats in this respect is chicken. While poultry is generally regarded as healthier than 'red' meats, such as beef and lamb, this is not necessarily the case. Most chickens are kept in miserable circumstances and loaded with growth-promoting antibiotics during their brief lives. Some chicken processors go on to add proteins from other animals (such as cows and pigs) to the meat to help its retention of added water. Chicken is one meat that is almost certainly worth eating in its organic, free-range form. The same is also true of pork, which is another intensively reared meat. While organic is the best option for other meats such as lamb and beef, this is generally less of a concern as these animals are usually less intensively reared (particularly sheep).

The processing of meat is another potential concern. There is a big difference between an unadulterated organic chicken breast and a chicken nugget. The latter is likely to contain poor quality meat, a range of additives and some particularly unhealthy trans fatty acids too. Also, processed meats such as hot dogs may contain curing chemicals such as nitrites that have been linked with an increased risk of brain tumours.[5] Unwanted chemicals – and way too much salt – may also be found in sausages and hamburgers too. One way of exercising some control over what goes into your child is to make your own burgers. Another option is to develop a relationship with a trusty butcher who may already be doing a good job of producing sausages and burgers that are made with decent meat and little else.

Dairy products

Dairy products such as milk, cheese, fromage frais and yoghurt are generally taken to be essential dietary items for growing kids. One of the major boons that dairy products offer is their high content of calcium. It is true that adequate amounts of calcium are important for bone growth, though parents reading this book might be interested to know that after maturity, the amount of calcium in the diet seems to have very little bearing on bone strength.[6] Milk is also a source of protein, vitamins B2, B6, B12, A, C, D and E, and the minerals magnesium, phosphorus and zinc.

Despite the wholesome reputation of milk and other dairy products, I do not share the enthusiasm the dietetic establishment has for them. Much of my disquiet is based on the observation that they are a common cause of food sensitivity reactions. Dairy products are a relatively recent addition to the human diet (see page 6 for more details), and some scientists believe that pasteurisation makes milk proteins more difficult to digest and more likely to cause unwanted reactions. Conditions that seem to be frequently connected with dairy sensitivity include nasal congestion, post-nasal drip, glue ear, ear infections, frequent colds, asthma, eczema and recurrent tonsillitis and sore throat. More details about food sensitivity and how to identify problem foods can be found on pages 211–21.

In general, experience shows that children are less likely to react to dairy products that come from other species of animal such as goats and sheep, rather than cows. Goat's milk and cheeses and yoghurts based on goat's and sheep's milk are becoming increasingly available, and are a good alternative to cow's products.

From a nutritional perspective, I think yoghurts are a better dairy product than milk or cheese. The bacterial fermentation process that turns milk into yoghurt seems to help the digestibility of milk proteins, which in turn appears to reduce the risk of food sensitivity problems. Also, many yoghurts are 'live', which means they contain bacteria that are generally good for the gut and help digestive function. However, most 'fruit' yoghurts (and also fromage frais) generally contain too much sugar, and some contain artificial sweeteners too. I recommend plain yoghurt, though this may be jazzed up with a little honey and some fresh or dried fruit if need be.

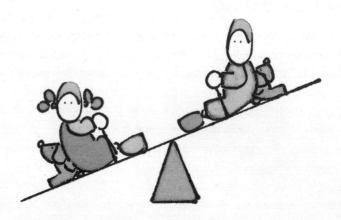

Dairy alternatives

Soya milk is generally seen as a good alternative to cow's milk, and soya yoghurt and cheese are popular too. Clinical experience and some research suggest that soya-based foods are better tolerated than regular dairy products. However, it is also true that soya can be quite a common cause of food sensitivity problems too. Soya is also rich in hormone-like substances called phytoestrogens, which may possibly pose health risks for children if taken in quantity in the long term. These issues are discussed in more depth on page 249.

If a parent is looking for an alternative to cow's milk, I generally recommend rice milk. This tends to be far less likely than soya to provoke food sensitivity reactions and is not loaded with phytoestrogens either.

Will my child get enough calcium?

Calcium is important to growing bones, but the evidence suggests many other nutrients are important too. For more details about this, see the section on bone health entitled 'broken bones'. Also, it's worth bearing in mind that the human is the only species on this planet that chooses to drink the milk of another animal, and this is something that is actually quite a recent development in terms of our evolution. Some populations (the Chinese, for instance) consume little or no dairy products after weaning, but there is no evidence that this causes problems with growth and development.

In general, I think the value of dairy foods for bone development may well be overstated. However, children who are not consuming regular dairy products still need to get this nutrient from somewhere. Good sources of calcium include calcium fortified rice milk, sardines, tinned salmon, nuts and seeds and green leafy vegetables.

Eggs

Not so long ago, the humble egg was viewed as a cheap, nutritious and versatile food. But, today, a general paranoia over their content of saturated fat and cholesterol means that we are often advised to avoid eating too many eggs. However, the evidence suggests that eating eggs does not put up levels of cholesterol in the bloodstream. One study found that feeding men and women two extra eggs each day for 12 weeks did not lead to a significant increase in their cholesterol levels.[7]

Similarly, despite the scares surrounding saturated fat, the wealth of evidence suggests that this dietary component is not a significant factor in either heart disease or obesity (see pages 154–7). Also, eggs actually contain more monounsaturated fat than saturated fat. They are a good source of protein, too, and contain other useful nutrients, including vitamins D and A. All-in-all, eggs do seem to have a place in a healthy balanced diet.

Some eggs boast a high omega-3 content. The chickens from which these eggs come are fed food rich in omega-3 fats, which then boost levels of omega-3 fats (essentially DHA – see page 229) in the egg. Consuming omega-3-rich eggs is likely to have health advantages over more common-or-garden egg varieties.

Butter and margarine

One dairy product that I do recommend over its commonly found alternative is butter. The problems with sensitivity to dairy foods seems to lie mainly in the proteins that they contain. Butter contains very little protein as it is made almost exclusively of fat. The mainly saturated fat that is found in butter is something that has been part of the human diet (in the form of meat) for a very long time and is therefore something we seem to be well adapted to. Also, as discussed, the supposed perils of saturated fat seems to have been somewhat overstated. While I do not recommend children gorge themselves on butter, I do see it as a natural and relatively unprocessed food, which can take some place in the diet.

I have very different views on margarine, however. While it is often recommended for its cholesterol-reducing effects, it is unlikely that a heavily processed, chemicalised food could really have a healthy edge over the essentially natural and untainted food that is butter. Most margarines are rich in trans fats, which are being increasingly linked with ill-health, including an increased risk of heart disease (see page 157). Increasing concerns about trans fats have led some margarine manufacturers to look for alternative ingredients for their products. As a result, some spreads are now based on what is known as interesterified fat. These are fats that have been chopped up chemically and then reassembled into novel fats. The long-term effects of interesterified fats remain unknown, but I am always nervous about eating any food that is fundamentally new to the human species. Whatever the margarine manufacturers claim, my opinion is that butter really is better.

Cooking oils

Cooking oils are generally made from seeds or grains, such as sunflower seeds or corn. Most oils are heavily refined, which may damage the fatty molecules they contain and impart some undesirable properties on them. The best oils for use in salad dressings and for cooking are those that are what is known as 'cold pressed'. This means the oil has been extracted by pressure alone, something which helps ensure an oil retains all of its health-giving properties.

One commonly available cold pressed oil is olive oil. Olive oil is rich in monounsaturated fat, a type of fat that is believed to help prevent heart disease and stroke. Olive oil also contains other disease-protective nutrients including oleuropein and squalene. Coldpressed olive oil is an ideal oil for salads and cooking. Other good options include cold pressed avocado and sunflower oil (these can be found in health food stores). If using an oil for frying, avoid heating it to a temperature that causes it to 'smoke' (this is a sign that the oil is being damaged).

Water

Water is an essential component of a healthy diet, but evidence suggests that many children don't drink enough of it. The National Diet and Nutrition Survey of young people in the year 2000 found that four out of ten primary-aged children did not drink any plain water during the course of a week. Rather disturbingly, the consumption of soft drinks by four to six year olds was found to be ten times higher than plain water consumption and children aged seven to ten years drank about seven times as much soft drinks as plain water.[8]

How much water does a child need?

As a rough guide, a child should consume about 30 ml of fluid for each kg of his body weight per day. However, even within these guidelines, a child's requirements can vary according to factors such as temperature and activity.

There is evidence that a good guide to our state of hydration is the colour of our urine.[9] The aim is to consume enough water to keep his or her urine pale yellow or very pale yellow throughout the course of the day. Obviously, the more water a child drinks, the more he or she will need to pass water. Having a child needing the loo every half-hour or so can get very frustrating during a long motorway journey or visit to the cinema. It's fine to cut back on how much water goes into your child at these times, but do make sure he or she gets plenty when this is more convenient.

Bottled or tap?

Some parents are concerned that tap water may contain harmful chemicals that should be avoided or filtered out. There is evidence that these concerns are valid. The regulatory bodies here in the UK claim that tap water is every bit as good as bottled water. However, the main disinfecting agent used in the production of tap water is chlorine. Chlorine is what is known as an oxidising agent, and can induce chemical changes that, at least in theory, should increase the risk of disease, including cancer. Tap water may also contain compounds related to chlorine called trihalomethanes, which are also thought to have cancer-inducing potential. A review of ten studies that examined the link between chlorine and its by-products found that exposure to these harmful chemicals increased the risk of bladder cancer by 21 per cent and rectal cancer by 38 per cent.[10] Another study found that exposure to chlorine or trihalomethanes was associated with an increased risk of brain tumours.[11] Other research has linked drinking trihalomethane-contaminated water during pregnancy with a range of disorders including birth defects and low birth weight.[12]

Aluminium, another potential contaminant in tap water, is believed to have the potential to be toxic to nervous tissue, and there is some evidence that it might increase the risk of Alzheimer's disease and dementia.[13]

In some areas, fluoride is added to the municipal water supply. It is commonly believed that this practice is highly effective in preventing tooth decay in children. However, the largest review to date on water fluoridation found that the practice is based on weak scientific evidence.[14] The study found that just one in six people drinking fluoridated water appears to benefit from this practice – far less than previously thought. Not only that, but almost half of children drinking fluoridated water at permissible levels exhibit a condition known as dental fluorosis – a mottling and discoloration of the teeth caused by fluoride toxicity. Some dentists have questioned the wisdom of preventing dental disease in one in six people, only to cause it in one in two.

Personally, I also question the practice of adding a supposedly medicinal agent into the water supplies of men, women and children irrespective of sex, weight, health and medical history. The fact that the dose of fluoride is not controlled, but is essentially dictated by thirst, is another worry. I am generally less concerned about fluoridated toothpastes and mouthwashes on the basis that the doses of fluoride are more measured and little of this is likely to be ingested. However, I do think there are very real medical and ethical question marks over the practice of water fluoridation. Currently, about 10 per cent of the UK water supply is treated with fluoride, though there are moves afoot to expand the practice.

I suggest that children are not given water straight out of the tap to drink. At the very least, I recommend filtering it first, either through a jug filter or plumbed-in system. Another option, of course, is to drink mineral water. According to European law, mineral waters must emerge from the ground in a state fit to drink, and must be bottled at source. Mineral water must also be protected from pollution to ensure its purity.

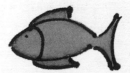

Soft drinks and squashes

My strong advice is to avoid most soft drinks and squashes. Canned soft drinks are full of refined sugar. One study found that drinking each additional can of sugared soft drink increased the risk of obesity by a staggering 60 per cent.[15] I do not regard artificially sweetened drinks (in cans or otherwise) as healthy alternatives. The reasons for this are covered on page 161. The additives that many of these drinks contain is another cause for concern (see pages 159–61).

Many health food stores, farm shops and supermarkets sell squashes and cordials based on fruits or other things such as elderflower or ginger, but are free from additional additives such as colouring and preservatives. The main thing going against these drinks is their intensely sugary nature. However, when well diluted with water, they are almost certainly OK to have in moderation in the diet.

Fast and processed food

Fast and processed foods come in a variety of forms, including burgers, chips, pizzas and ready-meals. In many ways, these foods epitomise the worst elements of the modern-day diet. It's best not to dwell too much on this sort of food, but their notable constituents include partially hydrogenated and trans fatty acids, refined sugars and starches, salt and artificial additives. While it is not essential to ban these sorts of foods from the diet, the less that your child eats of them, the better. Also, occasional indiscretions can be 'balanced' and made up for by ensuring a good intake of healthy food at other times.

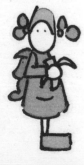

Crisps and other savoury snacks

Crisps and many other savoury snacks are based on potato, potato starch or refined grains (such as wheat or corn). These are all relatively un-nutritious starting materials for a food and all of them tend to release sugar quite quickly into the bloodstream (see page 204 for information on the hazards this may pose for the body). Also, these products will often contain damaged fats that are toxic to the body. The addition of salt does not help matters either. In addition, some savoury snacks contain artificial flavourings. An alternative to crisps and other savoury snacks is nuts (see page 175). For kids that will eat them, olives are another good option (see olive oil, page 181).

Chocolate

The essential ingredient in all types of chocolate is the cocoa bean, which comprises two basic components; a protein-rich part (cocoa) that gives chocolate its characteristic colour and taste, and a fatty part known as cocoa butter. Laboratory analysis reveals that the cocoa in chocolate is surprisingly loaded in minerals, such as potassium, magnesium and copper. Cocoa is rich in a class of plant substances called polyphenols. Also found in foodstuffs such as red wine, tea, apples and onions, polyphenols have the capacity to combat ageing and disease-promoting substances called free radicals. Polyphenols have been particularly linked with a reduced risk of heart disease.

Although some people are wary of the fat content of chocolate, cocoa butter's two main constituents, oleic acid (the predominant fat in olive oil) and stearic acid, have been shown to reduce cholesterol levels in the blood. However, it is important to bear in mind that the varying amounts of cocoa, cocoa butter, milk and sugar used to make chocolate have a bearing on the nutritional properties of the final product. From a health perspective, the best type of chocolate is plain. One benefit of plain chocolate is that it is generally lower in sugar than milk and white chocolate varieties. Plus, the darker the chocolate, the more cocoa there is, and the more it provides in the way of polyphenols. Brands that boast 60 or 70 per cent cocoa solid content are the healthiest.

COOKING METHODS

It makes sense to keep a child's diet as natural as possible, but I believe the same is true for how it is prepared. Ever since we discovered fire, we have been cooking food through the use of what is called 'radiant' heat. Traditional means of cooking, from the campfires of early man to modern-day electric ovens and halogen hobs essentially all do the same thing, and cook food from the outside in. All forms of cooking, such as baking, grilling and frying, are roughly equivalent. If food is being fried, however, I recommend using a good quality olive oil (extra virgin) and avoiding heating this to a temperature at which it starts to smoke. This is a sign that the oil is being damaged, which will detract from its healthy properties.

MICROWAVE COOKING

The last 30 years have seen the rise and rise of the microwave oven in family food preparation. There is no doubt that these devices are quick and convenient and there is a growing number of foods and ready-meals available that are designed specifically for the microwave. However, microwaves heat food in a very different way to conventional cooking methods, and eating foods cooked in this way may have undesirable effects on the body. Microwave ovens generate what is known as an alternating current, the effect of which is to cause food molecules to gyrate quite unnaturally, billions of times each second. All this movement creates frictional heat, effectively cooking the food not from the outside in, but from the inside out.

Of particular concern is the apparent ability of microwaves to change the molecular structure of food. For instance, one study found that the microwaving of milk led to structural changes in the proteins that might well pose hazards for the body.[16] Some scientists have suggested that one amino acid formed in this way (D-proline) is toxic to the nervous system, kidneys and liver.

Swiss research has revealed that consuming food thawed and/or cooked in a microwave oven could cause undesirable changes in blood chemistry. Two notable effects were a reduction in the level of the blood pigment haemoglobin (predisposing to anaemia) and an increase in the overall number of immune cells in the bloodstream (generally taken to be a sign of stress, infection or inflammation in the body). Also, exposing light-emitting (luminescent) bacteria to blood drawn after the consumption of microwaved food caused them to glow more brightly. The suggestion is that microwaves may lead to unnatural energetic changes in food that could pass to those who eat it. Sorry, but my advice is to avoid the use of microwave ovens.

Meal and snack suggestions

This part of the chapter contains eating suggestions for the main meals of the day, together with information on snacks – to be eaten both at home and in lunchboxes.

Breakfast

They say that breakfast is the most important meal of the day and children eating breakfast has been associated with a number of particular benefits, including better school attendance and improved academic performance. The benefits of breakfast are explored in more depth in the next chapter. These days, however, many children's breakfasts are centred around sweetened cereals and toast. Unfortunately, these very starch-and sugar-based breakfasts are not ideal for many kids. One major problem with them is that they will generally give rise to considerable surges in blood sugar levels, that may have short and long term consequences to a child's health and wellbeing – this is covered in depth on pages 204–11. Also, this type of breakfast generally means eating a lot of wheat, which is one of the most common causes of health issues related to something called food sensitivity (see pages 211–21). Wheat, in the refined form it often comes at breakfast time, offers little in the way of fibre and nutrients too.

At breakfast, it will help a child to eat something that is more likely to give a sustained release of sugar into the bloodstream. Keeping starches as whole as possible (e.g. porridge oats, 100 per cent wholemeal bread, whole rye toast), will help with this and will also help provide a more nutritious breakfast. Another thing that can help with blood sugar control is for a child to eat a bit less cereal and toast and a bit more protein in the form of eggs, plain yoghurt, nuts or even peanut butter. Giving a variety of food, including those that do not contain wheat, can only help matters. If you can manage to graft some fresh fruit somewhere into the breakfast, even better.

Healthy breakfast suggestions
- Porridge sweetened with a little honey
- Unsweetened, oat-based muesli topped with natural yoghurt and some fresh fruit
- Wholegrain, unsweetened cereal with milk and topped with some fresh fruit
- Natural yoghurt with nuts and dried or fresh fruit sweetened with a little honey
- A boiled or poached egg with a slice of wholemeal or whole rye toast
- Wholegrain (preferably rye) toast with some peanut butter and some fresh fruit

Main meals

Many parents have busy lives, and so gravitate to foods that are convenient and get eaten! Hence processed foods such as fish fingers, chicken nuggets and baked beans will feature in most kids' diets. But processed foods may contain trans fatty acids, sugar, salt and other additives and so are not ideal to be eaten in quantity. One particular type of food that seems to be used more and more with children is pasta: it's cheap, quick and has a reputation for being low in fat and nutritious. However, the refined flour used in pasta is relatively low in nutrients and tends to be quite upsetting for blood sugar balance, so I suggest keeping pasta meals to a minimum or putting more emphasis on using wholewheat pasta. The nutritional failings of regular pasta are also true for other refined carbs (e.g. white rice, couscous and white bread) and potatoes, and there are other foods that are not ideal for kids (or adults!).

The trick is not necessarily to cut these sorts of food out of the diet, but to down-play them in favour of other, more nutritious, fare. I suggest making these foods an accompaniment to a meal, similar to how you might view, say, a portion of vegetables. Protein is important for growing kids, so include it in main meals in the form of meat, fish, eggs, nuts, beans or pulses. If at all possible, vegetables should feature at main meals too, either raw (e.g. as salad or crudités) or cooked.

Healthy main meal suggestions

- Home-made chicken nuggets (chicken coated in flour and fried in olive oil) served with salad or vegetables and some boiled new potatoes
- Bean stew served with fresh vegetables
- Spanish omelette and salad
- Home-made beef burger served with fresh vegetables
- Lamb chop (fried, grilled or baked) served with salad dressed with olive oil and vinegar (e.g. balsamic vinegar)
- High quality sausages served with mashed potato and peas
- Home-made fish goujons (fish covered in breadcrumbs) served with green vegetables and brown rice
- Grilled salmon or trout served with pasta and tomato salad
- Small baked potato filled with tinned salmon served with salad or vegetables
- Lentil curry served with brown rice
- Chicken/prawn/vegetable stir-fry served with brown rice

Lunchboxes and snacks

According to the Department of Education, most children do not eat school meals. Because of this, lunchboxes are now the only option for most younger children. For older kids, a packed lunch offers a potentially healthy alternative to the generally unhealthy foods to be found in fast food joints and chip shops. Most parents would like to believe their child is going off to school with something balanced and sustaining in their rucksacks and satchels. However, this is generally easier said than done. In an effort to lend a helping hand, I have included here some potential lunchbox items with a brief description of their nutritional attributes. In general, the quality of foods increases the further down the list you go. As I shall explore in the next chapter, it seems the best way to get a child to eat more healthily is through gradual changes made with a minimum of fuss. So, if your child is a relatively picky eater, it might help to start with some suggestions at the top of the list (the least nutritious but most kid-friendly) and work your way towards items lower on the list in time.

The items in this list can also be used as snacks for children. While eating between meals is usually discouraged by the dietetic establishment, there is a considerable amount of evidence that it can help stabilise the body's chemistry and promote health. The benefits of snacking are explored on page 196. However, the quality of the snack is important. Currently, it seems as though children in the UK left to their own devices tend to snack on pretty awful stuff. In 2000, a *Times* survey of almost 1400 children's purchasing choices showed most money was spent on edible items. The box opposite is a summary of the findings.

The study found that the average child spends £6 per week on sweets, crisps and fizzy drinks, a rise of 42 per cent since the 1998 survey. Giving your child healthy snacks is no guarantee that he or she will eat them. However, if he or she has at least some of what you make easily available, the chances are that less healthy foods will naturally fall by the wayside. Plus, providing a child with healthier options at least helps educate them about nutrition and may encourage them to make better choices in the long term.

Items bought on the way to school	Items bought on the way home from school
Sweets 40%	Sweets 45%
Crisps or savoury snacks 38%	Canned or fizzy drinks 26%
Canned or fizzy drinks 26%	Chocolate 27%
Chocolate 25%	Crisps or savoury snacks 21%
Chewing gum 14%	Other soft drinks 10%
Other soft drinks 9%	Chewing gum 6%
Pokemon 5%	Ice lollies 6%
Chips 4%	Ice cream 5%
Stickers 2%	Comics/magazines 4%
Water 2%	Chips 4%
Cigarettes 2%	Pokemon 2%
Cakes 2%	Stickers 2%
Comics/magazines 2%	Water 2%
Biscuits 1%	Cakes 1%

HEALTHY LUNCHBOX AND SNACK ITEM SUGGESTIONS

Peanut butter sandwich (white bread)

The grain in this bread is low in fibre and nutrients and will also tend to release sugar very quickly into the system. However, the protein-rich peanut butter in this sandwich will help temper the blood sugar surges from this bread and offers some useful nutrients, such as monounsaturated (heart-healthy) fat, potassium, magnesium and fibre.

Nut bar

Many health food stores and some supermarkets sell bars made predominantly of nuts. They can be quite sweet, but nevertheless make a better option than common-or-garden confectionery or starch-based muesli bars.

Dried fruit (raisins or figs)

Dried fruit is not as good as fresh, but is much, much better than confectionery. Many kids, even picky ones, will eat raisins, though dried figs, dried apricots (unsulphured, preferably) and dried apple are other options.

Freshly squeezed fruit juice

Fruit juice is not as good as whole fruit, mainly on account of the fact that fibre and other potentially useful nutrients can get left behind during the juicing process. However, this freshly squeezed juice is miles ahead of carbonated drinks, fruit drinks and fruit-flavoured drinks.

Organic dark chocolate

This chocolate is much lower in sugar than regular confectionery. It is also rich in substances called flavonols, which are believed to have benefits for the heart.

Chicken salad sandwich on granary bread

The chicken in this sandwich will help provide the protein that is very important for growing bodies, and the granary bread is a nutritional step up from white. Putting some cucumber, lettuce or tomato in this sandwich will also help to enhance the nutritional value of this food.

Bag of dried fruit and nuts

Bags of dried fruit and nuts represent a healthy lunchbox or snack item, and are much more preferable to a packet of crisps.

Hard-boiled egg

For all the scare mongering about eggs, they are a good (and relatively cheap) source of protein and other nutrients, and the evidence suggests that they can form part of a healthy diet. Recent years have seen the introduction of eggs rich in omega-3 fat (see page 180), and these probably have a nutritional edge over regular varieties.

Smoothie

Smoothies are generally better than fruit juice, as they tend to contain pulped (whole) fruit that may retain nutritional qualities lost during juicing.

These can also be a good option for kids who won't eat whole fruit.

Salmon salad on wholemeal bread
Compared to more refined varieties, 100 per cent wholemeal breads release sugar more slowly into the bloodstream and are richer in fibre and nutrients too. The salmon in this sandwich is rich in omega-3 fats, which have been linked with better brain function and behaviour. Sardine or mackerel are other omega-3 rich fish that make good sandwich fillings.

Fresh fruit
Children with adventurous palates would do well to eat a variety of fruits rotated through the week.

Crudités (e.g. carrot, cucumber and celery) Many kids, even little ones, will eat raw veggies once they're cut up into child-friendly fingers.

Mineral water
The predominant fluid in any child's diet should be water (and preferably not from the tap). However, if mineral water seems like a stretch, fill a water bottle with tap water that has at least been filtered first.

Key points

- Fruit is rich in fibre and nutrients and represents very healthy food. Dried fruit is not as healthy as fresh, but is much better than other sweet treats, such as sweets and confectionery.
- Fruit juice is not as healthy as fresh fruit and is rich in fructose, which can pose hazards to health. The best juice is freshly squeezed, but this is best diluted with water before drinking.
- Fruit drinks and fruit-flavoured drinks are not healthy on account of their low fruit content and the fact that they generally contain significant quantities of artificial additives and sugar and/or artificial sweeteners.
- Vegetables, other than the potato, are generally highly nutritious food in both their raw and cooked state.
- Agrochemical residues may pose hazards to health. Thorough washing of fruit and vegetables will help to remove these chemicals.
- Organic produce appears to offer significant advantages over conventionally grown food.
- Generally, wholegrain starches such as wholemeal bread, brown rice and oats, should be eaten in preference to refined starches, such as white bread, white rice and pasta.

- Beans and lentils give slow release of sugar into the bloodstream and are rich in fibre and nutrients.
- Nuts and seeds are highly nutritious foods and are especially rich in healthy fats and other heart-health nutrients.
- Fish and seafood are healthy, particularly oily fish (such as salmon, trout, mackerel and sardine), which is rich in very healthy omega-3 fats.
- Meat, in as natural a form as possible, is a nutritious food. Chicken is generally very intensively reared and is best bought organic. Processed meat is best avoided.
- Dairy products are reasonably nutritious, though significant numbers of children are sensitive to them. Butter is generally very well tolerated.
- Margarine is based on unnatural fats and is generally rich in additives. Butter, a relatively natural and untainted food, is better.
- The best vegetable oils are those that have been minimally processed. Cold-pressed olive oil is ideal for salads and cooking. Generally, a child should drink enough water to keep his or her urine pale yellow throughout the course of the day.
- Soft drinks and squashes are generally rich in sugar and/or artificial sweeteners and additives and are best avoided. Natural cordials are much better.
- Crisps and most other savoury snacks are un-nutritious and generally rich in salt and processed vegetable oils. Nuts make a much better snack food.
- Dark chocolate is relatively low in sugar and rich in substances called flavonols, which may have health-giving properties. Milk and white chocolates should be kept to a minimum.
- Microwave ovens can induce unnatural changes in food and may have health effects. It is best to stick to more traditional cooking methods.
- Forget trying to create a 'perfect' diet for your child. It is what he or she eats most of the time (not some of it) that will determine health and wellbeing in the long term.

Chapter 3
Food and meal culture

The previous two chapters explored some of the fundamentals of nutrition and highlighted the value of eating a diet based on mainly natural and unprocessed foods. However, as a parent, you won't need me to tell you that offering nutritious food to children is one thing, getting them to eat it is another. This chapter is designed to help with the practicalities of feeding children healthily. This chapter is not about what to feed your kids, but how to feed them.

It is natural for parents to want to exert some control over their child's diet. However, as we shall see, if this is done too vigorously, it can compound the problem. Studies show that attempting to coerce a child into eating a healthy food generally ups the repulsion factor and may feed a child's rebellious streak. Also, forbidding foods tends to lead to children wanting them more, and may cause them to eat more of them when they have the opportunity.

This chapter explores how to upgrade the quality of your child's diet using gradual change and more subversive tactics that tend not to cause stress and upset. Generally, the earlier these techniques are started, the better. Specific advice about the feeding and weaning of babies and toddlers can be found in Chapter 6. This chapter also looks at the role that family meals have in helping ensure a child eats a healthy, balanced diet, and the particular importance of breakfast.

The importance of family meals

Statistics show that over the last few decades there has been a steady decline in the percentage of meals that children eat at home. This trend may have important consequences for the overall quality of a child's diet, and may have important implications for their health in the long term too.

Not surprisingly, eating family meals has been associated with better nutrition in kids. In one study, the frequency of family meals and quality of the overall diet were assessed in almost 5000 children.[1] More frequent family meals were found to be associated with an increased intake of healthy foods, including fruits and vegetables, and a more modest consumption of soft drinks (which, by the way, have strong links with obesity in kids). Children eating more meals with the family were found to have generally higher intakes of protein and calcium (important dietary elements for growing boys and girls), as well as other key nutrients, including iron, folate and vitamins A, C and E.

Other research has found that eating evening meals at home was associated with an increased consumption of fruit and vegetables, and healthier eating habits overall.[2] Interestingly, this study also discovered that parental participation at the evening meal seemed to increase the likelihood of children eating breakfast the following morning. Why this should be is unclear, but it is significant because there is evidence that having breakfast may boost mental powers and has been linked with improved performance at school (see opposite). Other evidence also links the eating of family meals with better learning.[3–4]

Yet another benefit of the family meal is that it appears to have the capacity to instil some food awareness in children. At least two studies have found that the more frequent family dinners are, the more likely kids are to discuss and gain learning about matters of a nutritional nature.[5–6] Another study found that adolescents reported feeling more confident about making healthy food choices at family meals, rather than at other eating opportunities.[7]

It's not always going to be possible for the whole family to sit down together for meals. Many children have after-school and evening activities that make this difficult, and parents' commitments and ever-increasing working hours don't help. However, old fashioned and rather traditional though this concept may be, there is overwhelming evidence to suggest that when it comes to giving our kids nutritious diets, and some awareness of what it means to eat healthily, there really is no place like home.

The benefits of breakfast

One meal that has been the subject of several studies in children is breakfast. The first meal of the day helps to ensure adequate fuel for both body and brain. This is important because many children may go ten or more hours between their last meal of the day and the next morning. With such a long gap between fuel stops, it is not uncommon for blood sugar levels to drop to sub-normal levels overnight. This can cause a child to be tired and grumpy in the morning, and can certainly take the edge off even the sharpest of minds. A number of studies have found that when children skip the first meal of the day, memory, verbal fluency and mathematical dexterity may suffer.[8]

By restoring blood sugar levels after the overnight fast, eating breakfast helps ensure a child has a productive morning in the classroom. Regular breakfasting may have important long-term benefits as well, by helping to ensure your child gets the nutrients needed for a growing body and mind. This is likely to reap dividends in terms of general physical wellbeing and mental functioning.

To date, there have been three studies that have examined the impact of eating breakfast on children's behaviour and learning.[9] Interestingly, these studies found that children who did not skip breakfast were less likely to skip school too. So, the evidence suggests that eating breakfast not only helps learning, but may also increase the amount of learning a child is subjected to! It comes as no surprise, therefore, that the studies that have been conducted in this area found that eating breakfast is associated with better performance in a variety of scholastic tests. Ideas for healthy breakfasts can be found on pages 187–8.

Snacking

In today's culture, snacking has a generally negative image. It is often viewed as something that increases the amount we eat in a day and can therefore pose problems to our weight. However, despite its unhealthy reputation, there is good evidence that snacking can actually have significant benefits for health. One of the major advantages of snacking is that it can help to reduce the amount of food had at any one sitting. This is important because large meals tend to lead to correspondingly large rises in blood sugar levels. In response to this, the body tends to secrete more of the hormone insulin, which, in excess, can have a number of undesirable effects, including an ability to convert sugar in the body into fat.

Smaller, more frequent meals help to balance the body's chemistry and seem to have a number of benefits. Studies have linked more regular eating with less risk of excess weight, and also lower levels of unhealthy blood fats, such as cholesterol and triglycerides. The overwhelming evidence suggests that snacking is healthy, but the type of snack is clearly important too. Ideas for nutritious snacks can be found on pages 190–1.

Gradual changes are best

Reading through the previous chapter, you might feel inclined to purge your kitchen of some of the unhealthy foods that may be lurking there. While it might be tempting to take this sort of short-sharp-shock tactic, it may not have the desired effect. Children tend to notice sudden changes to the foods that are available, and may well rebel against these changes.

One study found that restricting access to specific foods focuses children's attention on those foods, and at the same time increases their desire to get hold of those foods.[10] This research also found that highly controlling approaches to child feeding undermine a child's ability to exercise self-control over eating – trying too hard to restrict foods can encourage a tendency for a child to overeat. In another study, children whose parents tended not to restrict their child's food intake responded more appropriately to internal cues of feeling full following a meal. Interestingly, the children in this study were also found to eat few unhealthy snack foods. Basically, children who are fed in an unrestricted way judge better when they are full, tend not to eat more than they need, and eat better too. In contrast, children whose mothers restricted their intake were more likely to eat 'forbidden' foods, even when they were not hungry.[11]

What these studies suggest is that it helps not to make an issue of food and, in particular, it seems it is useful not to be seen to be laying down the law about what your child should and should not eat. What seems to help, however, is for children to get clear and consistent messages about what represents healthy food, and what doesn't. The aim is to instill in your child a degree of food awareness and knowledge. Family meals (see page 195) have the potential to play a part here.

> **Avoid using food as a reward**
> One tactic that parents sometimes use to get a child to eat healthy foods is to use other more palatable foods as a reward. For instance, some parents may cajole a child into eating vegetables by dangling a dessert or some chocolate as a carrot. However, studies have shown that children generally learn to dislike foods eaten to obtain rewards[12] and learn to prefer foods given as rewards.[13]
>
> Sometimes, 'treats' are used to modify a child's behaviour. For instance, a parent may offer the reward of some ice cream in return for a child tidying his or her room or doing the washing up. However, there is evidence that using food to change a child's behaviour seems to increase the risk of obesity by interfering with a child's ability to regulate his or her own food intake.[14] The message is clear – avoid using food as a reward. Encouraging the consumption of healthy foods, including fruit and vegetables, is best done using other tactics – see below.

Encouraging kids to eat fruit and veg

Whatever wonderful properties they may possess, unfortunately not all children take to fruit and vegetables. Even when these foods are made abundantly available to kids, they may simply not want to eat them. However, a few simple tactics can help here.

- As a general rule, playing to a child's strengths is a good idea. Even if a child likes only a limited number of fruits or vegetables these should be provided in quantity. For instance, if a child is keen on fruit but not vegetables, keeping a well-stocked fruit bowl may reap more dividends than force-feeding him or her with spinach and broccoli.
- Likewise, if a child likes some vegetables but not others, giving those he or she likes and not making an issue of any pet hates is a good long-term strategy. It's worth bearing in mind that most children go through picky-eating phases, but these very rarely persist for too long. Besides, as discussed above, attempting to ply a child with unwanted foods can reinforce the problem and encourage the development of some serious mental barriers to specific foods.
- One useful trick for getting a child to eat more fruit and veg is disguise. For instance, a child who won't eat fresh fruit may nonetheless be very

happy to drink blended fruit in the form of a smoothie. Zizzing up a banana with some berries (e.g. strawberries, raspberries, blueberries) and a little water and ice makes a tasty and nutritious drink for children of practically all ages. An added dollop or two of yoghurt can often give added appeal too.

- Blending can also be a useful tactic for getting more vegetables into a child. For instance, puréeing some carrots for addition into a pasta sauce can add real nutritional value to a meal without registering a blip on a child's food radar.
- Some children are keener on raw vegetables, particularly when supplied with a favourite dip. Many kids find raw carrots, celery or cucumber dipped into hummus or guacamole a surprisingly attractive proposition, and make a good option as an 'appetiser' before the main meal starts in earnest.
- It can help to bear in mind, too, that vegetables may taste a lot better to a child once they've been dressed up a bit. So the addition of some olive oil and balsamic vinegar may make a child more inclined to tuck into a salad. A bit of butter on the carrots or broccoli may help to get these vegetables to slip down.

A lot of children can be intimidated by food. For young children, in particular, start by serving small portions of vegetables (especially if it's a new food to them), and cut it up small too.

Parents often find that the more they involve their child in food preparation the more likely they are to eat those foods. Even small children can be encouraged to wash fruit and vegetables, or add them to a pot or blender. And one final thing; studies show that parents who eat plenty of fruit and veg are more likely to have children who do the same, and generally require little in the way of coercion to do so. As far as healthy eating goes, as with most things in life, it helps to lead by example.

Encouraging children to drink water

Along with fruit and vegetables, another foodstuff many children could
do with consuming more of is water. Making plenty of water available (for
instance, giving your child a bottle of water to take to school and having a jug
of water on the kitchen table) will generally help to ensure your child gets more
water than he or she would otherwise. Young children very often respond to
the notion that while water is good for cleaning the outside of the body, it's
good for keeping the inside nice and clean too.

If at first you don't succeed ...

Not all children take to a new food first off. A child screwing up his or her face
and spitting food out may make parents reluctant to serve that food again.
However, research suggests that repeated offerings of a food (best done
without coercion and nagging) often gets there in the end. Studies have found
that giving a child multiple opportunities to sample a new food can change
rejection into acceptance.[15-16] It seems that as far as getting children to eat
new foods is concerned, persistence pays.

In the supermarket

Many foods are branded and specifically marketed to children. Most supermarkets
are full of attractively packaged and enticing kids' food, but there is usually no case
to be made for them from a nutritional perspective. Shopping with children can be
an endurance exercise in itself. However, it most certainly is not made any easier
by a child's persistent demands for foods that you'd rather they wouldn't eat.

One approach that tends to work well when out shopping for food is to
ensure your kids are not hungry (this works well for adults too, by the way).
The hungrier a child is, the more likely he is to want to eat the unhealthiest
of foods on offer in a supermarket. Before embarking on a shopping trip,
I suggest feeding kids a good meal or at least some healthy snacks.

Another tactic that tends to work well is to agree a set number of treats
(I suggest one or two) that a child can choose on each outing. Children usually
respond well to the element of choice afforded to them in this scheme.
Crucially, however, this approach puts a predetermined ceiling on the amount
of rubbish that ends up in the shopping trolley.

The most common arena for the food feuds that can go on between children and their parents is the supermarket, as these are notorious for having temptation all over the shop. If possible, I suggest avoiding taking kids into this environment at all. The absence of children clearly dissolves much of the potential for the battle of wills that the supermarket setting tends to induce. Not all parents have the luxury of being able to extricate themselves from their kids when the shopping needs doing. However, if two grown-ups are on hand, an option might be for one to take on the mantle of child-minding duties while the other does the supermarket shop.

Speciality and farm shops

An even better tactic, though, might be to junk the supermarket altogether. Making use of the farm shops, farmers' markets or the high street butcher, fishmonger, baker and greengrocer may be preferable for a variety of reasons, including support of local businesses, and possibly some local producers too. Importantly, however, these shops are generally bereft of unhealthy, processed foods marketed directly at children. For some people, the idea of multi-stop shopping may seem unnecessarily arduous compared to the convenience of the supermarket. However, many find this more traditional way of purchasing food an altogether more wholesome experience, and one that can make countering unhealthy influences on their children much easier.

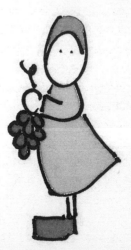

Key points

- What you feed your child is important, but how that food is fed may be critical to what your child actually eats.
- Family meals have been linked with a variety of benefits, including a higher intake of nutrients, lower intake of unhealthy foods and better knowledge and awareness of nutritional matters.
- Eating breakfast has been associated with better school attendance and scholastic performance.
- Snacking is generally viewed as unhealthy, but can help to stabilise the body's chemistry and reduce the risk of overeating.
- Avoid attempting to control your child's diet too vigorously. Gradual changes are best.
- Children tend to learn to dislike foods eaten to obtain a reward. Also, giving food as a reward may upset a child's ability to regulate food intake and may increase the risk of overweight and obesity.
- Give your child the fruits and/or vegetables he or she likes.
- With new foods, serve small portions and cut them up small.
- Vegetables can be blended into soups and sauces, and may be more likely to be eaten if jazzed up with something else like hummus or a dab of butter.
- Repeated offerings of food (without coercion) will help to get a child to accept a food in the long term.
- Feed your child before you go shopping.
- Speciality and farm shops may provide a more wholesome shopping experience for you and your child.

Chapter 4
Common childhood
problems

A balanced and nutritious diet can go a very long way towards ensuring that a child grows up fit and well. The strategies outlined in the preceding chapters represent important foundation stones for your child's physical and mental wellbeing. However, sometimes a child may have one or more imbalances that are at the root of his or her symptoms or condition. In this situation, a more specific dietary approach may be called for.

This chapter sets out the most common imbalances seen in children, namely:
- **Blood sugar imbalance**
- **Food sensitivity**
- **Yeast overgrowth**
- **A deficiency or imbalance in beneficial fats in the body**

Identifying and correcting one or more of them in your child can lead to a quantum leap in health and wellbeing. The specific imbalances detailed in this chapter may be an underlying feature of a great many conditions, including fatigue, migraine, eczema, asthma and acne. Where relevant, advice on individual ailments may refer back to the information contained in this chapter. For each of the major imbalances, a questionnaire is included that is designed to help you identify a specific problem in your child. Practical information and advice on how to correct the imbalance is also given.

Blood sugar balance and health

The body is constantly adjusting and balancing its internal environment using a process that is referred to as homeostasis. One very important component of homeostasis is the regulation of the level of sugar in the bloodstream. However, some children can be prone to swings in blood sugar levels that can be quite disruptive to their health. In the short term, imbalance in the blood sugar level can give rise to symptoms such as fluctuating energy, mood swings and cravings for sweet and starchy foods. In the long term, this issue is believed to increase the risk of longer-term health problems, such as weight gain and diabetes.

Blood sugar balance in the body

Carbohydrates (sugars and starches) are absorbed from the gut in the form of sugar. As blood sugar levels rise (see opposite) the body secretes a hormone called insulin from an organ in the abdomen known as the pancreas. One of the chief effects of insulin is to transport sugar out of the bloodstream and into the body's cells. In this way, blood sugar is lowered again, preventing the accumulation of sugar in the bloodstream. In general, the body copes well with foods that release sugar quite slowly into the bloodstream. However, if the blood sugar level rises very quickly, the body tends to secrete a lot of insulin in response. The problem here is that this may drive blood sugar levels lower than normal, a condition that is termed 'hypoglycaemia'.

The symptoms of low blood sugar

An adequate level of sugar in the bloodstream is an essential fuel for both body and brain. So, if blood sugar levels dip, it can cause physical and mental energies to stall. A typical time for problems in this respect is the mid–late afternoon, as a result of the trough of blood sugar that can come after the peak that follows lunch. Fluctuating blood sugar levels often cause fluctuating mood, and this can manifest as deep depression and temper tantrums (and everything in between).

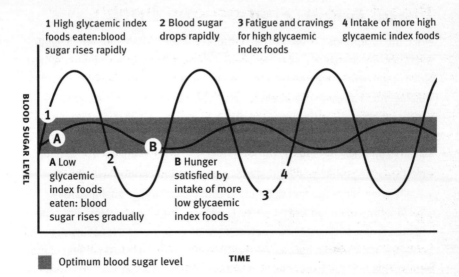

1 High glycaemic index foods eaten:blood sugar rises rapidly

2 Blood sugar drops rapidly

3 Fatigue and cravings for high glycaemic index foods

4 Intake of more high glycaemic index foods

A Low glycaemic index foods eaten: blood sugar rises gradually

B Hunger satisfied by intake of more low glycaemic index foods

BLOOD SUGAR LEVEL

TIME

Optimum blood sugar level

Another common symptom of low blood sugar is food cravings. When a child's blood sugar levels get low, it is natural for the body to crave foods that will replenish sugar quickly into the bloodstream. A child that 'needs' sweet foods, such as biscuits, chocolate or highly sugared drinks, from time to time is normally struggling with a blood sugar issue. In some children, blood sugar levels can drop during the night, which can cause the body to secrete the hormone adrenaline in an effort to get blood sugar levels to rise (by stimulating its release from the liver). Surges of adrenaline may disrupt sleep, however, and may cause some children to wake in the night, sometimes in an agitated state.

The problems of excess insulin

While the symptoms of blood sugar imbalance are most obvious when sugar levels are low, high blood sugar levels have hazards too. In response to a high blood sugar level, the body secretes insulin. While insulin is important for keeping blood sugar in check, excess amounts of this hormone can pose significant hazards in the body. One of insulin's effects is to stimulate the conversion of sugar into a starch-like substance called 'glycogen' in the liver and muscle. However, when the glycogen stores in the body are full, insulin stimulates the production of substances called 'triglycerides', which is actually fancy language for fat. Children with blood sugar imbalance may therefore tend to put on weight. In the long term, high levels of insulin in the body can increase the risk of diabetes. If the body secretes a lot of insulin over many years, then it can become increasingly less sensitive to the effect of that insulin. This may lead to a condition known as Type II diabetes (also known as non-insulin dependent diabetes).

Getting blood sugar back in balance

Children who have symptoms and signs of blood sugar imbalance can generally expect to have more stable levels of mood and energy when steps are taken to correct this. A loss of excess weight, if this is an issue, is very likely too.

One important factor in getting blood sugar back in balance is to eat a diet based on foods that give a controlled release of sugar into the body. The speed and extent to which a food increases blood sugar can be quantified using something called the glycaemic index scale. Here, the speed and extent of a food's sugar release into the bloodstream is compared with glucose (the fastest releasing food), which is given a value of 100. The higher a food's glycaemic index, the faster it releases sugar into the bloodstream, and the worse it tends to be for a child's health. In the box opposite is a list of the commonly eaten carbohydrates and their respective glycaemic indices.

IS YOUR CHILD SUFFERING FROM A BLOOD SUGAR IMBALANCE?

The following questionnaire is designed to help you to assess whether blood sugar imbalance is a factor in your child's health. Score each question as indicated and then add up your total score.

1 Does your child's energy tend to fluctuate during the day?

No – 0 points

Occasional or mild symptoms – 2 points

Frequent or severe problems – 4 points

2 Do you find that eating something can often pick up his or her energy levels?

No – 0 points

Occasionally – 2 points

Frequently – 4 points

3 Does your child often feel tired or unable to concentrate in the mid–late afternoon?

No – 0 points

Occasional or mild problems – 2 points

Frequent or severe problems – 4 points

4 Does your child tend to be cranky at this time, and need something to eat?

No – 0 points

Occasional or mild problems – 2 points

Frequent or severe problems – 4 points

5 Does your child tend to wake in the middle of the night, sometimes feeling anxious or nervy?

No – 0 points

Occasional or mild problems – 3 points

Frequent or severe problems – 5 points

6 Is your child prone to mood swings and/or irritability, especially if a meal is skipped?

No – 0 points

Occasional or mild problems – 2 points

Frequent or severe problems – 4 points

7 Does your child crave sweet or starchy foods from time to time?

No – 0 points

Occasional or mild symptoms – 3 points

Frequent or severe symptoms – 5 points

8 Do you have a history of Type II diabetes in your family?

No – 0 points

Yes – 4 points

Interpreting your child's score

0–7: *Blood sugar imbalance is unlikely.*

8–16: *Blood sugar imbalance is quite likely and measures taken to stabilise blood sugar are likely to be of benefit.*

17 and above: *Blood sugar imbalance is likely and measures taken to stabilise blood sugar are highly recommended.*

High glycaemic index foods (with glycaemic indices greater than 50)[1]

Glucose	100	Cantaloupe melon	65
French baguette	95	High Fibre Rye Crispbread	65
Lucozade	95	Couscous	65
Baked potato	85	Bread – rye	64
Cornflakes	83	Muffin	62
Rice Crispies	82	Muesli Bar	61
Pretzels	81	Ice cream	61
Rice cakes	77	Pizza (cheese)	60
Cocopops	77	Rice (white)	58
Doughnut	76	Pitta bread (white)	57
French fries	75	Potato (new)	57
Corn chips	74	Muesli	56
Potato (mashed)	73	Popcorn	55
Bagel (white)	72	Rice – brown	55
Sultana Bran	71	Pasta (durum wheat)	55
Bread (wheat, white)	71	Sweetcorn	55
Shredded Wheat	69	Sweet potato	54
Bread (wheat, wholemeal)	69	Banana	54
Croissant	67	Special K	54
Gnocchi	67	Kiwi fruit	53
Pineapple	66	Orange juice	52

Low glycaemic index foods (with glycaemic indices up to 50)

Pumpernickel	50	Pear	37
Porridge	49	Chick peas	33
Baked beans	48	Butter beans	31
Grape	46	Apricots (dried)	31
Orange	44	Soya milk	30
All-bran	42	Kidney beans	29
Apple juice	41	Lentils	29
Apple	38	Grapefruit	25
Pasta (wholemeal)	37	Cherries	22

For a long time, traditional nutritional wisdom has dictated that foods rich in sugar produce rapid rises in blood sugar, while starches, because they need to be broken down to sugar prior to absorption, release more slowly into the bloodstream. However, the glycaemic index list on the previous page reveals that this is far from the truth. While some starches, e.g. oat porridge, release sugar relatively slowly, others, notably pasta, potato, bread, rice and sweetcorn, do not. Bearing in mind the preponderance of fast-releasing foods in many children's diets, it is perhaps no surprise that we are seeing increasing problems with behaviour, learning, excess weight and diabetes.

Getting decent control over blood sugar and insulin levels is a key aspect of health, and a crucial part of this is a diet based on low GI foods. It is not necessarily important to get higher GI foods right out of the diet, and neither is this realistic. However, what this is about is balance. It's about emphasising healthier, slower-releasing foods, while at the same time pulling back on the faster-releasing stuff.

The importance of protein

One thing that seems to be particularly important for blood sugar control is that there is adequate protein in the diet. Protein stimulates the production of a hormone called 'glucagon', which has the opposite effect to insulin, and thereby helps to stabilise blood sugar levels. Increasing the amount of healthy proteins in your child's diet can make a big difference to blood sugar levels. Good sources of protein in the diet include meat and fish. Eggs are another protein rich food, and may be a good choice for vegetarian children. Vegans may find their protein in beans and pulses, nuts, seeds and soya-based products such as tofu. See page 153 for more information about the role of protein in the body.

Mixing meals for better balance

One practical way of establishing better blood sugar in your child is to make sure that if he or she is eating a fast-releasing food, that plenty of slower-releasing food is eaten with it. Protein helps here, as we have already discussed. Another approach would be to add plenty of slow-releasing vegetables to a meal. For example, let's say your child is going to eat a meal that contains white rice. White rice has a high glycaemic index and is therefore not ideal from a blood sugar balance point of view. However, if that white rice is eaten as part of a meal that also contains some fish or lean meat, or beans and pulses with plenty of fresh, steamed vegetables such as broccoli and French beans, then it is much more likely that there will be a controlled release of sugar into the bloodstream. Studies show that the overall glycaemic index of a meal comes from a balance of the speed of sugar release of its components and their relative amounts.

Eating patterns and the benefits of snacking

In Chapter 3 I looked at some of the benefits to be had from snacking. Snacking has particular significance to blood sugar control. Whatever it is that a child eats, eating small amounts of it more frequently will generally lead to a more stable level of sugar and insulin compared to eating that food in two or three big meals. Regular meals are important for children, but healthy snacks in between can be extremely useful too. Fresh and dried fruit, cut up raw veggies, as well nuts and seeds all make eminently nutritious snacks that help keep hunger at bay, but may also help to keep blood sugar levels on an even keel. More ideas for snack foods can be found on page 190.

Supplements for blood sugar control

Several nutrients are known to be involved in the processes that regulate the level of sugar in the body. Some of the key nutrients are the B-vitamins (particularly B3), magnesium and chromium. It can therefore help a child who is suffering from blood sugar imbalance to take a good quality multivitamin and mineral supplement that contains a comprehensive range of nutrients, which will help with balance in the body. More details about specific supplements can be found on pages 14–17.

Food sensitivity

While food can have health-giving and healing properties, it can also cause considerable health issues too. Food has the capacity to cause unwanted reactions in the body that are often referred to as 'food sensitivity'. Food sensitivity does seem to be a common problem in children and may manifest as one or more of a wide variety of symptoms, including frequent colds, a runny nose, headaches and migraine, abdominal bloating, eczema and asthma. The identification and elimination of problem foods from the diet can often make a major change to a child's health and wellbeing.

What is food sensitivity?

Conventional medical wisdom dictates that before food is absorbed through the gut wall into the bloodstream, it is first broken down into its smallest molecular constituents. In other words, fats are broken down into fatty acids, starches are broken down into individual sugar molecules, and proteins are broken down into amino acids. The basic building blocks of foods have limited potential to cause adverse reactions in the body, as these are simply too small to be seen as foreign by the body.

However, contrary to received wisdom, food can sometimes make its way through the gut wall into the body in a partially digested form. Once in the body, the body may see these undigested food molecules as 'foreign', as it would, say, a bacterium or virus. It is the body's reactions to food that are believed to be at the root of food sensitivity problems.

Food allergy and intolerance

Many food sensitivity reactions are mediated through the body's immune system and involve the production of substances called antibodies (also known as immunoglobulins). Antibodies help the body to neutralise or destroy invading organisms or foreign substances. Antibodies come in five different forms, two of which are immunoglobulin E (IgE) and immunoglobulin G (IgG). It is IgE and IgG that concern us with regard to food sensitivity.

IgE sensitivity

IgE can trigger the release of a substance called histamine. Histamine is the substance that causes the sneezing and runny eyes characteristic of hay fever. In hay fever, IgE production and histamine release is a response to pollen, but sometimes, these reactions can be triggered by food. If an individual eats a strawberry and quickly develops a red rash, this is almost definitely an IgE reaction. Another example of an IgE sensitivity is peanut (or other nuts) allergy, in which severe reactions can lead to something known as anaphylactic shock (see page 31), which can have potentially fatal consequences. In reality, childhood food sensitivities that are IgE related are very rare and tests for this (see pages 212–19) can be useful in identifying a problem. However, the immune system may react to foods in a way that does not involve IgE, but IgG antibodies.

IgG sensitivity

If blood samples are drawn from food sensitive individuals, it is often possible to detect IgG antibodies to specific foods. There is a theory that the IgG antibodies produced to foods can also cause the immune response to spill over into the body's own tissues, and it is this process that is often at the root of many chronic health conditions. IgG food reactions tend to come on much more slowly than IgE reactions. While IgE reactions are pretty much immediate, IgG reactions can take two or more days to show themselves. Also, while the symptoms of IgE sensitivity tend to be quite obvious (e.g. vomiting, rash), those related to IgG tend to be more subtle.

It is not uncommon for IgG reactions to produce vague symptoms of fatigue or general feelings of malaise. Sometimes, though, IgG sensitivity can manifest as quite specific symptoms, which include colic (in babies), glue ear, ear infections, eczema, asthma or recurrent tonsillitis, excess mucus or catarrh formation, hyperactivity, food cravings (particularly for things such as bread and cheese), dark circles under the eyes, irritable bowel syndrome (IBS), hives or rash and abdominal bloating. Drawing a distinction between IgE and IgG sensitivity is important, as many conventional tests look at only IgE, and may therefore fail to identify the cause of a child's problems. This is discussed in more depth later in this chapter on pages 212–19.

DOES MY CHILD HAVE A FOOD SENSITIVITY?

The following questionnaire is designed to help you to assess whether food sensitivity is a factor in your child's health. Score each question as indicated and then add up your total score.

1 Does your child seem to feel tired and lethargic soon after eating?
No – 0 points
Occasional or mild problems – 2 points
Frequent or severe problems – 4 points

2 Can your child seem 'hyper' after eating?
No – 0 points
Occasional or mild problems – 2 points
Frequent or severe problems – 4 points

3 Does your child have recurrent, unexplained symptoms?
No – 0 points
Occasional or mild problems – 2 points
Frequent or severe problems – 4 points

4 Does your child suffer from (or did your child suffer from) colic, glue ear, ear infections, eczema, asthma or recurrent tonsillitis or sore throats?
No – 0 points
Yes, occasional problems – 3 points
Yes, frequent and/or severe problems – 5 points

5 Does your child suffer from excess mucus or catarrh formation in the nose or throat?
No – 0 points
Occasional or mild problems – 2 points
Frequent or severe problems – 4 points

6 Does your child seem particularly drawn to certain foods such as bread or cheese?
No – 0 points
Occasionally – 2 points
Frequently – 4 points

7 Does your child have dark circles under his eyes?
No – 0 points
Yes – 5 points

8 Does your child have a horizontal crease on his nose and tend to wipe his nose on the back of his wrist or hand?
No – 0 points
Yes – 5 points

9 Does your child suffer from abdominal bloating or irritable bowel syndrome?
No – 0 points
Occasional or mild problems – 2 points
Frequent or severe problems – 4 points

10 Does your child suffer from eczema, hives (urticaria) or undiagnosed rash?
No – 0 points
Occasional or mild problems – 2 points
Frequent or severe problems – 4 points

Interpreting your score
0 – 9: *Food sensitivity is unlikely.*
10 – 25: *Food sensitivity is quite likely.*
26 and above: *Food sensitivity is very likely.*

Testing for food sensitivity

If you suspect your child might be food sensitive, then the next step might be to identify which specific foods or foods are the problem. There are a variety of tests available for food sensitivity, which include:

SCRATCH TESTING AND IgE BLOOD TESTING

The scratch test, also known as the prick test or patch test, involves breaching the outer layer of the skin and introducing a tiny amount of the food or other substance (e.g. animal hair, pollen) to be tested. Redness and swelling at the site of the test indicate a sensitivity to whatever is being tested. Blood tests also exist that detect IgE to specific foods. These tests can be useful in finding a food sensitivity reaction that is related to IgE. If one of these tests comes up as negative for a specific food, then many doctors will assume that there is no problem with that food. However, because the immune system can react to foods in ways that do not involve IgE, the possibility of a problem remains even if tests for IgE-type sensitivity are normal. Also, it is possible that a child may react adversely to a food in a way that does not involve the immune system at all. The bottom line is that IgE-based tests are simply not reliable for diagnosing all the foods a child may have problems with.

THE CYTOTOXIC AND ALCAT TEST

The cytotoxic test is performed by mixing immune cells with individual food extracts and then ascertaining which foods caused reactions in the immune cells. This test is usually interpreted by a technician who uses a microscope to assess whether the immune cells have reacted and to what degree. In this sense, the test may be affected by human error and there is much doubt about the reproducibility and consistency of these tests. I don't generally recommend them.

A better option is probably the ALCAT blood test. ALCAT stands for the 'antigen leucocyte cellular antibody test'. It is quite similar to the cytotoxic test, except that the white cells' reactions to foodstuffs is measured by a sophisticated piece of laboratory equipment rather than a technician. ALCAT is probably more accurate than cytotoxic testing, but it's usually more expensive too.

IGG TESTING

Blood tests for IgG antibodies are available, and tend to give relatively consistent and useful results. There are two basic techniques used, RAST (radioallergosorbent test) and ELISA (enzyme-linked immunoserological assay). It is believed that ELISA is more sensitive than RAST, and it's generally cheaper too. Of all the blood tests for non-IgE related food sensitivity, this is probably the best one.

ELECTRO-DERMAL TESTING

Practitioners of Chinese medicine believe that energy flows down tracts known as meridians in the body. In the 1950s a German doctor by the name of Reinholdt Voll discovered that you could derive much information about the health status of the body by measuring the electrical current flowing through the acupuncture points. Electro-dermal testing involves measuring the electrical current that flows through an acupuncture point, and then detecting any changes in this as the body is challenged with individual foods. In this form of testing, foods are often tested by putting them in a very low-voltage electrical circuit, which is passed through the subject being tested. If the presence of the food in the circuit changes the amount of current flowing through the individual, then this suggests that there is a problem with the food. Some more sophisticated devices have foods stored on a computer in the form of the electromagnetic 'fingerprint' of that food.

In skilled hands, this method seems to give good results, which are instantaneous. Electro-dermal testing is relatively cheap compared to the blood tests that are available for diagnosing food sensitivity. Because it is economical and instantaneous, I like this form of testing, but I think it helps to find a practitioner who has had plenty of testing experience.

APPLIED KINESIOLOGY

This is similar to electro-dermal testing except that the practitioner measures muscle strength in response to foods rather than the electrical current flowing through the body. Typically, muscle strength is first ascertained by the practitioner pressing down on the subject's outstretched arm. This is repeated while challenging the subject with foods either by having them hold them close to their body or by putting samples of food under the tongue. Like electro-dermal testing, the results are thought to be relatively accurate in skilled hands and the results are instantaneous. Again, testing tends to be inexpensive compared to blood tests for food intolerance. It's also a good choice for kids because it circumvents the need for a blood sample to be drawn.

THE ELIMINATION DIET

The elimination diet is regarded by many practitioners of nutritional medicine as the most accurate way of testing for food sensitivity. The concept is simple: all likely problem foods are removed from the diet for a period of time. Once the symptoms or conditions being treated reduce or disappear, foods are added back into the diet, one at a time, and a note is made of which foods cause a recurrence of the symptoms.

Knowing which foods to eliminate from the diet is an art in itself. Sometimes it can help to keep a food diary. This involves making a note of everything that passes your child's lips for a week or so. Record the time that each item is eaten or drunk, along with the approximate quantities, on the left-hand side of a piece of paper or notebook. On the right-hand page, record any symptoms you notice, the time they occur and how long they last. Obviously this is easier with older children, who will be able to tell you how they feel, or may even keep the diary themselves. With younger children you may want to note down any obvious changes in behaviour, any rashes or hives that might appear, any changes in bowel movements, or anything unusual.

At the end of a week or so, go through the diary, looking for recurring patterns. You may notice that your child becomes slightly moody after having cereal in the morning, or suffers a headache after eating a piece of cheese. However, while food diaries may help pinpoint foods for testing, they have limitations. One major problem is that reactions to foods can be very delayed – often by a few hours, and maybe by even a day or two. This makes looking for associations between food and symptoms difficult. Also, a child may be eating or drinking a problem food several times a day (e.g. wheat or milk) with the result that the symptoms are so frequent as to make looking for a pattern quite impossible.

REMOVING FOODS FROM A DIET

Sometimes, the best thing is to simply take foods out of a child's diet to see what effect this has. With kids, I recommend starting with the following foods:

- Dairy products such as milk, cheese, yoghurt and ice cream
- Wheat (including bread, pasta, pastry, biscuits, wheat-based snacks, wheat-containing cereal bars, cakes and wheat-based or wheat-containing breakfast cereals)
- Any food your child craves or doesn't seem to be able to do without.

The rationale behind removing these foods from the diet is as follows:

Dairy products

Dairy products are a common cause of food sensitivity in children (and adults). Be particularly suspicious of a problem if your child suffered colic as a baby, or suffers from frequent colds, a runny nose, ear problems or sore throats and/or tonsillitis. While we generally accept the idea of drinking milk and eating dairy products, these foods are relatively new to the human species in terms of our evolution (we have consumed milk for about only the last 10,000 years of our two or more million years on this planet). It's worth bearing in mind that cow's milk (and milk from any species other than human beings for that matter) is not designed for our consumption, which helps to explain why many of us do not seem to tolerate it that well. The main problem with dairy foods seems to be the protein molecules within them. Pasteurisation is believed to change the nature of dairy proteins, which does seem to increase the likelihood of us having a reaction to them. In addition, some people may react to the milk sugar (lactose) found in milk, and to a lesser degree, in ice cream, yoghurt and cheese. For more details about this condition (lactose intolerance), see pages 104–5. One dairy product that tends to be well tolerated is butter, which may be because it contains relatively low levels of both protein and lactose.

Wheat

Like dairy products, wheat is a relatively recent addition to the human diet (about 10,000 years). Not only that, but wheat is one grain that has been modified over the years using plant breeding techniques. In other words, the type of wheat we eat now is often quite different from the wheat we originally started eating all those years ago.

It seems to be true that the more of a food we eat, the more likely we are to develop a sensitivity to it. These days, it's not uncommon for a child to eat wheat in significant quantity several times a day. The same, by the way, is often true for dairy products too.

Food cravings

Children sometimes crave and become quite wedded to the very foods that they are sensitive to. A child, for instance, who loves bread and pasta is quite likely to be wheat sensitive. One that loves milk and must have some before bedtime, is probably harbouring a dairy problem. What causes this phenomenon is not known for sure, though it's probably not too dissimilar from the cravings that individuals can get for other things that are not good for the body such as nicotine, alcohol and caffeine.

Finding alternative foods

Taking foods out of the diet is one thing, finding something to replace it with is another. The chart below includes a list of the most common food sensitivities, and some viable alternatives.

REPLACEMENT FOODS FOR COMMON SENSITIVITIES	
Problem foodstuff	**Alternative**
Wheat-based bread	100 per cent rye bread / Rye crackers Rye pumpernickel bread / Rice cakes / Oat cakes
Wheat-based breakfast cereals	Oat muesli / Porridge (oatmeal)/ Cornflakes / Puffed rice Multi-grain cereals based on non-wheat grains such as amaranth, millet and rice
Pasta (durum wheat)	Vegetable, rice and corn-based pasta
Egg noodles	Rice noodles
Gluten-containing food	Rice cakes / Rice / Rice noodles
(wheat, oats, rye and barley)	Vegetable, rice and corn-based pasta Potato / Polenta (corn meal)
Cow's milk	Goat's milk / Rice milk
Cow's cheese	Goat's cheese / Sheep's cheese (e.g. feta) / Buffalo mozzarella
Cow's yoghurt	Sheep's yoghurt / Goat's yoghurt / Soya yoghurt

If your child does suffer from a food sensitivity, he or she may well be feeling much better after a week or two on this regime. Many children (and, indeed, adults) whose health issues are linked with food sensitivity find they experience a sudden improvement in their condition, along with increased energy, enhanced mental clarity and less problematic digestive function.

As is the case with general detoxification, it is not uncommon for sensitive children to experience withdrawal reactions during the initial phase of an elimination diet. A gnawing hunger, nasal stuffiness, inability to concentrate, fatigue, grumpiness, insomnia and nervousness are not uncommon symptoms of this. These reactions normally last for a few days and very rarely longer than a week. The symptoms can often be lessened if a child takes some vitamin C (250–500 mg every couple of hours or so).

Re-testing foods

If your child is feeling better after a couple of weeks on the elimination diet, it's time to start testing foods. Take one of the foods that has been eliminated, and offer a substantial portion of it one morning. A glass of milk at breakfast is an example. Over the next few hours, you will need to look out for any symptoms that suggest food sensitivity. These include headache, itching, depression, fatigue, irritability and foggy thinking. If you see any reaction, make a note that the provoking food is one of your child's sensitivities, and eliminate it again from his or her diet. If there is no reaction to the first exposure to the food, try it again at lunch and dinner. If by the following morning your child is totally free from symptoms, add it provisionally to your safe list of foods.

For the next three days, re-eliminate the food and keep a watchful eye out for any symptoms that suggest a food reaction. It is possible that the symptoms of a reaction can come on two or three days after a food or drink is consumed. If such a reaction occurs, then you should suspect this food. If your child still feels well after the three-day break, you can be pretty sure the foodstuff you are testing is fine. In this way, proceed through the major foods you have eliminated, making a note of safe and unsafe foods as you go.

Overcoming food sensitivities

The first step in overcoming food sensitivities is to avoid the problem foodstuff(s). In normal circumstances, it is wise for problem foods to be excluded from your child's diet for at least a month. Two months is better if you can manage it. Abstaining from a food for a period of time can make the body more tolerant to the food in the long term. However, with regard to food reintroduction, there are a few things that need to be borne in mind:

1 INITIALLY, FOOD REACTIONS CAN BE WORSE, NOT BETTER, THAN BEFORE

For some time (often a month or two) after the point of exclusion, it is common for an adverse reaction to a foodstuff to be worse than it was before. This is often referred to as 'hypersensitivity'. Care needs to be taken, therefore, when dealing with potentially serious medical conditions such as asthma. Elimination and reintroduction of foods is sometimes better done under the supervision of a nutritionally oriented doctor for this reason.

2 WHEN A FOOD IS REINTRODUCED, IT IS BEST NOT TO SERVE TOO MUCH OF IT, TOO FREQUENTLY

It is usually possible to reintroduce a problem food back into the diet and not have problems with it. However, if that food is eaten in relatively large quantities and/or is eaten quite frequently, then this increases the risk of the original problems recurring. It is a good idea when reintroducing problem foods to eat them in 'rotation'. What this means is only offering the food once every three or four days. So, for example, toast for breakfast on Sunday followed by a pasta supper on Wednesday but no other wheat in between is unlikely to re-ignite the original symptoms that led to you excluding wheat in the first place.

While occasional eating of problem foods is unlikely to cause problems, it's a good idea not to push it as this generally leads to a re-emergence of the original problem. In general, my advice is to avoid your child having problem foods when you can, and not to worry about it when you can't.

3 IN THE LONG TERM, FOOD SENSITIVITIES CAN BE REDUCED BY IMPROVING DIGESTION

The better a child digests food, the less likely he is to absorb it in a partially digested form, and the lower his risk of food sensitivity. Two simple strategies for improving overall digestion are:

CHEWING FOOD THOROUGHLY

Proper chewing is essential for proper digestion. Chewing stimulates the secretion of acid and digestive enzymes. Chewing also mixes food with saliva, which contains an enzyme important for the digestion of starchy foods such as bread, potatoes, rice and pasta. And perhaps most importantly of all, chewing breaks food up, massively increasing the surface area available for contact with the digestive juices. This increases the efficiency of digestion by giving digestive enzymes the opportunity to penetrate the food and do their digestive work. Encouraging your child to chew mouthfuls of food to a cream before swallowing will help reduce the risk of food sensitivity, and will also help him or her get maximum nutritional value from the food being eaten. Family meals (see page 195) are a good forum for teaching the art of thorough chewing.

AVOID DRINKING WITH MEALS

Some children tend to drink quite a lot of fluid with meals and believe this can only help to 'wash food down'. The reality is quite the reverse. Drinking with meals dilutes the acid and enzymes that do the digestive work, and does nothing to help the process of digestion. The odd glass of water with a meal is unlikely to present any problem. However, encourage your child to do the bulk of his or her drinking between meals, and not at meal time.

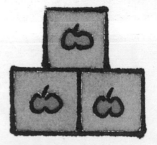

SUPPLEMENTS FOR FOOD SENSITIVITY

Multivitamins and minerals

Children with food sensitivity issues will often benefit from supplementation with a good quality multivitamin and mineral. This helps nourish the lining of the digestive tract and make it less prone to leaking partially digested food into the bloodstream where it may provoke food sensitivity reactions. Another benefit of supplementation is that it can help ensure a child does not run into problems in the long term as a result of the nutrient deficiencies related to a more restricted diet. More details about appropriate multivitamin and mineral supplements can be found on pages 14–16.

Probiotics

Probiotic (healthy gut bacteria) supplements are useful too, as these can help improve digestive function and enhance the health of the gut wall. Children with food sensitivity issues are often helped by taking a probiotic supplement for two to three months. More details about probiotic supplements for children can be found on pages 16–17.

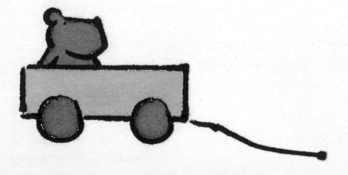

Yeast overgrowth

The inside of the gut is not a sterile environment, but full of dozens of different organisms, mostly bacteria that are beneficial for the digestive tract and for general health. In fact, the adult gut contains about 1.5–2 kg (3–4 lb) of bacteria, which assist in digestion, keep unhealthy organisms at bay, and also help to ensure that the lining of the gut remains healthy. Another type of organism that might be found in the digestive tract is yeast (including a species known as *Candida albicans*). In healthy individuals, levels of yeast in the gut are low and it may not even be present at all. However, under certain circumstances yeast can overgrow in a child's gut and this may give rise to a number of symptoms including abdominal bloating, wind, fatigue, sweet or starch cravings, thrush (vaginal yeast infection) and athlete's foot. In children with food sensitivity issues (see above), yeast overgrowth is a common problem too. One reason for this could be that yeast overgrowth may impair the digestion of food and increase the likelihood of 'leakiness' in the gut wall – both factors that would tend to make reactions to food more likely.

Yeast overgrowth (sometimes referred to as candida) is not a diagnosis that is commonly made in conventional medicine. In fact, many doctors dismiss the notion of yeast overgrowth as the stuff of fantasy. Nevertheless, I do see it as quite a common problem in children and one that often responds well to a natural approach.

What causes yeast overgrowth?

Antibiotics are a major, perhaps the major factor, in candida overgrowth. Designed to kill harmful bacteria in the body, they can kill healthy bacteria too. Yet, they do not kill yeast. As a result, antibiotics can lead to a predominance of yeast in the gut. While recent years have seen doctors exercising a little bit more caution and restraint in their prescribing of antibiotics, the fact remains that they are still a mainstay treatment for common childhood ailments. Yeast overgrowth is believed to be a relatively modern-day complaint, which is almost certainly linked to the antibiotic age in which we live.

DOES YOUR CHILD HAVE CANDIDA?

The following questionnaire is designed to help you ascertain whether yeast overgrowth is a factor in your child. Score each question as indicated, and then add up your total score.

1 Are your child's bowel movements somewhat erratic, perhaps constipated some of the time, and on the loose side at others?

No – 0 points
Occasional or mild problems – 2 points
Frequent or severe problems – 4 points

2 Does your child appear to suffer from excessive wind and flatulence?

No – 0 points
Occasional or mild problems – 2 points
Frequent or severe problems – 4 points

3 Does your child suffer from significant abdominal bloating?

No – 0 points
Occasional or mild problems – 2 points
Frequent or severe problems – 4 points

4 Does your child suffer from anal itching, not related to worms (see page 43)?

No – 0 points
Occasional or mild problems – 2 points
Frequent or severe problems – 4 points

5 If your child is a girl, has she ever had a vaginal yeast infection (thrush)?

No – 0 points
Occasional or mild problems – 3 points
Frequent or severe problems – 6 points

6 Does your child suffer from episodes of poor concentration, mental fatigue, low mood or irritability?

No – 0 points
Occasional or mild problems – 2 points
Frequent or severe problems – 4 points

7 Does your child suffer from skin problems such as athlete's foot, generalised itching or a rash between his buttocks or in his groin?

No – 0 points
Occasional or mild problems – 3 points
Frequent or severe problems – 6 points

8 Does your child crave sugar, sugary foods such as chocolate, biscuits or cakes, or yeasty foods such as cheese, bread or vinegar?

No – 0 points
Occasional or mild problems – 2 points
Frequent or severe problems – 4 points

9 How would you describe your child's antibiotic consumption in the past?

Very few antibiotics generally – 0 points
Moderate use for occasional infections such as winter infections, chest infections, etc. – 5 points
Frequent and/or extended use for problems such as acne, recurrent urinary tract infections, chronic sinusitis, tonsillitis, ear infections, etc. – 10 points

10 Has your child ever had inhaled steroids (usually for asthma) such as Becotide for three months or more?
No – 0 points
Yes – 4 points

11 Does your child have a number of vague health problems that no one has been able to explain?
No – 0 points
Yes – 4 points

Interpreting the score
0 – 7: *Yeast overgrowth is unlikely.*
8 – 18: *Yeast overgrowth should be considered as a possibility and further testing or a trial of the anti-candida regime is likely to be worthwhile.*
19 – 29: *Yeast overgrowth is likely, and steps taken to combat yeast are very likely to help improve weight loss and general health.*
30 and above: *Yeast overgrowth is very likely, and steps taken to combat this are almost certainly going to improve weight loss and general health.*

If your child has scored highly or moderately on the questionnaire, you may wish to confirm whether or not your child has a yeast problem with some sort of testing. There are several different types, including blood and stool tests, as well as dowsing and applied kinesiology. Although these tests all have their own merits, particularly if the assessment is carried out by an experienced and skilled practitioner, it is usually possible to diagnose yeast overgrowth by looking carefully for the symptoms and underlying factors that are typical in the condition.

The anti-yeast diet

The cornerstone of the anti-yeast approach is a diet that helps starve this organism out of the system. This means no foods that feed yeast directly, or encourage yeast by being yeasty, mouldy or fermented in their own right. It might sound a bit strict for the average child, but given that they will not have had as long for the condition to become deep-seated, the diet should probably only need to be undertaken for a month or two to get good results. Also, the diet does not generally need to be strictly enforced for it to work.

YEAST-FEEDING FOODS TO AVOID
- Sugar
- Sweetening agents such as maple syrup, molasses, honey and malt syrup
- Sugar containing foods such as biscuits, cakes, confectionery, ice cream, pastries, sugared breakfast cereals, soft drinks and fruit juice
- White flour products including white bread, crackers, pizza and pasta

YEASTY, MOULDY OR FERMENTED FOODS TO AVOID
- Bread and other yeast-raised items
- Yeast extract spreads such as Marmite and Vegemite
- Alcoholic drinks, particularly beer and wine, which are very yeasty (this may be relevant for older teenagers and adolescents)
- Gravy mixes (most contain brewer's yeast)
- Vinegar and vinegar containing foods such as ketchup (which also contains sugar), mustard, mayonnaise and many prepared salad dressings
- Pickles, miso, tempeh and soy sauce (all fermented)
- Aged cheeses including Cheddar, Stilton, Swiss, Brie and Camembert (cheese is inherently mouldy)
- Peanuts (and peanut butter) and pistachios (tend to harbour yeast)
- Mushrooms (mushrooms are mould!)
- Dried fruit (are intensely sugary and tend to harbour mould)
- Yeast-containing foods such as soups and pre-packaged foods

Individuals who have a yeast overgrowth problem are likely to have food sensitivities, particularly to wheat and/or dairy products (see pages 211–22). The safest bet, therefore, is for these foods to be minimised too while a child is on the anti-yeast diet.

FOODS TO EAT FREELY

The foods that are generally very safe to eat on an anti-yeast regime are listed below.

Protein foods
- Eggs
- Fish including naturally smoked fish
- Shellfish
- Chicken
- Turkey
- Lamb
- Beef
- Pork
- Duck
- Tofu (soya bean curd)

Vegetables
- Lettuce
- Tomato
- Cucumber
- Celery
- Cabbage
- Broccoli
- Cauliflower
- Spinach
- Chard
- Kale
- Watercress

- Brussels sprouts
- Asparagus
- Onion
- Leek
- Green beans
- Parsnips
- Aubergine
- Artichoke
- Avocado

FOODS TO BE EATEN IN MODERATION

Certain foods such as grains, high-starch vegetables, legumes or pulses can be eaten on an anti-candida regime, but it's best not to offer masses of them because they do tend to have some fermentation potential. The bulk of the diet should be based around the foods that can be eaten freely, supplemented with more limited amounts of the foods that follow in this list:

High starch vegetables
- Potatoes
- Sweet potatoes
- Squash (e.g. butternut)
- Pulses
- Lentils
- Split peas
- Kidney beans
- Navy beans
- Lima beans
- Black beans
- Adzuki beans

Grains
- Yeast-free rye bread
- Rye crackers
- Brown rice
- Wild rice
- Rice cakes
- Barley
- Millet
- Corn
- Rye
- Oats, oat cakes and oat-based breakfast cereals

- Buckwheat
- Quinoa
- Spelt
- Brown rice cakes

WHAT ABOUT FRUIT?

Whether or not fruit is advisable on an anti-yeast regime is a real moot point. Some practitioners say it can be eaten freely, others say it should be completely excluded, at least to begin with. I have to say, I take the middle ground, partly because kids need the nutrients from fruit (and they are less likely to want to get key vitamins and minerals from vegetables) and also because they represent an easy way to encourage good nutrition in kids. My experience is that one or two pieces of fruit a day are generally very well tolerated, though I'm no fan of grapes, which are intensely sugary and usually covered in a mouldy bloom. All fruit that you're not going to peel prior to eating should be washed thoroughly. Dried fruits, as mentioned before, are out.

SUPPLEMENTS FOR COMBATING YEAST

Probiotics

Probiotics (healthy gut bacteria) are extreme useful in helping eradicate yeast from the body. One effect they seem to have is to 'crowd out' the yeast in the gut. They are also essential for replacing the bacteria whose loss is often the starting point for yeast overgrowth in the gut. I recommend probiotics for three to four months. Advice on and recommendations for specific supplements can be found on pages 15–16.

Multivitamins and minerals

In addition, it also helps for children to take a multivitamin and mineral supplement. This helps nourish the lining of the digestive tract and reduces the risk of any nutrient deficiencies that may come as a result of a restricted diet. More details about specific multivitamin and mineral formulations can be found on pages 16–17.

Fatty acid imbalance

In Chapter 1, I explored the role of the different sorts of dietary fats in health. In particular, I looked at the potentially health-giving effects of fats known as polyunsaturated fats in the diet. Just to re-cap, polyunsaturated fats are found in two main types in the diet: omega-3 fatty acids and omega-6 fatty acids. The major omega-6 fatty acid in the diet is known as linoleic acid, which is found most abundantly in plant oils such as hemp, pumpkin, sunflower, safflower, sesame, corn, walnut and soya oil. The major omega-3 fatty acids in the diet come in the form of alpha-linolenic acid (from plant sources such as flaxseed) and fats known as eicosapentaenoic acid (EPA) and docosahexaenoic acid (DHA), which are mainly found in oily varieties of fish. Linoleic acid, alpha linolenic acid, EPA and DHA are often referred to as essential fatty acids (EFAs).

Both omega-3 and omega-6 fats have important roles to play in the body, though their actions are roughly antagonistic. What this means is that the relative amounts of these two main types of fat in the body are critical to health. Some scientists believe that the ideal ratio of omega-6:omega-3 fats in the diet is 1:1. However, there is evidence that many children may be deficient in essential fatty acids. In particular, children may suffer from a relative deficiency of omega-3 compared to omega-6 fatty acids, and this may have profound implications for health.

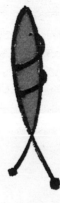

IS YOUR CHILD SUFFERING FROM AN OMEGA-3 DEFICIENCY?

Apart from the learning and behavioural problems, such as dyslexia and hyperactivity, there are other tell-tale signs of a deficiency in the omega-3 essential fats. The following questionnaire is designed to help identify a deficiency in your child.

1 If your child is an adolescent girl, does she suffer from PMS or breast pain?

No – 0 points

Occasional or mild symptoms – 2 points

Frequent or severe problems – 4 points

2 Does your child suffer from eczema or dry skin?

No – 0 points

Occasional or mild symptoms – 2 points

Frequent or severe problems – 4 points

3 Does your child suffer from dry eyes?

No – 0 points

Occasional or mild symptoms – 2 points

Frequent or severe problems – 4 points

4 Does your child suffer from dry hair?

No – 0 points

Occasional or mild symptoms – 2 points

Frequent or severe problems – 4 points

5 Does your child suffer from excessive thirst?

No – 0 points

Occasional or mild symptoms – 2 points

Frequent or severe problems – 4 points

6 Does your child suffer from water retention?

No – 0 points

Occasional or mild symptoms – 2 points

Frequent or severe problems – 4 points

7 Does your child suffer from a learning or behavioural disorder?

No – 0 points

Occasional or mild symptoms – 3 points

Frequent or severe problems – 6 points

8 Does your child suffer from lack of coordination?

No – 0 points

Occasional or mild symptoms – 3 points

Frequent or severe problems – 6 points

Interpreting the score

0 – 10: *EFA imbalance is unlikely.*

11 – 20: *EFA imbalance is likely.*

21 and above: *EFA imbalance is very likely.*

What are the problems associated with a deficiency of omega-3 fats?

One of the fundamental roles of omega-3 fats is in the structure and function of the brain. DHA is believed to be important in the building of the brain during pregnancy and in maintaining its growth and development after birth. EPA is also important and seems to play some role in the day-to-day running of the brain.

A deficiency of omega-3 fats can manifest in a number of ways including dyslexia (see page 77), dyspraxia (see page 78) and attention deficit hyperactivity disorder (see pages 38–41). In the long term, a deficiency of omega-3 fats is thought to lead to potential problems with inflammation in the body (e.g. arthritis) and an increased risk of circulatory diseases such as heart disease and stroke.

What causes essential fatty acid imbalance?

Essential fatty acid imbalance appears to be a relatively new phenomenon and may reflect changes in food manufacturing, methods of animal rearing and food choices. The last half-century has seen an explosion of the use of partially hydrogenated fats and trans fatty acids in processed foods (see pages 156–7 for more details about these fats). These fats are unhealthy in their own right, but also seem to interfere with the body's ability to utilise whatever healthy EFAs it gets in the diet.

The way animals are farmed and reared these days also does not bode well for our intake of EFAs. Wild and grass-fed animals tend to be quite rich in omega-3 fats. However, more intensively reared and grain-fed animals tend to contain much less in the way of omega-3 fats, and more omega-6 in their flesh. Farmed fish are also generally lower in omega-3 than wild varieties.

Another gradual but profound change in our diet in recent decades has been a reduction in consumption in foods rich in omega-3 fats (such as oily fish) coupled with a significant increase in foods rich in omega-6 fats (such as fast and processed foods). Another critical factor in the balance of EFAs in a child's body relates to how it is fed early on in life. Breast milk is generally rich in omega-3 fats, while formula feed is not. Problems can even start before birth, for instance if a mother's intake of omega-3 fats is low during pregnancy (Chapters 5 and 6 deal with these issues in more detail).

Correcting an EFA imbalance

For many children, ensuring a greater intake of omega-3 fats is key to improving and maintaining their health. Good sources of omega 3-oils include oily fish such as salmon, trout, mackerel, herring and sardine. Including these in the diet (say, twice a week) is a good idea if a child will eat them.

Fish oil supplementation

Concentrated fish oil supplements (which contain EPA and DHA) are probably the best bet for non-vegetarian children. It's not always easy getting kids to take fish oils, however. The capsules tend to be large and may be difficult to swallow. BioCare make a small children's capsule that contains 79 mg of DHA and 52 mg of EPA. For younger children, the capsules may be opened into food each day. EPA and DHA have a fishy odour and are therefore best added to strong tasting food such as a soup, stew or casserole.

Two capsules of this supplement each day will provide a good long-term dose for children. However, if there are signs of EFA imbalance, and particularly if the child has learning or behavioural difficulties, four to six capsules a day is a better dose for two to three months in order to get omega-3 levels up in the body. (For more details, see Useful contacts and information – under BioCare.)

For vegetarian children

Vegetarian children for whom oily fish and fish oil supplements are not options have other alternatives.

Vegetarian DHA: Vegetarian DHA (derived from algae) do exist. One suitable supplement is Healthspan's Cerebrum vegetarian DHA. (For more details, see Useful contacts and information.)

Flaxseed oil: Flaxseed oil is rich in alpha-linolenic acid, which may then be converted to EPA and DHA in the body. However, it is believed that this conversion can be slow in many individuals. Nutrients may help this conversion, however, so in addition to supplementing with flaxseed oil, it can help to take a good quality multivitamin and mineral supplement each day too. Advice on specific supplements can be found on pages 15–16. A good dose for children is 10–15 ml (2–3 tsp) of flaxseed oil a day.

Hemp seed oil: Hemp seed oil (oil from the seeds of the hemp plant) is also rich in alpha-linolenic acid, but is actually richer in linoleic acid (an omega-6 fatty acid). I find hemp seed oil particularly useful for remedying dry skin and eczema. Cold-pressed hemp seed oil is available from Fitzsimmons Herbals. (For more details, see Useful contacts and information.) I recommend giving 10–15 ml (2–3 tsp) per day.

Key points

- Blood sugar imbalance, food sensitivity, yeast overgrowth and an imbalance in certain healthy fats (essential fatty acids) in the diet are common problems in children and may be at the root of many specific symptoms or conditions.
- Blood sugar imbalance may manifest as fluctuating energy levels, mood swings and cravings for sweet foods.
- The basic dietary approach to this problem is to eat a diet based on foods that release sugar slowly into the bloodstream (low glycaemic index foods).
- Regular meals, perhaps with healthy snacks in between, will also help blood sugar stability.
- Supplementing with nutrients may help to improve blood sugar balance.
- Food sensitivity can cause a wide range of symptoms, including ear infections, throat infections, eczema, asthma and irritable bowel syndrome.
- The most common foods to cause problem are dairy products and wheat.
- After identification and elimination of problems foods, it is usually possible for a child to eat them in moderation without ill effect.
- Improving digestion and nourishing the gut may help reduce the risk of food sensitivity in the long term.
- Yeast overgrowth in the body is common after treatment with antibiotics, and can give rise to problems with abdominal bloating, fatigue and fungal skin infections.
- The main dietary approach to this problem is to starve yeast out of the body by avoiding foods such as sugar, refined carbohydrates and yeasty, mouldy or fermented foods.
- At the same time, it generally helps to take a supplement of healthy gut bacteria (probiotic).
- A deficiency of healthy fats in the diet (particularly omega-3 fatty acids) may manifest in a variety of ways, including behavioural or learning problems, dry skin, dry hair and excessive thirst.
- Emphasising plenty of essential fatty acids in the diet, especially oily fish, will help to ensure a child gets adequate amounts of omega-3 fatty acids.
- Fish oil supplementation may be a useful adjunct or alternative to this.
- For vegetarian children, supplementation with vegetarian DHA, flaxseed oil or hemp seed oil are other options.

Chapter 5
Another baby?

Over the past 20 years or so there has been increasing interest in the role that nutrition plays in pregnancy. The raw materials that go into making a baby growing in the womb come from the mother's diet. While we are what we eat, a new-born baby is made of what his or her mother ate during pregnancy. Later in this chapter I look at the foods and nutrients that help make for a healthy baby, and a healthy pregnancy too.

While there is good evidence that diet plays a critical role during pregnancy, research also points to the importance of nutritional factors in the mother even before conception. For instance, certain dietary factors are known to influence fertility. Also, the supply of certain nutrients seems to be very important during the very early development of a foetus. Birth defects (for example, spina bifida) generally develop in the first few weeks of pregnancy and these may be prevented through adequate intakes of nutrients, such as folic acid. The role of this, and other nutrients, prior to pregnancy will be discussed here. This chapter starts with some of the most important nutritional considerations for women (and their partners) who are planning a pregnancy.

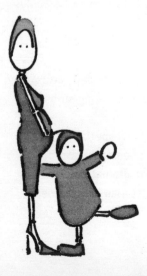

Why weight?

One of the health factors that may have a significant bearing on a woman's fertility and the progression of her pregnancy is her weight. It seems that both too much and too little in the way of body weight increase the risk of certain complications. A lot of the evidence for this comes from studies where scientists have looked at the relationship between weight and the health of women and their children during pregnancy. These studies generally assess weight using a measurement known as the body mass index (BMI). I'm not a great fan of this sort of measurement, and believe that a healthy weight is better judged by personal criteria such as what an individual feels is right for her. Plus, the BMI tells us something about weight, but tells us nothing about body make-up. Someone who is of big build with reasonably well-developed muscles may turn out to have a raised BMI despite not having much in the way of body fat. Nevertheless, the studies I'm going to refer to are based on the BMI, so it's useful for you to know what this is – see below.

BODY MASS INDEX

The BMI is a popular method for assessing weight, and is thought to be a big improvement on the height and weight tables that originated in the 1950s. The BMI is calculated by dividing an individual's weight in kilograms by the square of their height in metres.

weight in kg $\div$ (height in m)^2

The higher the BMI, the heavier a person is. BMI results have been split into bands. BMIs of between 20 and 25 are generally regarded as healthy. BMIs of less than 19 (underweight) or more than 25 (overweight) are generally regarded as unhealthy. The chart opposite allows you to calculate your BMI and the band you're in.

HEIGHT (CM)

BMI (BODY MASS INDEX)

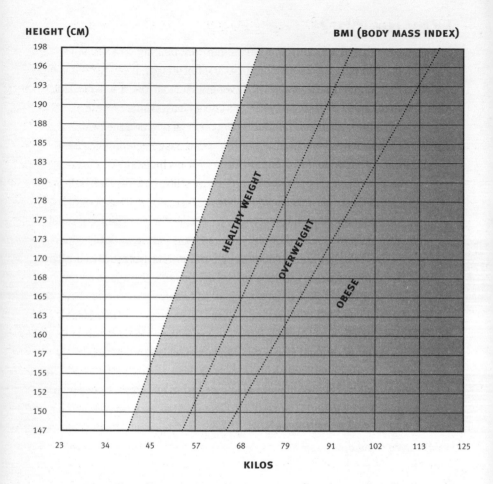

KILOS

Overweight and pregnancy

Carrying more weight than is ideal during pregnancy has been associated with a number of complications. Excess weight is associated with an increased risk of infertility. Also, there is evidence that even after successful conception with an infertility treatment such as IVF (*in vitro* fertilisation), overweight women are less likely to carry this pregnancy to term.[1] Also, even if the pregnancy proceeds successfully, excess maternal weight appears to increase the risk of the baby being born smaller than average.[2] A child born with low birth weight seems to be at increased risk of a number of health issues in later life, including heart disease and diabetes (see page 73). There are now several studies showing that overweight women are at increased risk of having children with neural tube defects (such as spina bifida) and other birth defects.[3] One study found that taking folic acid (usually effective in preventing neural tube defects) did not appear to reduce the risk of defects in children born to obese women.[4]

Excess weight has potential consequences not just for the child, but the mother also. Even moderate levels of excess weight (a BMI in excess of 25) appear to be a risk factor for several pregnancy-related problems including:
- Gestational diabetes (diabetes in pregnancy)
- Pregnancy induced hypertension (high blood pressure in pregnancy)
- Increased risk of problems with sugar metabolism and/or blood pressure later in life
- Pre-eclampsia (see page 125)
- Abnormal labour
- Emergency Caesarean section.[5]

While the evidence shows that too much weight is not ideal for a healthy pregnancy, too little weight poses hazards too.

Underweight and pregnancy

In a culture that celebrates the physique of the super-model, it is sometimes hard to imagine that being stick-thin is anything but desirable. However, one major problem with low maternal weight is that it can reflect on the weight of the baby. In short, women with low BMIs are at increased risk of having a low birth weight baby.[6] One study found that women who were underweight prior to conception who achieved good weight gain during the pregnancy itself, still had a significantly increased risk of having a low birth weight baby.[7]

Several studies have found that low birth weight is a risk factor for high blood pressure in children, and even in subsequent adulthood too. This is important because high blood pressure (hypertension) is a risk factor for other conditions, including heart disease and stroke. There is also a link between low birth weight and the risk of developing diabetes later in life (Type II diabetes).[8]

Weight control prior to pregnancy

Attaining a healthy weight prior to pregnancy appears to have a number of benefits, including enhanced fertility, a reduced risk of complications in pregnancy and labour, and a healthier baby too. The core approach to healthy weight regulation is a healthy diet. In recent years, the dietetic establishment has advocated that we eat a diet based around carbohydrate foods such as bread, potatoes, rice, pasta and cereals. However, there are significant problems associated with eating too many carbs, especially those that release sugar quickly into the bloodstream (see pages 149–51). Experiments in both animals and humans show, for instance, that carbohydrate eating can lead to changes in the body's metabolism, which can lead to weight gain in the long term.[9]

Equally, for those wanting to gain weight healthily, a carbohydrate rich diet is not a necessarily good thing either. Eating a carb-rich diet has been linked with a variety of problems including heart disease and diabetes.[10] Also, many of the starches commonly eaten in the diet are refined and offer relatively low levels of fibre and nutrients. In general, I think the value of potatoes and grain-based starches in the diet has been seriously over-stated.

While we have generally been encouraged to base our diet on carbohydrate, we have also been warned of the perils of eating too much fat. However, what often gets lost in this message is that some fats, such as those found in oily fish, extra virgin olive oil, nuts, seeds and avocado, are positively healthy. Some of these fats have been linked with better foetal growth and brain development during pregnancy (see pages 245–6). Also, contrary to popular opinion, there seems to be little or no relationship between dietary fat and body weight.[11] As far as general health goes, the research suggests that it's the quality of the fat in the diet that is important, not the quantity. Plenty of healthy fats in the diet is a good thing, and moderate amounts of saturated fat (e.g. red meat, butter) seem compatible with a healthy diet too. The fats to avoid are the so-called trans fatty acids (also known as partially hydrogenated fats) found in many margarines and in most processed and fast foods. More about these thoroughly unhealthy man-made fats can be found on pages 157–8.

Whether you are seeking to lose weight, gain it, or neither, the best dietary approach is to eat a diet based on whole, natural foods, in as unprocessed and unadulterated a form as possible. More details about fundamentals of a healthy diet can be found in Chapters 1 and 2.

Fine-tuning approaches for pre-conceptual weight loss

While eating as natural a diet as possible is often effective in reducing weight, specific approaches are sometimes necessary. More details about the role of diet (and exercise) in weight control can be found in the section on childhood obesity (see pages 119–23). The recommendations in this section are utterly relevant to adults too.

Sometimes, however, I find that very specific issues can be causing problems with weight gain. Try as they might, some women do find losing weight difficult despite doing all the right things. If this sounds like you, then it is just possible that you may have one or more of these specific issues that can contribute to a weight problem.

1 Blood sugar imbalance

Peaks of blood sugar generally stimulate the body to secrete copious quantities of the hormone insulin, which can convert sugar in the body into fat. Symptoms suggestive of blood sugar imbalance include fluctuating energy with lethargy being a particular problem in the mid–late afternoon and cravings for sweet foods. Individuals with this issue are often simply eating too much carbohydrate. Taking steps to stabilise blood sugar levels can be very effective in bringing down weight. More information on how to go about doing this can be found on pages 204–11.

2 Food sensitivity

Some individuals react to foods in a way that can cause unwanted symptoms, including weight gain. Any food, in theory, might do this, but wheat is a very common culprit. Some individuals get wedded to the very foods that are causing problems for them. For instance, individuals with wheat sensitivity may love pasta and/or bread. See pages 211–22 for more details about the diagnosis and treatment of food sensitivity issues.

3 Yeast overgrowth

In certain circumstances (particularly after treatment with antibiotics), yeast organisms such as candida can overgrow in the gut and elsewhere in the body, and this often causes problems with weight. Symptoms suggestive of yeast overgrowth include abdominal bloating and yeast infections such as vaginal thrush and athlete's foot. More details about this and how to treat it can be found on pages 223–8.

4 Low thyroid function

The thyroid gland is the chief gland responsible for regulating the body's metabolism. Low thyroid function seems to be quite common in women and can lead to weight gain (which is often very resistant to normal methods of weight loss). Other symptoms suggestive of low thyroid function include sensitivity to cold, cold hands and feet, fatigue and dry skin and hair. In conventional medicine, low thyroid function is diagnosed with a blood test. However, for a variety of reasons, the blood tests are by no means foolproof, and often fail to identify individuals with a real problem. If you have some symptoms suggestive of low thyroid function (even if a blood test for this has come back as 'normal'), log onto www.thyroiduk.org. This self-help website is a mine of information about the diagnosis and treatment of low thyroid function.

Supplementation prior to pregnancy

Research shows that good intakes of certain nutrients, notably folic acid, help to maintain a healthy pregnancy and reduce the risk of abnormalities. However, risk of the formation of birth defects is greatest during the very early stages of pregnancy. Often, it is some weeks before a woman realises she is pregnant. Supplementation at this stage may be beneficial, but may also have missed the time when adequate levels of certain nutrients are most critical. What this means is that, for the best protection, supplementation should be started before conception.

The importance of folic acid

Folic acid, perhaps more than any other nutrient, is recommended for pregnant women. One of folic acid's chief roles is to ensure the normal functioning of DNA: the component in the body's cells that carries our genetic code. Normal function of DNA is especially important during pregnancy. If DNA goes awry at this time, problems with the development of the foetus are more likely. By helping to ensure DNA does its job without mishap, folic acid helps reduce the risk of genetic problems such as spina bifida (failure of the spinal column to close during development) and anencephaly (abnormal development of the skull and/or brain). These sorts of problems are collectively referred to as neural tube defects (NTDs). One study found that folic acid supplementation reduced the incidence of neural-tube defects by 70 per cent.[12]

NTDs form early in pregnancy – within a month of conception – which is why it's important, if possible, to start supplementation of this nutrient prior to pregnancy. Currently, the recommended daily intake of folic acid for women is 400 µg (micrograms). For women who have a previous history of having a child with an NTD, 5000 µg (5 mg) per day is recommended.

Other important nutrients

Folic acid is not the only important nutrient during the early development of the foetus. Other nutrients that are involved in DNA function include vitamin B12 and zinc. A deficiency in the nutrient copper in early pregnancy also seems to have the potential to cause abnormalities.[13] Another nutrient that seems to have an important role in pregnancy is selenium – levels of which have fallen significantly in the UK diet in recent time (see below). There is some evidence that selenium deficiency may contribute to miscarriage.[14]

The value of supplementation

While the core nutritional approach to preparing for a healthy pregnancy is best centred around a healthy diet, there seems little doubt that supplementation offers considerable benefits too. Unfortunately, our diet cannot always be relied upon to give us optimal amounts of nutrients. Over the last 60 years the vitamin and mineral content of foods such as fruits and vegetables has shown a distinct downward trend. Intensive farming methods, the extensive use of agrochemicals, and modern ripening and storage systems appear to be eroding the nutritional content of our diet. The average consumption of the trace mineral selenium, for instance, has fallen by a third in the last 30 years alone. Government statistics show that significant numbers of women are not getting enough of essential nutrients such as folic acid, copper, zinc, vitamin A, vitamin C, calcium, magnesium, iron or iodine in their diets.

In studies, multi-nutrient supplementation has been found to have a range of positive effects on the outcome of pregnancy. One study examined the effects of giving a variety of nutrients starting three months prior to conception and continuing for the first few months of pregnancy.[15] This research found several benefits, which included:

- Significantly reduced risk of neural tube defects
- Significantly reduced risk of defects in the urinary tract (e.g. the kidneys and bladder)
- Significantly reduced risk of cardiovascular defects (such as heart defects)
- A reduced rate of limb deficiencies
- A reduced risk of a condition known as congenital hypertrophic pyloric stenosis (a condition in which the outlet to the stomach becomes blocked in the first few weeks of life causing projectile vomiting and dehydration).

Another study found that women who took vitamin and mineral tablets before and during pregnancy appeared to reduce the risk that their baby would develop a certain type of cancer of the nervous system called neuroblastoma.[16] Daily vitamin and mineral use in the month before pregnancy and throughout pregnancy was associated with a 30–40 per cent reduction in the risk of this cancer.

Vitamin A in pregnancy

There is some evidence in the scientific literature that supplementing with vitamin A at doses of around 3000 mcg a day or more during pregnancy may increase the risk of birth defects.[17] However, more recent evidence suggests that vitamin A can be taken in higher doses quite safely.[18–19] Nevertheless, it seems the most sensible thing to do is err on the side of caution with this. I recommend that women who are pregnant or planning pregnancy should not supplement with vitamin A at doses exceeding 3000 mcg per day.

Specific supplements

Pregnancy and Lactation Formula contains a blend of nutrients important during pregnancy (including folic acid, vitamin B12 and zinc), at dosages generally recommended at this time. Take one capsule a day. (For more details, see Useful contacts and information – under BioCare.) (Pregnancy and Lactation Formula contains 700 mcg (2333 IU) of vitamin A per capsule – see Vitamin A box, opposite.)

Eating for a healthy pregnancy

Because babies are essentially made out of raw materials supplied by the mother's diet, what a woman eats during pregnancy can have a profound influence on the health of her child. Not only that, I sometimes think not enough is said about what a tremendous drain pregnancy can be on a woman. To ensure the survival of the species, it makes sense that we should have evolved to ensure that the foetus gets a preferential supply of nutrients. This can leave a pregnant mum short on a variety of things, which can affect her during pregnancy and also leave her in not the best of shape after birth too.

The maternal diet during pregnancy seems to have the potential to make a big difference to the health of a child not just immediately after birth, but for many years to come. It seems the seeds for conditions such as heart disease, high blood pressure and Type II diabetes can be sown in the womb, and are particularly related to impaired growth and development of the foetus.[20] It is believed that poor foetal growth may reflect inadequate nutritional supply during pregnancy. There is a theory that a lack of certain nutrients at such an early stage in life can have long-lasting effects on an individual's structure, physiology and biochemistry. In other words, nutrient deficiency may 'programme' the body for ill health, which might only manifest years or even decades later. The fundamentals of a healthy pregnancy diet can be found in the general section on nutrition in Chapter 1. Again, the basic approach here is to eat as natural a diet as possible. Just to summarise, the foods to emphasise in the diet include:

- Fruit
- Vegetables (both raw and cooked)
- Meat (preferably organic) and fish (preferably wild)
- Nuts and seeds
- Eggs
- Butter and extra virgin olive oil
- Natural yoghurt and butter
- Water

Foods to limit in the diet include:
- Processed foods, such as ready meals and canned food
- Foods containing 'trans' fats, including fast foods and margarine
- Refined grains, such as white bread, white rice and pasta
- Foods sweetened with sugar (including fructose)
- Foods containing artificial additives
- Foods containing artificial sweeteners, including aspartame
- Soft drinks

Eat a varied diet

As wide a variety of healthy foods should be eaten as possible. This will help provide the range of nutrients needed for the healthy development of your baby. However, one other benefit of eating a varied diet is that it may help your child eat more healthily once he or she is born. The flavours from the mother's diet eaten during pregnancy are transmitted to amniotic fluid and swallowed by the foetus. Later, some of these flavours may be experienced in breast milk. There is evidence that foods commonly eaten during pregnancy are more likely to be accepted by young babies than those that were not.[21] The study concluded that flavours chosen during pregnancy may affect a baby's food preferences. Eating a wide variety of foods in pregnancy may therefore help prevent faddy eating later on.

DIETARY GUIDELINES SPECIFIC TO PREGNANCY

In addition to these general guidelines, it is important to focus on specific dietary elements that seem to have a particular bearing on pregnancy. These include caffeine, alcohol and healthy fats known as omega-3 fatty acids.

CAFFEINE IN PREGNANCY

Another dietary factor that might affect risk of miscarriage is caffeine. One study found that pregnant women who consumed more than 100 mg of caffeine (which is roughly equivalent to a cup of coffee or two small cups of tea) were more likely to miscarry between six and twelve weeks of pregnancy than those who consumed less than this.[22]

In another study, drinking four to seven cups of coffee a day was found to be associated with a 40 per cent increase in the risk of stillbirth.[23] In this study, drinking eight or more cups of coffee a day appeared to more than double the risk. However, while this research showed that quite a lot of coffee may increase the risk of stillbirth, a small amount appeared to have the opposite effect: women drinking one to three cups of coffee a day were actually 40 per cent less likely to suffer a stillbirth compared to women drinking no coffee at all. All things considered, the current evidence suggests that drinking a cup of coffee or tea each day is generally safe for expectant mums and their babies.

ALCOHOL AND PREGNANCY

There is considerable evidence that excessive alcohol consumption during pregnancy can increase the risk of birth defects. One of the potential consequences of heavy drinking in pregnancy is a condition known as foetal alcohol syndrome (FAS). Children born with FAS tend to be small at birth and may suffer from a range of learning and developmental problems as they age. While excessive amounts of alcohol in pregnancy should be avoided, not all the news about alcohol is bad. There is evidence that very moderate alcohol consumption is not associated with problems in pregnancy.[24] In one study, women drinking 10–14 or more units of alcohol each week were found to be at increased risk of early labour.[25] However, up to nine units a week was associated with a reduced risk of this pre-term delivery. Intakes of 15 ml (1 ½ units) of alcohol or more each day have been found to be associated with an increased risk of low birth weight.[26] Taken as a whole, the evidence suggests it is generally safe for women to consume up to about one unit of alcohol per day (e.g. one small beer or small glass of wine).

THE OMEGA-3 FATS IN PREGNANCY

The omega-3 fats are a particular class of 'healthy' fats to be found in certain nuts and seeds (as alpha-linolenic acid) and in oily fish such as salmon, trout and sardine (as eicosapentaenoic acid (EPA) and docosahexaenoic acid (DHA)). Research over the last 20 years has linked the so-called omega-3 fats with a range of benefits, including a reduced risk of heart disease, stroke and certain forms of cancer. However, there is also a considerable amount of evidence that the omega-3 fats, DHA in particular, can have very important benefits for the growing foetus.

DHA seems to be particularly important for the visual function and the normal development of the brain. Levels of DHA in the mother tend to decline in pregnancy, which is taken as a sign that this nutrient is important for foetal development. Also, it has been noted that babies born with a low birth weight or born prematurely tend to be deficient in DHA.[27] Interestingly, higher levels of DHA are associated with healthier weight, length and head size of babies at birth.[28] Other evidence points to omega-3 fats being important for preventing premature birth and low birth weight.[29]

The benefits of DHA seem to extend beyond pregnancy too. Babies born to mothers with high DHA levels in their blood have been found to have well developed nervous systems, and are better sleepers.[30] And the benefits of omega-3 fats seem to extend to the mother too. Higher DHA levels during pregnancy appear to reduce the risk of post-natal depression.[31]

Keeping up a good intake of DHA

- DHA is found most abundantly in oily fish such as salmon, trout, mackerel, herring and sardine.
- Including two or three servings of this in the diet each week during pregnancy may have a variety of benefits.
- Historically, tuna has been recommended to pregnant mums on the basis of its omega-3 content. Actually, the omega-3 content is quite low. Also, tuna is one fish that tends to be contaminated with mercury, and exposure to this during pregnancy has been linked with problems with the neurological development of the foetus. My advice is to avoid tuna during pregnancy, along with other fish that tend to be tainted with mercury, such as marlin and swordfish.

SUPPLEMENTATION WITH OMEGA-3 FATS DURING PREGNANCY

Individuals who don't eat fish have the option of taking concentrated fish oil supplements that contain DHA. These will generally also contain another omega-3 fat found in fish known as EPA (eicosapentaenoic acid). I recommend 1 g of concentrated fish oil each day.

Fish oils are obviously not suitable for vegetarians. Another option is to supplement with flaxseed oil. This is rich in a fat known as alpha-linolenic acid, which can convert to DHA in the body. However, there is evidence that this conversion is slow and inefficient, which means taking flaxseed oil does not ensure good levels of DHA in the body. However, I suggest anyone keen to take this approach should take 15ml (1 tbsp) of flaxseed oil a day throughout pregnancy. Another option is to use a DHA supplement that has not been derived from fish. Such supplements do exist, as DHA can also be extracted from algae. One suitable supplement is Healthspan's Cerebrum vegetarian DHA. (For more details, see Useful contacts and information.)

OTHER SUPPLEMENTS DURING PREGNANCY

In the section on pre-conceptual nutrition (pages 240–2), I highlighted the importance of getting good levels of nutrients including folic acid, copper and selenium to help ensure a healthy pregnancy and baby. Other nutrients that seem to be particularly important during pregnancy include iron, calcium, and zinc. All-in-all, 14 key nutrients have been identified which, if deficient, increase the risk of low birth weight. These are:

• Biotin	• Iron	• Potassium	• Vitamin B6
• Calcium	• Magnesium	• Riboflavin B2	• Zinc[32]
• Copper	• Niacin B3	• Thiamine B1	
• Folic acid	• Phosphorus	• Vitamin B5	

While I believe very much in the potential of a healthy diet to provide good levels of these nutrients, I also pointed out on page 241 that the nutritional content of our diet is declining, and that many of us simply do not consume even the recommended daily amounts (which are lower than optimum, anyway) of key nutrients.

For those wanting to make sure there are no nutritional holes left by the diet, see the boxes 'Specific supplements' on page 259 and 'Vitamin A in pregnancy' on page 242.

Watch your weight during pregnancy

As discussed, maternal weight before pregnancy can affect the health of both mother and child. It is perhaps no surprise, therefore, that studies also show that the amount of weight a woman gains during pregnancy may also influence its outcome.

One study has found that the greatest risk of complications related to pregnancy comes if there is too little or too much in the way of weight gain during pregnancy.[33] Excess weight gain in pregnancy has been found to be associated with problems such as prolonged labour. Another study found that women gaining more than 20 kg during pregnancy had a higher risk of pregnancy and delivery complications compared to women gaining more than 11.5–20 kg.[34] The same study found that weight gain lower than this 11.5 kg was associated with low birth weight babies (weighing under 3.5 kg). Low birth weight is also associated with an increased risk of infant mortality.

Recent research has shown that the ideal weight gain associated with the lowest risk of foetal and neonatal deaths (deaths within four weeks of birth) depend on the mother's weight before pregnancy.[35-6] Official guidelines for weight gain during pregnancy are as outlined below.

OFFICIAL GUIDELINES FOR WEIGHT GAIN DURING PREGNANCY

BMI prior to pregnancy	Recommended weight gain
Under 19.8	12.5–18 kg
19.8–26	11.5–16 kg
26–29	7–11.5 kg
More than 29	6 kg (minimum)

The figures in the chart give a good general guide to healthy amounts of weight to amass during pregnancy. Following the healthy eating guidelines outlined in the chapter and elsewhere in this book should help ensure you gain adequate, but not excessive, amounts of weight during your pregnancy.

Key points

- Nutritional factors are important before and during pregnancy.
- Maintaining a healthy weight before and during pregnancy seems to be of particular importance.
- Alcohol and caffeine should be had only in moderation during pregnancy.
- Ensuring a good intake of omega-3 fats before and during pregnancy appears to be important for the brain development of the foetus.
- Supplementation with folic acid and other nutrients both before and during pregnancy appears to have benefits for both mother and child.

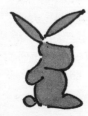

Chapter 6
Infant feeding and weaning

The last chapter explored the role of a nutritious diet in helping to ensure a trouble-free pregnancy and a healthy baby. However, once a child is born, nutrition remains a critical factor in health and wellbeing. What an infant is fed during the first few months of life, for instance, may influence growth and development. A lot of research has looked at the relative merits of breast-feeding and bottle-feeding. This chapter looks at the relative merits of these two forms of feeding, and gives practical suggestions for ensuring the healthy nutrition of your child, whichever you choose.

This chapter also covers a child's nutritional transition from milk to other foods, including more solid fare – the process that is commonly known as 'weaning'. There is evidence that giving children a wide variety of foods early on in their lives helps broaden their palates. However, introducing foods too early can increase the risk of health issues, including allergic-type illnesses. The chapter provides guidance on how to pick your way through this particular nutritional maze. The information should help ensure your child's nutritional needs are met at this critical time in his or her development.

Breast-feeding

Breast milk has been crucial to the survival and evolution of our species over millions of years. Analysis of human milk reveals that it contains a veritable cornucopia of nutrients and other elements that not only help to ensure the very best raw materials for a baby's development, but also appear to protect against a range of conditions and health issues.

What's in breast milk?

Breast milk contains proteins, carbohydrates, fats and a range of nutrients, including vitamins and minerals, which play important roles in the growth and wellbeing of a baby. It is, in essence, designed to give the right amounts of nutrients important for the early development of a human infant's body and brain. One critical difference between human milk and cow's milk is that it is relatively rich in fats (such as the omega-3 fat docosahexaenoic acid), which are believed to have many important functions, including supporting the development of the brain and visual function. In contrast, cow's milk (on which most formula-feeds are based) is pretty bereft of these crucial fats, and is generally richer in nutrients such as calcium and phosphorus. These minerals are important for bone-building, which has obvious significance for calves who are up on their hooves within a few minutes of being born. However, they have much more limited usefulness in human babies who generally won't be taking their first tentative steps for a year or more.

Another fundamental difference between human milk and cow's milk is the types of protein they contain. Some children may have difficulty digesting cow's milk protein and bottle-feeding is therefore more likely to give rise to problems often related to something called food sensitivity. Common manifestations of this include colic (see page 63) and eczema (see pages 81–2). More details about food sensitivity can be found on pages 211–22.

Crucially, breast milk is a 'live' food. Unprocessed in any way, it comes from the breast in a form that preserves all of its health-giving properties. In contrast, formula feeds are pasteurised and dried – processing techniques that can deplete the milk of many of its nourishing elements. Substances found in human breast milk that are not present in conventional formula feeds include enzymes, antibodies, immune cells, growth factors, hormones and substances that feed beneficial bacteria in a baby's gut.[1] With all this going for it, it's perhaps no surprise that feeding a child with breast milk has been found to be associated with so many benefits.

Benefits of breast-feeding

THE EMOTIONAL ANGLE

Before looking at the health benefits of breast milk, let us not forget that the act of breast-feeding can have important emotional elements too. Many women find breast-feeding an intensely enjoyable experience, and it seems that many babies get a lot from it too. The regular intimate contact it affords is generally believed to help cement the relationship between a mother and child in the first few weeks and months of life. During breast-feeding, mothers release a hormone called oxytocin, which some scientists believe actually promotes emotional attachment and bonding.

Oxytocin has some physical benefits, too, as it seems to reduce the bleeding directly after the birth and helps the recovery of the womb.[2] If you are planning to breast-feed, then putting your new baby to your breast as soon as is practically possible after the birth makes good sense. Studies show that mothers who breast-feed in the first hours of life choose to keep their infants longer in their rooms than mothers who have later contact. In addition, mothers who breast-feed are generally found to be less prone to anxiety and low mood after the birth.[3]

BOWEL BACTERIA

Breast milk contains elements that feed healthy bacteria in the gut of the new-born infant. Also, it has been shown that the bacteria in the faeces of breast-fed babies is quite different to those fed on formula,[4] and this may have important consequences for digestive and general health. One effect of having good amounts of the right sorts of organisms in the gut is a greater resistance to unwanted gastrointestinal infection. Studies show, for instance, that babies breast-fed for three or more months have a much lower risk of gastroenteritis compared to bottle-fed infants.[5]

THE IMMUNE SYSTEM

A baby's immune system is not fully developed at birth and will get added protection from antibodies and immune cells present in breast milk. The immune boost provided by breast-feeding helps to prevent a variety of different infections, including diarrhoea, respiratory tract infections, ear infections, urinary tract infections (cystitis and kidney infections) and septicaemia (infection of the blood).[6] What is more, this added protection lasts for years after breast-feeding has stopped and therefore has longer-term health benefits for your child.

ALLERGIC CONDITIONS

There is evidence that asthma and other allergies can be prevented or at least partially protected against through breast-feeding.[7–8] This protective effect may be related to the fact that allergic conditions in children are often related to food sensitivity, and breast-feeding helps prevent this problem through a variety of mechanisms. In particular, delaying the introduction of cow's milk proteins (in the form of formula) seems to reduce the risk that a child will develop a sensitivity to milk and perhaps other dairy products. Breast-feeding also helps to ensure the right amount of healthy bacteria in the gut – something that will help improve digestion and reduce the risk of undigested food 'leaking' through the gut wall. The concept of food sensitivity is discussed on pages 211–22.

LEARNING

As mentioned a little earlier in this chapter, breast milk is relatively rich in certain fats (including docosahexaenoic acid) that are important for brain development. Apart from these healthy fats, it is likely that the mixture of nutritional factors and growth hormones that breast milk contains also contribute to better brain development. A long-term study of 1000 children found breast-fed children had consistent and statistically significant increases in:

- Intelligence quotient (IQ) at age eight and nine years
- Reading comprehension, mathematical ability and scholastic ability assessed at 10–13 years of age
- Teacher ratings of reading and mathematics assessed at 8 and 12 years
- Better performance in examinations.[9]

Another study showed that breast-fed babies went on to have higher IQs in childhood, and this seemed to translate into higher intelligence in adulthood.[10] The authors of the study suggested that the bond between a mother and child that develops during breast-feeding might also play a role by stimulating brain development.

OBESITY

There is some evidence that breast-feeding lowers the risk of childhood obesity and may also protect against obesity in later life.[11] Why this should be is not clear, though it is important bearing in mind the epidemic of childhood obesity we're seeing in the West.

PROTECTION AGAINST OTHER DISEASES

Many studies have found that breast-feeding appears to protect against other conditions too, including:

- Sudden infant death syndrome (cot death)[12-14]
- Insulin-dependent (Type I) diabetes [15]
- Crohn's disease (see page 68–9)[16-18]
- Ulcerative colitis[19]

While breast-feeding seems to have clear advantages over bottle-feeding for a child's health, the benefits do not end there: studies suggest that it may have important implications for the mother too.

Maternal health

As already mentioned, breast-feeding increases levels of the hormone oxytocin in the mother, which seems to reduce blood loss and enhance recovery.[20] During breast-feeding, a woman's periods are unlikely to return. Pregnancy can be a quite a drain on a woman's body and this is not helped by menstruation. By holding off menstruation, breast-feeding helps to preserve some nutrients (for example iron) in a woman's body. Also, breast-feeding is a natural contraceptive, which helps give women a natural 'breather' between pregnancies.[21-2]

Many women are keen to lose weight that they might have put on during pregnancy. Research shows that women who breast-feed tend to return to their pre-pregnant weight earlier than those who don't.[23] Looking at the longer term, it has been found that women who breast-feed are also at a reduced risk of osteoporosis,[24] and cancer of the ovary and breast.[25-7]

The importance of the mother's diet

Breast milk really is the best first food for babies, but it needs to be borne in mind that it is made from raw materials that come from the mother's diet. What this means is that the more nutritious a mother's diet, the more nutritious her baby's will be too. The basics of what constitutes a healthy diet are covered in the previous chapter, with the emphasis placed on unprocessed, whole, unrefined foods with some oily fish, if possible (for the omega-3 fats).

One nutrient that may be in short supply in breast milk is vitamin K. Vitamin

K is necessary for blood clotting and a lack of this nutrient is believed to increase the risk of a condition known as haemorrhagic disease of the newborn, characterised by bleeding, which can have potentially serious, even fatal, consequences. About 2 per cent of breast-fed babies develop this condition, but it is almost never found in bottle-fed babies. For this reason, a vitamin K injection is generally given to new-born babies to ensure they do not have problems with this condition. Breast-feeding mothers might like to consider supplementing with vitamin K. One study found that taking a daily dose of 5 mg of vitamin K increased the level of this nutrient in breast milk,[28] and this is likely to reduce the risk of abnormal bleeding in a new-born baby.

Supplementation during breast-feeding

Nutrient supplementation in the mother during breast-feeding can help boost the levels of nutrients in the breast milk, and can only enhance the benefits breast milk has to offer. One supplement that has been specifically formulated for this purpose is BioCare's Pregnancy and Lactation Formula. It contains a blend of nutrients in the amounts generally recommended during pregnancy and breast-feeding. Take one capsule a day. (For more details, see Useful contacts and information – under BioCare.)

Problems with breast-feeding

Even with the best will in the world, breast-feeding may not be free of problems. Many mothers find that they, or their child, simply do not 'take' to breast-feeding. While there are many different reasons for this, it seems that the position of a baby relative to the breast is a critically important factor. Ideally, breast-feeding infants should have their mouth filled with breast, with the result that the nipple itself is at the back of the mouth near the throat. This ensures the baby is well latched onto the breast, and is important for him or her to be able to suck effectively. If a baby is incorrectly positioned, it may not be able to get the necessary milk, which many mothers interpret as a problem with milk supply. Actually, almost all women (even those with small breasts) make enough milk, but positioning is critical if the baby is to get it. Incorrect position also seems to be why some women have problems with persistently cracked and sore nipples.

Although breast-feeding is a natural process, there seems little doubt that it is a skill to be learnt too for some women. However, it is not uncommon for new mothers to have had little or no instruction in or experience of breast-feeding before they are suddenly faced with the prospect of breast-feeding themselves. If this applies to you, then it may help to spend some time with nursing mothers before the birth, observing breast-feeding and perhaps getting tips from women in the know! After the birth, such women may provide valuable support too. An experienced breast-feeding-friendly midwife is another potential resource, as is the La Leche League – a group devoted to promoting breast-feeding, and the National Childbirth Trust. (For more details, see Useful contacts and information.)

There's no doubt that breast-feeding is time-consuming and can be downright inconvenient too. Some women may want to get back to work or have other commitments that make breast-feeding impractical. If this is the case, it might be worth considering expressing breast-milk, which can be given to your child via a conventional bottle. More details about the practicalities of this can be obtained from the La Leche League and the National Childbirth Trust.

Is my baby getting enough?

In the first few days, the breasts produce a rich, yellow milk called colostrum. After this, breast milk thins out, turning slightly blue in colour. Breast milk has a thinner consistency than formula feeds and cow's milk. However, despite its somewhat watery constitution, don't forget it is designed with all your baby's nutritional needs in mind. It is, however, important that your child gets enough of it. Signs that your baby is hungry include mouthing or the pressing of the mouth in the general direction of your breasts. Your child may cry only once it is very hungry, so being watchful for early signs of hunger can nip problems in the bud. As a rule of thumb, new-born babies generally need to feed about 8–12 times each day, and most will not want to go more than four hours between feeds, even in the night. Each feed should ideally be until they are satisfied, which generally is about 10–15 minutes on each breast.

Signs that your baby is getting enough milk
- He is alert and bright-eyed
- He wants to feed every two to three hours and is satisfied between feeds
- He has at least five wet nappies per day

After the first week, your baby should ideally:
- Be happy during and after feeding
- Gain about 115–200 g (4–7 oz) per week (there is often a small loss of weight during the first week)
- Have five or more pale-coloured, wet nappies in 24 hours
- Have 4–12 stools in 24 hours
- Be alert and bright-eyed

Once a child is established on regular feeds, things normally proceed quite smoothly. However, you may want to contact your doctor, midwife, health visitor or breast-feeding counsellor if:
- Your baby sucks only briefly, very softly or irregularly
- Your baby becomes jaundiced (yellowing of the skin and whites of the eyes)
- You have severe nipple pain that is not getting better
- You have breast pain and a temperature (this may be a sign of mastitis)
- Your baby fights the breast or cries after a minute or two
- Your baby has fewer than five wet nappies a day
- Your baby has little or no stool, or has dark green mucus stools
- Your baby seems weak, tired or not interested in feeding.[29]

How long should I breast-feed for?
Exclusive breast-feeding is believed to offer optimal nutrition for growth and development during about the six months after birth. After this, other foods may be introduced, though gradual phasing out of breast-feeding up until a child is about a year of age will help to ensure they get plenty of nutritional support in this still critical time. If you want to continue feeding longer than this, so much the better. While some health professionals frown on this, it's worth bearing in mind that in developing countries, the average age of weaning is about two-and-a-half years. Again, if you have to go back to work and cannot keep up the regular feeds, you might want to consider expressing and freezing milk. Another option might be to feed in the morning and evening.

Bottle-feeding

About a third of women choose not to, or are unable to, breast-feed. Even of those who do, about 40 per cent have stopped by six weeks after the birth. There is no doubt that bottle-feeding represents a viable and practical alternative to breast-feeding. The vast majority of formulas are based on cow's milk. However, some babies do not process the proteins in cow's milk very well, and may suffer from colic (see page 64) or other problems, such as eczema (see page 81) as a result. In such situations it may be worthwhile considering switching to an alternative formula based on goat's milk. Another option is to try a cow's milk formula that has been treated to break up the protein molecules to make them more digestible (these are called hydrosylates). A knowledgeable midwife or health visitor should be able to help you choose the right product for your baby.

One type of infant formula I do not recommend, however, is those based on soya. These are quite often advocated as an alternative to cow's-milk-based products. Infants may not be particularly well-equipped to deal with cow's milk, but the same could also be said to be true for products rich in soya . In fact, soya is rich in substances called phytoestrogens (plant substances that have an action in the body similar to, though far weaker than, the hormone oestrogen), which might possibly have detrimental effects in the body. One study estimated that the daily exposure of infants to isoflavones in soy infant-formulas is 6–11 times higher on a bodyweight basis than the dose an adult may get from consuming soy foods.[30] There has been some concern that phytoestrogens from soy may impair the function of the thyroid gland.[31] Other concerns have been expressed over the high levels of aluminium and manganese (two metals that can have adverse effects on health) in soy-based infant formula. There simply has not been enough work on the health effects of soy-based formulas in infants to judge their long-term effects. However, in my opinion, there is good reason to view them with suspicion. Unless there is an express medical need or the child is vegan, I recommend avoiding using soy-based formula in your child.

'Enriched' formulas

It is now possible to get formula feeds that have been enriched with fats
believed to be important for brain development, such as docosahexaenoic
acid (DHA) and something known as arachidonic acid (AA). Some formulations
contain healthy gut bacteria (known as probiotics) as well as substances that
feed that bacteria (known as prebiotics). I do think these represent a healthier
alternative to common-or-garden varieties of formula feed.

Making your own enriched formula

Another option is to 'enrich' your
formula feed yourself. Capsules of
concentrated fish oil (which is rich in
DHA) can be opened into made-up
formula. I recommend adding 500 mg
of concentrated fish oil a day. In
addition, you might also like to add a
product INT B1 to your child formula.
INT B1 is rich in the strain of bacteria
found most plentifully in the guts of
breast-fed babies (*Bifidobacterium
infantis*) along with a prebiotic by the
name of fructo-oligosaccharide. Add
⅛ of a teaspoon of this to your child's
feed, once or twice a day. (For more
details, see Useful contacts and
information – under BioCare.)
In one study, adding a probiotic to a
formula feed improved the levels of
healthy fats in the baby's body. It is
believed that the healthy gut bacteria
may help the digestion and absorption
of beneficial fats from the formula.
The overall effect of the addition of
the probiotic to the infant formula
was to reduce the tendency to
inflammation and protect against
allergic conditions such as eczema.[32]

Another benefit of supplementing
your child with a probiotic is that it
may also help protect against infection,
especially of the gut. Adding INT B1 to
the formula each day will help keep the
digestive tract well stocked with
bacteria, which can help keep
unhealthy organisms at bay.

Microwaves and bottle-feeding

Microwave ovens are a quick and convenient way of heating infant feeds. However, I have great reservations about the use of microwaves for the use of cooking, heating and thawing food, which are outlined on page 192. Of particular relevance to the heating of formula feeds is one study that found the microwaving of milk led to structural changes in some elements in milk that might pose hazards for the body.[33] Some scientists have suggested that one amino acid formed in this way (D-proline) is toxic to the nervous system, kidneys and liver. My advice is to avoid microwaves for the warming of formula feeds.

Bottle feeding and dental decay

Bottle-feeding has also been linked to increased dental caries (cavities and decay). This may be because the milk tends to pool around the teeth, and also because the lactose (milk sugar) contained within it can feed bacteria, which may damage the enamel. The best way to avoid this is to offer formula in a bottle only until the age of six months (when many children get their first teeth), and then switch to a beaker or cup. Avoid putting your baby (or toddler) to bed with a bottle containing any liquid other than water.

When should I wean?

There comes a time when a child must start to make the transition from milk to more varied fare. The introduction of food into a child's life is a natural progression, but if done too soon seems to increase the likelihood of a variety of problems, including food sensitivity and excess weight (see opposite). While a child seems satisfied with the milk he or she is getting, there is no reason at all to give anything else. If you are bottle-feeding, you may wish to switch to a brand designed for older, hungrier babies.

One of the most important reasons for this is that the gut in babies is immature at birth and takes time to develop before it can handle proper food. Enzymes for digesting protein only get going after about three months, and those for carbohydrate digestion may not come for more than a year.[34] Nutrients are also more efficiently absorbed by the intestines as your baby grows older. Breast milk (and formula) are much more easily digested and absorbed by the body, and breast milk also contains enzymes that help to digest other foods, which is one good reason to keep some breast-feeding up while you are weaning.

Secondly, a baby's gut is very porous and the lining only 'closes' properly around four or five months of age. Before this, large molecules of food are able to escape into the bloodstream, which can lead the body to recognise them as invaders and set up an immune or other response. This is referred to as food sensitivity (or food intolerance) and can manifest as a wide range of problems, including eczema and asthma. One study found that persistent coughs, respiratory illness and eczema were more common in babies who had been given solid food before 12 weeks, compared to those who were introduced to solids at an older age.[35]

Another study found that feeding of solids at 15 weeks was associated with an increased risk of wheezing during childhood and also seemed to increase the likelihood of weight problems.[36] The authors of the study concluded that the likelihood of a child experiencing respiratory problems at any point in childhood was significantly reduced if he or she was fed exclusively breast milk for 15 weeks, and recommended that no solid foods were introduced during this time.

Yet another study found a link between early weaning and an increased risk of eczema. Babies exposed to solid foods in the first four months of life seemed to be 60 per cent more likely to develop eczema than babies who were given solids later.[37] This study found that early introduction of foods seems to dramatically increase the risk of eczema in later childhood too.

I suggest that no solid foods be given to children before four or five months of age. If you have a family history of allergic conditions, such as asthma and eczema, then holding off for even longer (six months, if your child can manage it) is preferable. It seems the longer introduction of solids is left, the less likely it is to lead to health problems in children.

GENERAL TIPS ON WEANING

The whole point of the weaning process, ultimately, is to have your child eat and enjoy a wide variety of foods. Specific tactics that tend to make weaning a more successful and enjoyable process include the following ideas.

• **Give only one new food at a time**
New foods are best introduced one at a time. A variety of new foods offered at one time ups the risk of a child feeling overwhelmed and rejecting the whole lot.

• **Introduce new foods when you and your child are relaxed**
The more relaxed and harmonious you both are, the more likely a child is to accept a new food. Avoid trying new foods if there's any tension in the air or if your child seems tired or at all fractious.

• **Introduce new foods at lunch**
A bad reaction to a new food at suppertime may disrupt his or her sleeping and keep you both up at night. For this reason, it is best to introduce new foods at lunch.

• **Avoid force-feeding your child**
However much you want a child to eat a food, avoid cajoling him or her into eating it. Studies show that attempting to force a child to eat a food often causes them to dislike it more.

• **Let your baby play**
Small children can see meal times as play time. Although this may be messy, it can also help a child become accustomed to and feel comfortable with new foods. Small children put toys in their mouths, so don't be too surprised if some cucumber or carrot goes in too. Even if he or she doesn't eat it, the experience of having the taste of the food may help the child grow accustomed to it.

• **Offer small amounts of a new food and cut it up small**
This reduces the risk of a child feeling intimidated by a new food

• **Offer the food repeatedly**
When a child rejects a food, it's easy to be put off offering it again. However, research suggests that repeated offerings of a food (best done without coercion and nagging) often gets there in the end (see page 208).

• **Avoid offering alternatives**
If your child refuses a new food, avoid offering something you know will be eaten as an alternative. Otherwise, your child may just learn that saying no gets what he or she wants.

• **Avoid encouraging overeating in your child**
We live in a culture in which overeating is generally regarded as undesirable and unhealthy, and some even see it as a sign of a weak will and lack of self-control. The reality is, however, that, from an early age, we can encourage

our children to eat more than they want. Small children are often cajoled into eating 'just one more spoonful' of food, even when they clearly do not want any more. A potential problem here is that a child may learn to 'override' the internal signals he or she is getting that he or she is full, and this may lead to overeating later in life. Once your child seems full, resist the urge to continue feeding him or her.

Beginning weaning

6–9 MONTHS

The main aim of the early stages of weaning is to accustom your baby to taking food from a spoon, and to provide different tastes and textures. I suggest sticking to foods that are nutritious and relatively easily digested, such as:
• Apple, pear, peaches, apricots, bananas
• Parsnips, swede, green beans, squash, sweet potato, cauliflower, carrots, peas, broccoli

These foods are generally safe for small children and are unlikely to bring on problems with food sensitivity. At this stage, avoid giving your child baby rice or potatoes, or other grains such as wheat oats and barley. A baby's digestive system is not really ready for these concentrated carbohydrate sources at this stage, and they do not provide much in the way of nutritional value anyway. Also, there is growing concern about the effects grain-based carbohydrates may have on health in the long term, which are discussed on pages 176–7 and 214–20.

9–12 MONTHS

Once your baby has become accustomed to eating fruits and vegetables from a spoon, you can begin to introduce other tastes and textures.
• Pulses (such as lentils and black beans) can be puréed with other vegetables.
• Dried fruits can also be soaked and puréed.
• Small amounts of other foods, including millet, chickpeas and mangoes, are a good addition at this point, as is a little meat or fish.
Everything should be puréed or mashed to a manageable form. Don't be too

worried about small lumps – the sooner your baby gets used to different textures, the better.

If you can, avoid offering commercially prepared baby foods as these tend to be bland and similarly textured. Plus, food prepared from fresh is likely to offer more in the way of nutrients compared to processed stuff. Making food in batches and freezing can cut down on the workload considerably. Try to make your baby's diet as varied as possible, as this is likely to ensure he or she has a broad palate later on. He or she may be putting foods into his or her mouth now, so you might like to try finger foods, such as cooked green beans, carrots, bananas, pears and other soft fruits.

At this stage, avoid giving too much in the way of wheat-based foods (e.g. bread, wheat-based breakfast cereals, crackers) and dairy products, such as cow's milk, cheese and yoghurt. These are very common causes of food sensitivity problems and introducing them in quantity at this stage increases the risk of having problems with them now or later on.

1 YEAR +

This stage of weaning marks progression to the more mature diet outlined in Chapter 1. The emphasis, as ever, should be on whole, unrefined and unprocessed food. Some meat and fish, plenty of fruits and vegetables, beans, pulses and wholegrains (e.g. wholemeal bread, brown rice and oats) should form the bulk of the diet.

At this stage, a child is likely to be drinking milk. This may be fine, but it is important to bear in mind that sensitivity to milk is quite common in small children. If your child seems to make a lot of mucus or gets frequent colds, milk sensitivity is a likely problem. Goat's milk or calcium-fortified rice milk are generally better options. More information about food sensitivity can be found on pages 222–35.

Apart from milk (whatever form that comes in), the other principal fluid in a young child's diet should be water. The last 20 years have seen an increasing vogue for giving squashes and fruit juices to toddlers. However, there are many reasons why this may not be a good idea. Generally, these drinks are way too sugary for small bodies. Apart from problems with dental decay, sugar can upset the body's chemistry and lead to a range of problems, including mood changes, weight gain and an increased risk of diabetes. Although the main sugar in fruit juices (fructose) is often said to be a 'healthy' sugar, there are significant health hazards associated with it. The health problems associated with sugary drinks (including fruit juice) are covered on page 173.

Early experiences with food and food preferences in later life

Another major problem with giving sweet drinks to young children is that it can give them a taste for sugar. Research shows that most flavours and food preferences are not predetermined, but are acquired through a child's experience of food and his or her environment.[38-9] The giving of sweet drinks early in life is likely to lead a child to want more sweet foods and drinks in the long term.

Of course, sweet drinks are not the only cause of problems in this respect. Biscuits, cakes, chocolate, rusks, sweet breakfast cereals and a whole host of other foods can all corrupt the taste buds too. The less a child eats of these and other unhealthy foods early in life, the less likely they are to want them later on.

Supplementing small children

With the declining nutritional content of the modern-day diet, it is not easy to ensure children will get all the nutrients they need for healthy growth and development. While there may be no explicit need to give young children supplements, my belief is that they offer an important nutritional safety net. In practice, my preference is to use a multivitamin and mineral powder that can be mixed into a drink. The base ingredient in this product is freeze-dried banana. One scoop of this can be added to milk, or rice milk each day to make a very nourishing and tasty drink. The product is suitable for children of all ages, and is available from the manufacturer BioCare by mail order. (For more details, see Useful contacts and information.)

Feeding toddlers

Again, the fundamentals of what constitutes a healthy diet for children are covered in depth in Chapter 1. In addition to following these guidelines, it can be useful to be mindful of the importance of not just what you feed your toddler, but how you feed it too. Just like we can encourage babies to eat 'just one more spoonful', this is true also of toddlers and older children who may be put under pressure to 'finish everything up' or 'clean their plate', no matter how full they feel. Again, this type of force-feeding may encourage a tendency to ignore the cues a child's body is getting that tells him he is full.

Even the size of the portions we serve our children may have a bearing on how much they eat, and how well they respond to their own internal signals of how much is enough. In one study, researchers examined the effect portion size had on children's eating habits.[40] Researchers measured how much children (average age four years) ate when fed with a meal, the size of which was considered appropriate for their age. On another occasion, the researchers served the children a much larger portion of the same food, and found they ate significantly more than when offered the more modest portion. The study went on to assess the quantity of food consumed by children asked to serve themselves. Interestingly, left to their own devices, children ate portions about the same size as those deemed correct for their age. This study suggests that avoiding piling high our children's plates, or encouraging them to serve themselves, may help ensure they eat what they need, but no more.

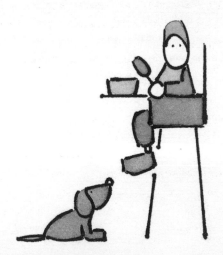

When a child refuses to eat

Many parents find mealtimes with a strong-willed toddler can be quite a battleground. Often, a child uses its refusal to eat as part of a control game or to get attention. Doing what you can to understand why your child is exhibiting this behaviour, and rectifying this, is a good basic tactic. However, it is generally best not to attempt to force-feed a child in these situations. This will generally cause stress and upset on both sides and will give your child a clear message about what it takes to wind you up or get your attention.

In practice, the best way for parents to play this particular game is not to play at all. Harsh though it sounds, if a child won't eat, a good approach is not to feed him or her. That way, it teaches the child that manipulation won't work. A child will eventually tell you he or she is hungry, at which point he or she can be fed with (hopefully) a minimum of fuss on both sides.

Flower essences can also help this situation, and the specific remedy that is indicated if rebellion is the issue is Holly. If attention seeking seems to be what your child is up to, try Heather. More details about flower essences can be found on pages 19–25.

Sometimes, a child may not eat because of physical reasons. One common underlying factor here is iron deficiency. Children deficient in this vital mineral tend to have poor appetites, and may be on the whiney and whingey side. If your child seems pale, this also points to iron deficiency. For more details about this, see 'Anaemia and iron deficiency' in the A-Z section of this book, pages 29–30.

Family meals

Research shows that another important influence on children is family meals. (For the benefits of eating as a family see pages 202–3.)

Key points

- Breast-feeding has been associated with a number of benefits for mother and child, including better bonding, improved immune function and learning, together with a reduced risk of a wide variety of conditions, including allergy, obesity and bowel disease.
- A healthy diet is important during breast-feeding, though nutrient supplementation at this time is likely to have additional benefits.
- If possible, exclusively breast-feed your child for at least four to six months after birth.
- While infant formulas are nutritionally inferior to breast milk, they can be 'enriched' using omega-3 fats and probiotics.
- Avoid heating formula feeds in the microwave.
- Introduce foods gradually during weaning.
- Tips for successful weaning include giving only one new food at a time, offering small amounts of new foods cut up small, repeated offering and avoiding offering too many alternatives.
- Avoid over-feeding your child and serve moderate portions (giving more if need be).
- Supplementing small children with nutrients is likely to help ensure their optimum health.

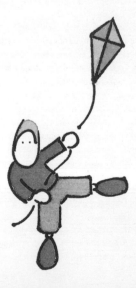

268

References

Introduction

[1] Clark LC, et al. 'Effects of selenium supplementation for cancer prevention in patients with carcinoma of the skin. A randomized controlled trial.' Nutritional Prevention of Cancer Study Group *Journal of the American Association* (1957–63, 96: 276(24))

A–Z of common complaints

[1] Cordain L, et al., 'Acne vulgaris: a disease of Western civilisation.' *Archives of Dermatology* (2002, 138(12): 1584–90)

[2] Hillstom L, et al. 'Comparison of oral treatment with zinc sulphate and placebo in acne vulgaris.' *British Journal of Dermatology* (1977, 97: 679–84)

[3] Michaelsson G, et al. 'A double blind study of the effect of zinc and oxytetracycline in acne vulgaris.' *British Journal of Dermatology* (1977, 97: 561–6)

[4] Snider B, et al. 'Pyridoxine therapy for premenstrual acne flare.' *Archives of Dermatology* (1974, 110: 130–1)

[5] Amann W. 'Improvement of acne vulgaris with Agnus castus (Agnolyt™).' *Therapie der Gegenwart* (1967, 106: 124–6)

[6] Safi-Kutti S. 'Oral zinc supplementation in anorexia nervosa.' *Acta Psychiatrica Scandinavia*, Supplement (1990, 361: 14–17)

[7] Birmingham CL, et al. 'Controlled trial of zinc supplementation in anorexia nervosa.' *International Journal of Eating Disorders* (1994, 15: 251–5)

[8] Brice CF, Smith AF. 'Effects of caffeine on mood and performance: a study of realistic consumption.' *Psychopharmacology* (2002, 164(2): 188–92)

[9] Lane JD, et al. 'Caffeine affects cardiovascular and neuroendocrine activation at work and home.' *Psychosomatic Medicine* (2002, 64: 595–603)

[10] Cryer PE. 'Symptoms of hypoglycaemia, thresholds for their occurrence, and hypoglycaemia unawareness.' *Endocrinology and Metabolism Clinics of North America* (1999, 28(3): 495–500)

[11] Seelig MS. 'Consequences of magnesium deficiency on the enhancement of stress reactions; preventive and therapeutic implications (a review).' *Journal of the American College of Nutrition* (1994, 13(5): 429–46)

[12] Hofle KH. 'Magnesium In Psychotherapy.' *Magnesium Research* (1988, 1: 99, 10th Hohenheim Magnesium Symposium)

[13] Benton D, Cook R. 'The impact of selenium supplementation on mood.' *Biological Psychiatry* (1991, 29(11): 1092–8)

[14] Carroll D. 'The effects of an oral multivitamin combination with calcium, magnesium, and zinc on psychological well-being in healthy young male volunteers: a double-blind placebo-controlled trial.' *Psychopharmacology* (2000, 150(2): 220–5)

[15] Adamidis D, et al., 'Fiber intake and childhood appendicitis.' *International Journal of Food Sciences and Nutrition* (2000, 51(3): 153–7)

[16] Ogle KA, et al, 'Children with allergic rhinitis and/or bronchial asthma treated with elimination diet.' *Annals of Allergy, Asthma, and immunology* (1977, 39: 8–11)

[17] Hodge L, et al, 'Increased consumption of polyunsaturated oils may be a cause of increased prevalence of childhood asthma.' *Australian New Zealand Journal of Medicine* (1994, 24: 727)

[18] Hodge L, et al, 'Consumption of oily fish and childhood asthma risk.' *Medical Journal of Australia* (1996, 164: 137–40)

[19] Burney PG, et al, 'The effect of changing dietary sodium on the bronchial response to histamine.' *Thorax* (1981, 44(1): 36–41)

[20] Durlach J. 'Magnesium and allergy: experimental and clinical relationships between magnesium and hypersensitivity.' *Rev Franc Allergol* (1975, 15: 133–46)

[21] Collipp PJ, et al. 'Pyridoxine treatment of childhood bronchial asthma.' *Annals of Allergy, Asthma, and Immunology* (1975, 35: 153–8)

[22] Ledezma E, et al. 'Efficacy of ajoene, an organosulphur derived from garlic, in the short-term therapy of tinea pedis.' *Mycoses* (1996, 39(9–10): 393–5)

[23] Satchell AC, et al. 'Treatment of interdigital tinea pedis with 25% and 50% tea tree oil solution: a randomized, placebo-controlled, blinded study.' *Australasian Journal of Dermatology* (2002, 43(3): 175–8)

[24] Carter CM, et al. 'Effects of a few food diet in attention deficit disorder.' *Archives of Disease in Childhood* (1993, 69: 564–8)

[25] Mitchell EA, et al. 'Clinical characteristics and serum essential fatty acid levels in hyperactive children.' *Clinical Pediatrics* (1987, 26: 406–11)

[26] Stevens, LJ, et al. 'Essential fatty acid metabolism in boys with attention-deficit hyperactivity disorder.' *American Journal of Clinical Nutrition* (1995, 62: 761–8)

[27] Richardson A and Ross MA. 'Fatty acid metabolism in neurodevelopmental disorder:

a new perspective on associations between ADHD, dyslexia, dyspraxia and the autistic spectrum.' *Prostaglandins Leukotrienes and Essential Fatty Acids* (2000, 63: 1–9)

[28] Richardson A, et al. 'Reduced behavioural and learning problems in children with specific learning difficulties after supplementation with highly unsaturated fatty acids.' *European Journal of Neuroscience* (2000, 12: supplement 11, 296)

[29] Richardson A and Puri B. 'A randomised double-blind, placebo-controlled study of the effects of supplementation with highly unsaturated fatty acids on ADHD-related symptoms in children with specific learning difficulties.' *Progress in Neuro-psychopharmacology and Biological Psychiatry* (2001, 26: 233–9)

[30] Starobrat-Hermelin B, et al. 'The effects of magnesium physiological supplementation on hyperactivity in children with attention deficit hyperactivity disorder (ADHD) Positive response to magnesium oral loading test.' *Magnesium Research* (1997, 10: 149–6)

[31] Knivsberg AM, et al. 'A randomised, controlled study of dietary intervention in autistic syndromes', *Nutritional Neuroscience* (2002, 5(4): 251–61)

[32] Knivsberg AM, et al. 'Reports on dietary intervention in autistic syndromes.' *Nutritional Neuroscience* (2001, 4(1): 25–37)

[33] Kidd PM. 'Autism, an extreme challenge to integrative medicine. Part 2: Medical management.' *Alternative Medicine Review* (2002, 7(6): 472–99)

[34] Kaplan BJ, et al. 'Dietary replacement in preschool-aged hyperactive boys.' *Pediatrics* (1989, 83(1): 7–17)

[35] Maizels MMD. 'Nocturnal enuresis: A logical approach.' *Hospital Medicine* (1990, 38–54)

[36] Egger J, et al. 'Effect of diet treatment on enuresis in children with migraine or hyperkinetic behavior.' *Clinical Pediatrics* (1992, 31(5): 302–7)

[37] Jalkut MW, et al. 'Enuresis.' *Pediatric Clinics of North America* (2001, 48(6): 1461–88)

[38] Cayan S, et al. 'The assessment of constipation in monosymptomatic primary nocturnal enuresis.' *International Urology and Nephrology* (2001, 33(3): 513–16)

[39] O'Regan S, et al. 'Constipation a commonly unrecognised cause of enuresis.' *American Journal of Diseases in Childhood* (1985, 140(3): 260–1)

[40] Moore SJ, et al. 'Field evaluation of three plant-based insect repellents against malaria vectors in Vaca Diez Province, the Bolivian Amazon.' *Journal of the American Mosquito Control Association* (2002, 18(2): 107–10)

[41] Stjernberg L, Berglund J. 'Garlic as an insect repellent.' *Journal of the American Association* (2000, 16;284(7): 831)

[42] Lindsay LR, et al. 'Evaluation of the efficacy of 3% citronella candles and 5% citronella incense for protection against field populations of Aedes mosquitoes.' *Journal of the American Mosquito Control Association* (1996, 12(2 Pt 1): 293–4)

[43] 'Berberine.' *Alternative Medicine Review* (2000, 5(2): 175–7)

[44] Watson NJ, et al. 'Education and debate Lesson of the Week: Vitamin A deficiency and xerophthalmia in the United Kingdom.' *British Medical Journal* (1995, 310: 1050–1)

[45] Brody I. 'Treatment of recurrent furunculosis with oral zinc.' *Lancet* (1997, 24–31; 2 (8052–3): 1358)

[46] 'Berberine.' *Alternative Medicine Review* (2000 5(2): 175–7)

[47] Daoud AS, et al. 'Effectiveness of iron therapy on breath-holding spells.' *Journal of Pediatrics* (1997, 130: 547–50)

[48] Tucker KL, et al. 'Diet patterns groups are related to bone mineral density: the Framingham Study.' *Journal of Bone and Mineral Research* (2000, 15: 222)

[49] New SA. 'The role of the skeleton in acid-base homeostasis.' *Proceedings of the Nutrition Society* (2002, 61: 151–64)

[50] Johnston C, et al. 'Calcium supplementation and increases in bone mineral density in children.' *The New England Journal of Medicine* (1992, 327(2): 82–7)

[51] Cashman K and Flynn A. 'Micronutrients: their role in bone health. In: ingredients, health and nutrition formulation.' *Markets and Technologies* (2001, 4: 10–15)

[52] Yilmaz C, et al. 'The contribution of vitamin C to healing of experimental fractures.' *Archives of Orthopaedic and Trauma Surgery* (2001, 121(7): 426–8)

[53] B. Sarisozen et al., 'The effects of vitamins E and C on fracture healing in rats.' *Journal of International Medical Research* (2002, 30(3): 309–13)

[54] Ruiz-Charles MG, et al. 'Risk factors associated with bronchiolitis in children under 2 years of age.' *Revista de Investigacion Clinica* (2002, 54(2): 125–32)

[55] Hunt C, et al. 'The clinical effects of vitamin C supplementation in elderly hospitalised patients with acute respiratory infections.' *International Journal for Vitamin and Nutrition Research* (1994, 64(3): 212–19)

[56] Evans AT, et al. 'Azithromycin for acute bronchitis: a randomised, double-blind, controlled trial.' *Lancet* (2002, 359(9318): 1648–54)

[57] Henneicke-von Zepelin H, et al, 'Efficacy and safety of a fixed combination phytomedicine in the treatment of the common cold (acute viral respiratory tract infection): results of a randomised, double blind, placebo controlled, multicentre study.' *Current Medical Research and Opinion* (1999, 15(3): 214–27)

[58] Grassi C, et al. 'A controlled trial of intermittent oral acetylcysteine in the long term treatment of chronic bronchitis.' *European Journal of Clinical Pharmacology* (1976, 9: 393–6)

[59] Schwartz J and Weiss ST. 'Dietary factors and their relation to respiratory symptoms. The Second National Health and Nutrition Examination Survey.' *American Journal of Epidemiology* (1990, 132(1): 67–76)

[60] Clemetson C. 'Vitamin C and bruising, low vitamin C status may predispose to bruising: Barlow's disease.' *Medical Hypotheses* (2002, 59(1): 52)

[61] Dalvit-McPhillips S. 'A dietary approach to bulimia.' *Physiology and Behavior* (1984, 33: 769–75)

[62] Mira M, et al. 'L-tryptophan as an adjunct to treatment of bulimia nervosa.' *Lancet* (1989, 2: 1162–3)

[63] Visuthikosol V, et al. 'Effect of aloe vera gel to healing of burn wound, a clinical and histologic study.' *Journal of the Medical Association of Thailand* (1995, 78(8): 403–9)

[64] Ozsoylu S, et al. 'Vitamin A for varicella.' *Journal of Pediatrics* (1994, 125: 1017–18)

[65] Endre L, Dolowschiak A. 'Effect of preparations combining trace-elements and vitamins on the frequency of illness among children attending kindergarten.' *Orvosti Hetilap* (2001, 142(6): 283–7)

[66] Behan PO, et al. 'Effect of high doses of essential fatty acids on the postviral fatigue syndrome.' *Acta Neurologica Scandinavia* (1990, 82: 209–16)

[67] Tamizi B, et al. 'Treatment of chronic fatigue syndrome by dietary supplementation with omega-3 fatty acids – a good idea?' *Medical Hypotheses* (2002, 58(3): 249–50)

[68] Kury PG, et al. 'The effect of prostaglandin E1 and E2 on the human erythrocyte as monitored by spin labels.' *Biochemical and Biophysical Research Communications* (1974, 56: 478–83)

[69] Kuratsune H, et al. 'Acylcarnitine and Chronic Fatigue Syndrome.' *Carnitine Today* (1997, 10: 195–213)

[70] Scholte HR, et al. 'Patients with chronic fatigue syndrome and children with complex regional pain syndrome have low plasma acylcarnitine. Some of the patients have a defect in the carnitine importer.' *Journal of Inheritable and Metabolic Diseases* (1998, 21: 58: 116)

[71] Heap LC, et al. 'Vitamin B status in patients with chronic fatigue syndrome.' *Journal of the Royal Society of Medicine* (1999, 92: 183–5)

[72] Seelig M. 'Presentation to the 37th Annual Meeting.' *American College of Nutrition* (October 13, 1996)

[73] Cox I, et al. 'Red blood cell magnesium and chronic fatigue syndrome.' *Lancet* (1991, 337: 757–60)

[74] Cox I, et al. 'Red blood cell magnesium and chronic fatigue syndrome.' *Lancet* (1991, 337: 757–60)

[75] Howard JM, et al. 'Magnesium and chronic fatigue syndrome.' *Lancet* (1992, 340: 426 (letter))

[76] Judy W. 'Southeastern Institute of Biomedical Research, Bradenton, Florida. Presentation to the 37th Annual Meeting.' *American College of Nutrition* (October 13, 1996)

[77] Janatuinen EK, et al. 'No harm from five year ingestion of oats in coeliac disease.' *Gut* (2002, 50(3): 332–5)

[78] Flodin NW. 'The metabolic roles, pharmacology, and toxicology of lysine.' *Journal of the American College of Nutrition* (1997, 16: 7–21)

[79] Terezhalmy GT, et al. 'The use of water-soluble bioflavonoid-ascorbic acid complex in the treatment of recurrent herpes labialis.' *Oral Surgery* (1978, 45: 56–62)

[80] Nead DE. 'Effective vitamin E treatment for ulcerative herpetic lesions.' *Dent Survey* (1976, 52(7): 50–1)

[81] Fink M, et al. 'Treatment of herpes simplex by alpha-tocopherol (vitamin E)' *British Dental Journal* (1980, 148: 246 (letter))

[82] Hovi T, et al. 'Topical treatment of recurrent mucocutaneous herpes with ascorbic acid-containing solution.' *Antiviral Research* (1995, 27(3): 263–70)

[83] Sanchez A, et al. 'Role of sugars in human neutrophilic phagacytosis.' *American Journal of Clinical Nutrition* (1973, 26: 180)

[84] Bernstein J, et al. 'Depression of lymphocyte transformation following oral glucose ingestion.' *American Journal of Clinical Nutrition* (1977, 30: 613)

[85] Anderson TW, et al. 'Vitamin C and the common cold: a double-blind trial.' *Canadian Medical Association Journal* (1972, 107: 503–8)

[86] Eby GA, et al. 'Reduction in duration of common colds by zinc gluconate lozenges in a double-blind study.' *Antimicrobial Agents and Chemotherapy* (1984, 25: 20–4)

[87] McElroy BH, Miller S. 'Effectiveness of zinc gluconate glycine lozenges (cold-eze) against the common cold in school-aged subjects: a retrospective chart review.' *American Journal of Therapeutics* (2002, 9(6): 472–5)

[88] Barret B, et al. 'Echinacea for upper respiratory infection.' *Journal of Family Practice* (1999, 48(8): 628–35)

[89] Schulten B, et al. 'Efficacy of Echinacea purpurea in patients with a common cold. A placebo-controlled, randomised, double-blind clinical trial.' *Arzneimittelforschung* (2001, 51(7): 563–8)

[90] Mumcuoglu M, et al. 'Inhibition of several strains of influenza virus and beneficial effect of Sambucol in the treatment of naturally occurring influenza B in a double-blind preliminary study.' 6th International Congress for Infectious Diseases, Prague (April 26–30 1994, Abstract 1271: 392)

[91] Lothe L, et al. 'Cow's milk whey protein elicits symptoms of infantile colic in colicky formula-fed infants: A double-blind crossover study.' *Pediatrics* (1989, 83(2): 262–6)

[92] Lothe L, et al. 'Cow's milk as a cause of infantile colic: A double-blind study.' *Pediatrics* (1982, 70(1): 7–10)

[93] Lindberg T. 'Infantile colic and small intestinal function: a nutritional problem?' *Acta Paediatrica*, Supplement (1999, 88(430): 58–60)

[94] Lust KD, et al. 'Maternal intake of cruciferous vegetables and other foods and colic symptoms in exclusively breast-fed infants.' *Journal of the American Diet Association* (1996, 96: 47–8)

[95] Sondergaard C, et al. 'Smoking during pregnancy and infantile colic.' *Pediatrics* (2001, 108(2): 342–6)

[96] Taubman B. 'Clinical trial of the treatment of colic by modification of parent-infant interaction.' *Pediatrics* (1984, 74: 998–1003)

[97] Hunziker UA, Barr RG. 'Increased carrying reduces infant crying: a randomized controlled trial.' *Pediatrics* (1986, 77(5): 641–8)

[98] Rankov BG. 'Vitamin A and carotene concentration in serum in persons with chronic conjunctivitis and pterygium.' *International Journal for Vitamin and Nutrition Research* (1976, 46(4): 454–7)

[99] 'Berberine.' *Alternative Medicine Review* (2000, 5(2): 175–7)

[100] Babbar OP, et al. 'Effect of berberine chloride eye drops on clinically positive trachoma patients.' *International Journal of Medical Research* (1982, 76: 83–8)

[101] Heine RG, et al. 'Cow's milk allergy in infancy.' *Current Opinions in Allergy and Clinical Immunology* (2002, 2(3): 217–25)

[102] Daher S, et al. 'Cow's milk protein intolerance and chronic constipation in children.' *Pediatric Allergy and Immunology* (2001, 12(6): 339–42)

[103] Anti M, et al. 'Water supplementation enhances the effect of high-fiber diet on stool frequency and laxative consumption in adult patients with functional constipation.' *Hepatogastroenterology* (1998, 45(21): 727–32)

[104] Marteau P and Boutron-Ruault MC. 'Nutritional advantages of probiotics and prebiotics.' *British Journal of Nutrition* (2002, 87 Suppl 2: 153–7)

[105] Heiner DC. 'Respiratory diseases and food allergy.' *Annals of Allergy, Asthma, and Immunology* (1984, 53(6): 657–64)

[106] Nisenson A. 'Seborrhoeic dermatitis of infants and Leiner's disease: a biotin deficiency.' *Journal of Pediatrics* (1957, 51: 537)

[107] Dahle LO, et al. 'The effect of oral magnesium substitution on pregnancy-induced leg cramps.' *American Journal of Obstetrics and Gynecology* (1995, 173: 175–80)

[108] Heaton KW, et al. 'Treatment of Crohn's disease with an unrefined carbohydrate, fibre rich diet.' *British Medical Journal* (1979, 2: 764–6)

[109] Riordan AM, et al. 'Treatment of active Crohn's disease by exclusion diet. East Anglian Multicentre Controlled Trial.' *Lancet* (1993, 342: 1131–4)

[110] Mate J, et al. 'Does dietary fish oil maintain the remission of Crohn's disease: a case control study.' *Gastroenterology* (1991, 100: A228)

[111] Hada T, et al. 'Comparison of the effects in vitro of tea tree oil and plaunotol on methicillin-susceptible and methicillin-resistant strains of Staphylococcus aureus.' *Microbios* (2001, 106 2: 133–41)

[112] Lusby PE, et al. 'Honey: A potent agent for wound healing?' *Journal of Wound, Ostomy and Continence Nursing* (2002, 29(6): 295–300)

[113] Molan PC. 'Re-introducing honey in the management of wounds and ulcers – theory and practice.' *Ostomy and Wound Management* (2002, 48(11): 28–40)

[114] Transkanen A, et al. 'Fish consumption and depressive symptoms in the general population in Finland.' *Psychiatric Services* (2001, 52: 529–31)

[115] Schmidt U, et al. 'St John's wort extract in the ambulatory therapy of depression. Attention and reaction ability are preserved.' *Fortschritte der*

Medizin (1993, 111(19): 339–42)

[116] Muller WE, et al. 'Effects of hypericum extract (LI 160) in biochemical models of antidepressant activity.' *Pharmacopsychiatry* (1997, 30: 102–7)

[117] Benton DA, et al. 'Vitamin supplementation for one year improves mood.' *Neuropsychobiology* (1995, 32: 98–105)

[118] Heseker 1990 cited in Benton DA, et al. 'Thiamine supplementation mood and cognitive functioning.' *Psychopharmacology* (1997, 129: 66–71)

[119] Alpert JE, Fava M. 'Nutrition and depression: the role of folate.' *Nutrition Reviews* (1997, 55: 145–9)

[120] Rayman M. 'The importance of selenium to human health.' *Lancet* (2000, 356: 233–41)

[121] Karjalainen J, et al. 'A bovine albumin peptide as a possible trigger of insulin-dependent diabetes mellitus.' *New England Journal of Medicine* (1992, 327: 302–7)

[122] Kostraba JN, et al. 'Early exposure to cow's milk and solid foods in infancy, genetic predisposition, and risk of IDDM.' *Diabetes* (1993, 42: 288–95)

[123] Fava D, et al. 'Relationship between dairy product consumption and incidence of IDDM in childhood in Italy.' *Diabetes Care* (1994, 17: 1488–90)

[124] The EURODIAB Substudy 2 Study Group, 'Vitamin D supplement in early childhood and risk for Type I (insulin-dependent) diabetes mellitus.' *Diabetologia* (1999, 42(1): 51–4)

[125] Hypponen E, et al. 'Intake of vitamin D and risk of Type I diabetes: a birth-cohort study.' *Lancet* (2001, 358(9292): 1500–3)

[126] Szajewska H, Mrukowicz JZ. 'Probiotics in the treatment and prevention of acute infectious diarrhoea in infants and children: a systematic review of published randomised, double-blind, placebo-controlled trials.' *Journal of Pediatric Gastroenterology and Nutrition* (2001, 33 2: 17–25)

[127] Szajewska H, et al. 'Efficacy of Lactobacillus GG in prevention of nosocomial diarrhoea in infants.' *Journal of Pediatrics* (2001, 138(3): 361–5)

[128] Strand TA, et al. 'Effectiveness and efficacy of zinc for the treatment of acute diarrhoea in young children.' *Pediatrics* (2002, 109(5): 898–903)

[129] O'Hare A, Khalid, S. 'The association of abnormal cerebellar function in children with developmental co-ordination disorder and reading difficulties.' *Dyslexia* (2002, 8(4): 234–48)

[130] Reynolds D, et al. 'Evaluation of an exercise-based treatment for children with reading difficulties.' *Dyslexia* (2003, 9(1): 48–71)

[131] Taylor KE, et al. 'Dyslexia in adults is associated with clinical signs of fatty acid deficiency.' *Prostaglandins, Leukotrienes and Essential Fatty Acids* (2000, 63(1–2): 75–8)

[132] Stordy J. 'Dark adaptation, motor skills, docosahexaenoic acid, and dyslexia.' *American Journal of Clinical Nutrition* (2000, 71; 323–6)

[133] Nsouli TM, et al. 'Role of food allergy in serous otitis media.' *Annals of Allergy, Asthma, and Immunology* (1994, 73: 215–19)

[134] Sampson HA. 'The immunologic role of food hypersensitivity in atopic dermatitis.' *Acta Dermao-venereologica*, Supplement (1992, 176: 34–7)

[135] Novembre E, Vierucci A. 'Milk allergy/intolerance and atopic dermatitis in infancy and childhood.' *Allergy* (2001, 56 67: 105–8)

[136] Horrobin DF. 'Essential fatty acid metabolism and its modification in atopic eczema.' *American Journal of Clinical Nutrition* (2000, 71: 367s–72s)

[137] Schalin-Karrila, et al., 'Evening primrose oil in the treatment of atopic eczema: effect on clinical status, plasma phospholipid fatty acids and circulating blood prostaglandins.' *British Journal of Dermatology* (1987, 117: 11–19)

[138] Gimenez-Arnau A, et al. 'Effects of linoleic acid supplements on atopic dermatitis.' *Advances in Experimental and Medical Biology* (1997, 433: 285–9)

[139] Kalliomaki M, et al. 'Probiotics in primary prevention of atopic disease: a randomised placebo-controlled trial.' *Lancet* (357: 1076–9)

[140] Isolauri E, et al. 'Probiotics in the management of atopic eczema.' *Clinical and Experimental Allergy* (2000, 30: 1604–10)

[141] Rier SE, et al.,'Endometriosis in rhesus monkeys following chronic exposure to 2, 3, 7, 8 tetrachlorodibenzo-p-dioxin.' *Fundamental and Applied Toxicology* (1993, 21: 433–41)

[142] Egger J, et al. 'Oligoantigenic diet treatment of children with epilepsy and migraine.' *Journal of Pediatrics* (1989, 114: 51–8)

[143] Hagberg B, et al. 'Tryptophan load tests and pyridoxal-5-phosphate levels in epileptic children. II. Cryptogenic epilepsy.' *Acta Psychiatrica Scandinavia* (1966, 55: 371–84)

[144] Ogunmekan, AO, et al. 'A randomized, double-blind, placebo-controlled clinical trial of d-alpha-tocopheryl acetate (vitamin E), as add-on therapy, for epilepsy in children.' *Epilepsia* (1989, 30: 84–9)

[145] Heseker H, et al. 'Psychological disorders as early symptoms of a mild-to-moderate vitamin deficiency.' *Annals of the New York Academy of Sciences* (1992, 669: 352–7)

[146] Seelig M. 'Presentation to the 37th Annual

Meeting.' *American College of Nutrition* (October 13, 1996)

[147] Meissner T, et al. 'Exercise induced hypoglycaemic hyperinsulinism.' *Archives of Disease in Childhood* (2001, 84(3): 254–7)

[148] El-Ashiry GM, et al. 'Local and systemic influences in periodontal disease. II. Effect of prophylaxis and natural and synthetic vitamin C upon gingivitis.' *Journal of Periodontology* (1964, 35: 250–9)

[149] Wilkinson EG, et al. 'Bioenergetics in clinical medicine. VI. Adjunctive treatment of periodontal disease with coenzyme Q10.' *Research Communications in Chemical Pathology and Pharmacology* (1976, 14: 715–19)

150 Holmes HM, et al. 'Hay fever and vitamin C.' *Science* (1942, 6: 497)

[151] Ruskin SL. 'High dose vitamin C in allergy.' *American Journal of Digestive Disorders* (1945, 12: 281)

[152] Bucca C, et al. 'Effect of vitamin C on histamine bronchial responsiveness of patients with allergic rhinitis.' *Annals of Allergy* (1990, 65: 311–14)

[153] Schwarts A, et al. 'Quercetin inhibition of the induction and function of cytotoxic T lymphocytes.' *Immunopharmacology* (1982, 4: 125–38)

[154] Wickens K, et al. 'Antibiotic use in early childhood and the development of asthma, hay fever and eczema.' *Clinical and Experimental Allergy* (1999, 29: 766–71)

[155] Eskenazi B, et al. 'Exposure of children to organophosphate pesticides and their potential adverse health effects.' *Environmental Health Perspectives* (1999, 107(3): 409–19)

[156] Henz BM, et al. 'Most chronic urticaria is food-dependent, not idiopathic.' *Experimental Dermatology* (1998, 7: 139–42)

[157] Lessof MH. 'Reactions to food additives.' *Clinical Experimental Allergy* (1995, 25(1): 27–8)

[158] Juhlin L. 'Additives and chronic urticaria.' *Annals of Allergy, Asthma, and Immunology* (1987, 59: 119–23)

[159] Kulczycki A Jr. 'Aspartame-induced urticaria.' *Annals of Internal Medicine* (1986, 104: 207–8)

[160] Al-Habbal MJ, et al. 'A double-blind controlled clinical trial of mastic and placebo in the treatment of duodenal ulcer.' *Journal of Clinical and Experimental Pharmacology and Physiology* (1984. 11: 541–4)

[161] Hollingworth HL, et al. 'The influence of caffeine on mental and motor efficiency.' *Archives of Psychology* (1912, 20: 1–66)

[162] Hicklin JA, et al. 'The effect of diet in rheumatoid

arthritis.' *Clinical Allergy* (1980, 10: 463)

[163] Leventhal LJ, et al. 'Treatment of rheumatoid arthritis with gamma-linolenic acid.' *Annals of Internal Medicine* (1993, 119: 867–73)

[164] Zurier RB, et al., 'Gamma-linolenic acid treatment of rheumatoid arthritis: A randomized, placebo-controlled trial.' *Arthritis and Rheumatism* (1996, 39: 1808–17)

[165] Leventhal LJ, et al. 'Treatment of rheumatoid arthritis with black currant seed oil.' *British Journal of Rheumatology* (1994, 33: 847–52)

[166] Brzeski M, et al. 'Evening primrose oil in patients with rheumatoid arthritis and side effects of non-steroidal antiinflammatory drugs.' *British Journal of Rheumatology* (1991, 30: 370–2)

[167] Jantti J, et al. 'Evening primrose oil and olive oil in the treatment of rheumatoid arthritis.' *Clinical Rheumatology* (1989, 8: 238–44)

[168] Kremer JM, et al. 'Fish oil fatty acid supplementation in patients with rheumatoid arthritis.' *Annals of Internal Medicine* (1987, 106(4): 497–503)

[169] Kremer JM, et al. 'Dietary fish oil and olive oil supplementation in patients with rheumatoid arthritis.' *Arthritis and Rheumatism* (1990, 33(6): 810–20)

[170] Geusens P, et al. 'Long-term effect of omega-3 fatty acid supplementation in active rheumatoid arthritis.' *Arthritis and Rheumatism* (1994, 37: 824–9)

[171] Van der Tempel H, et al. 'Effects of fish oil supplementation in rheumatoid arthritis.' *Annals of the Rheumatic Diseases* (1990. 49: 76–80)

[172] Cleland LG, et al. 'Clinical and biochemical effects of fish oil supplements in rheumatoid arthritis.' *Journal of Rheumatolgy* (1988, 15: 471–5)

[173] Kremer JM, et al. 'Effects of high dose fish oil on rheumatoid arthritis after stopping nonsteroidal antiinflammatory drugs.' *Arthritis and Rheumatism* (1995, 38: 1107–14)

[174] Gibson RG, et al. 'Perna canaliculus in the treatment of arthritis.' *Practitioner* (1980, 224: 955–60)

[175] de Vrese M, et al. 'Probiotics-compensation for lactase insufficiency.' *American Journal of Clinical Nutrition* (2001, 73(2): 421–9)

[176] Arrieta AC, et al. 'Vitamin A levels in children with measles in Long Beach, California.' *Journal of Pediatrics* (1992, 121(1): 75–8)

[177] Ross DA. 'Recommendations for vitamin A supplementation.' *Journal of Nutrition* (2002, 132: 2902–6)

[178] D'Souza RM, et al. 'Vitamin A for treating

measles in children.' *Cochrane Database Systematic Review* (2002, 1: CD001479)

[179] Sarker SA, et al. 'Prolonged depression of serum zinc concentrations in children following post-measles diarrhoea.' *Human Nutrition and Clinical Nutrition* (1985, 39: 411–17)

[180] Joffe MI, et al. 'Lymphocyte subsets in measles. Depressed helper/inducer subpopulation reversed by in vitro treatment with levamisole and ascorbic acid.' *Journal of Clinical Investigation* (1983, 72: 971–80)

[181] Lithgow DM, et al. 'Vitamin A in the treatment of menorrhagia.' *South African Medical Journal* (1977, 51: 191–3)

[182] Arvidsson B, et al. 'Iron prophylaxis in menorrhagia.' *Acta Obstetricia et Gynecologica Scandinavica* (1981, 60(2): 157–60)

[183] Ziaei S, et al. 'A randomised placebo-controlled trial to determine the effect of vitamin E in treatment of primary dysmenorrhoea.' *British Journal of Obstetrics and Gynaecology* (2001, 108(11): 1181–3)

[184] Joneja JM, et al. 'Outcome of a Histamine-Restricted Diet Based on Chart Audit.' *Journal of Nutritional and Environmental Medicine* (2001. 11: 249–62)

[185] Yang WH, et al. 'The monosodium glutamate symptom complex: assessment in a double-blind, placebo-controlled, randomized study.' *Journal of Allergy and Clinical Immunology* (1987, 99(1): 757–62)

[186] Van den Eeden SK, et al. 'Aspartame ingestion and headaches: a randomized, crossover trial.' *Neurology* (1994, 44: 1787–93)

[187] Mauskop A. 'Evidence linking magnesium deficiency to migraines.' *Cephalalgia* (1999, 19(9): 766–7)

[188] Murphy JJ, et al. 'Randomized double-blind placebo controlled trial of feverfew in migraine prevention.' *Lancet* (1988, ii: 189–92)

[189] Johnson ES, et al. 'Efficacy of feverfew as prophylactic treatment of migraine.' *British Medical Journal* (1985, 291: 569–73)

[190] Palevitch D, et al. 'Feverfew (*Tanacetum parthenium*) as a prophylactic treatment for migraine: A double-blind placebo-controlled study.' *Phytotherapy Research* (1997, 11: 508–11)

[191] George L, et al. 'Plasma folate levels and risk of spontaneous abortion.' *Journal of the American Association* (2002, 288(15): 1867–73)

[192] Barrington JW, et al. 'Selenium deficiency and miscarriage: a possible link?' *British Journal of Obstetrics and Gynaecology* (1996, 103(2): 130–2)

[193] Nelen WL, et al. 'Hyperhomocysteinemia and recurrent early pregnancy loss: a meta-analysis.' *Fertility and Sterility* (2000, 74(6): 1196–9)

[194] Nelen WL, et al. 'Homocysteine and folate levels as risk factors for recurrent early pregnancy loss.' *Obstetrics and Gynecology* (2000, 95(4): 519–24)

[195] Cnattingius S, et al. 'Caffeine intake and the risk of first-trimester spontaneous abortion.' *New England Journal of Medicine* (2000, 343(25): 1839–45)

[196] Wisborg K, et al. 'Maternal consumption of coffee during pregnancy and stillbirth and infant death in first year of life: prospective study.' *British Medical Journal* (2003, 22;326: 420)

[197] Li DK, et al. 'Exposure to non-steroidal anti-inflammatory drugs during pregnancy and risk of miscarriage: population based cohort study.' *British Medical Journal* (2003, 327(7411): 368)

[198] Craig LB, et al. 'Increased prevalence of insulin resistance in women with a history of recurrent pregnancy loss.' *Fertility and Sterility* (2002, 78(3): 487–90)

[199] Anderson AS. 'Managing pregnancy sickness and hyperemesis gravidarum.' *Professional Care of Mother and Child* (1994, 4: 13–15)

[200] Broussard CN, et al. 'Nausea and vomiting in pregnancy.' *Gastroenterology Clinics of North America* (1998, 27: 123–51)

[201] Iatrakis GM, et al. 'Vomiting and nausea in the first 12 weeks of pregnancy.' *Psychotherapy and Psychosomatics* (1988, 49: 22–4)

[202] Vutyavanich T, et al. 'Pyridoxine for nausea and vomiting of pregnancy: a randomized, double-blind, placebo-controlled trial.' *American Journal of Obstetrics and Gynecology* (1995, 173(3 Pt 1): 881–4)

[203] Vutyavanich T, et al. 'Ginger for nausea and vomiting in pregnancy: randomized, double-masked, placebo-controlled trial.' *Obstetrics and Gynecology* (2001, 97(4): 577–82)

[204] Herlofson BB, et al. 'The effect of two toothpaste detergents on the frequency of recurrent aphthous ulcers.' *Acta Odontologica Scandinavia* (1996, 54: 150–3)

[205] Porter SR, et al. 'Hematologic status in recurrent aphthous stomatitis compared to other oral disease.' *Oral Surgery, Oral Medicine and Oral Pathology* (1988, 66:41–4)

[206] Palopoli J, et al. 'Recurrent aphthous stomatitis and vitamin B12 deficiency.' *Southern Medical Journal* (1990, 83: 475–7)

[207] Wray D, et al. 'Nutritional deficiencies in recurrent aphthae.' *Journal of Oral Pathology and*

Medicine (1978, 7: 418–23)

[208] Ogura M, et al. 'A case-control study on food intake of patients with recurrent aphthous stomatitis.' *Oral Surgery, Oral Medicine, Oral Pathology, Oral Radiology and Endodontics* (2001, 91(1): 45–9)

[209] Das SK, et al. 'Deglycyrrhizinated liquorice in aphthous ulcers.' *Journal of the Association of Physicians of India* (1989, 37(10): 647)

[210] Hochman LG, et al. 'Brittle nails: response to daily biotin supplementation.' *Cutis* (1993, 51: 303–5)

211 Reid G, et al. 'Influence of lactobacilli on the adhesion of Staphylococcus aureus and Candida albicans to fibers and epithelial cells.' *Journal of Indian Microbiology* (1995, 15(3): 248–53)

[212] Davison KK, Birch LL. 'Weight status, parent reaction, and self-concept in five-year-old girls.' *Pediatrics* (2001, 107: 46–53)

[213] Strauss RS. 'Childhood obesity and self-esteem.' *Pediatrics* (2000, 105: 15)

[214] Harnack L, et al. 'Soft drink consumption among US children and adolescents: nutritional consequences.' *Journal of the American Dietetic Association* (1999, 99: 436–41)

[215] Ludwig DS, et al. 'Relation between consumption of sugar-sweetened drinks and childhood obesity: a prospective, observational analysis.' *Lancet* (2001, 357: 505–8)

[216] Jennifer O, et al. 'Children's bite size and intake of an entrée are greater with large portions than with age-appropriate or self-selected portions.' *American Journal of Clinical Nutrition* (2003, 77: 1164–70)

[217] Rolls BJ, et al. 'Serving portion size influences 5-year-old but not 3-year-old children's food intake.' *American Journal of Clinical Nutrition* (2000, 100: 232–4)

[218] Tremblay MS, et al. 'Is the Canadian childhood obesity epidemic related to physical inactivity?' *International Journal of Obesity and Related Metabolic Disorders* (2003, 27(9): 1100–5)

[219] Hernandez B, et al. 'Association of obesity with physical activity, television programs and other forms of video viewing among children in Mexico City.' *International Journal of Obesity* (1999, 23: 845–54)

[220] Tremblay MS, et al. 'Is the Canadian childhood obesity epidemic related to physical inactivity?' *International Journal of Obesity and Related Metabolic Disorders* (2003, 27(9): 1100–5)

[221] Robinson TN. 'Does television cause childhood obesity?' *Journal of the American Dietetic Association* (1998, 279: 959–60)

[222] Epstein LH, et al. 'Effects of manipulating sedentary behavior on physical activity and food intake.' *Journal of Pediatrics* (2002, 140: 334–9)

[223] Kotz K, Story M. 'Food advertisements during children's Saturday morning television programming: are they consistent with dietary recommendations?' *Journal of the American Dietetic Association* (1994, 94: 1296–1300)

[224] Lewis MK, Hill AJ. 'Food advertising on British children's television: a content analysis and experimental study with nine-year olds.' *International Journal of Obesity* (1998, 22: 206–14)

[225] Taras HL, Gage M. 'Advertised foods on children's television.' *Archives of Pediatrics and Adolescent Medicine* (1995, 149: 649–52)

[226] Borzekowski DLG, Robinson TN. 'The 30-second effect: an experiment revealing the impact of television commercials on food preferences of preschoolers.' *Journal of the American Dietetic Association* (2001, 101: 42–6)

[227] Dennison BA, et al. 'Television viewing and television in bedroom associated with overweight risk among low-income preschool children.' *Pediatrics* (2002, 109(6): 1028–35)

[228] Hemila H, Douglas RM. 'Vitamin C and acute respiratory infections.' *International Journal of Tuberculosis and Lung Disease* (1999, 3(9): 756–61)

[229] Bernard L, et al. 'Insulin resistance and polycystic ovary syndrome.' *Gynecology, Obstetrics and Fertility* (2003, 31(2): 109–16)

[230] Chappell, LC, et al. 'Effect of antioxidants on the occurrence of pre-eclampsia in women at increased risk: a randomised trial.' *Lancet* (1999, 354: 810–16)

[231] Benyo DF, et al. 'Hypoxia stimulates cytokine production by villous explants from the human placenta.' *Journal of Clinical Endocrinology Metabolism* (1997, 82: 1582–8)

[232] Chappell LC, et al. 'Effect of antioxidants on the occurrence of pre-eclampsia in women at increased risk: a randomised trial.' *Lancet* (1999, 354: 810–16)

[233] Han L, Zhou SM. 'Selenium supplement in the prevention of pregnancy induced hypertension.' *Chinese Medical Journal* (1994, 107(11): 870–1)

[234] Rossignol AM. 'Caffeine-containing beverages and premenstrual syndrome in young women.' *American Journal of Public Health* (1985, 75: 1337)

[235] Prior JC, et al. 'Conditioning exercise decreases premenstrual symptoms: a prospective, controlled 6-month trial.' *Fertility and Sterility* (1987, 47: 402–8)

[236] Berger D, et al. 'Efficacy of *Vitex agnus castus L.* extract Ze440 in patients with premenstrual

syndrome (PMS)' *Archives of Gynecology and Obstetrics* (2000, 264: 150–3)

[237] Halaska M, et al. 'Treatment of cyclical mastodynia using an extract of *Vitex agnus castus*: results of a double-blind comparison with a placebo.' *Ceska Gynekologie* (1998, 63: 388–92)

[238] Thys-Jacobs S, et al. 'Calcium carbonate and the premenstrual syndrome: effects on premenstrual and menstrual symptoms. Premenstrual Syndrome Study Group.' *American Journal of Obstetrics and Gynecology* (1998, 179: 444–52)

[239] Sherwood RA, et al. 'Magnesium and the premenstrual syndrome.' *Annals of Clinical Biochemistry* (1986, 23: 667–70)

[240] Facchinetti F, et al. 'Oral magnesium successfully relieves premenstrual mood changes.' *Obstetrics and Gynecology* (1991, 78: 177–81)

[241] Abraham GE, et al. 'Effect of vitamin B6 on premenstrual symptomatology in women with premenstrual tension syndrome: a double-blind crossover study.' *Infertility* (1980, 3: 155–65)

[242] Kerr GD. 'The management of premenstrual syndrome.' *Current Medical Research and Opinion* (1977, 4: 29–34)

[243] Ellis F. 'Ascorbic acid for prickly heat.' *Lancet* (1968, 20;2(7560): 173)

[244] Hindson TC. 'Ascorbic acid for prickly heat.' *Lancet* (1968, 22;1(7556): 1347–8)

[245] Vahlquist C, et al. 'The fatty-acid spectrum in plasma and adipose tissue in patients with psoriasis.' *Archives of Dermatology research* (1953, 278(2): 114–19)

[246] Mullet K, et al. 'The antipsoriatic Mahonia aquifolium and its active constituents; II. Antiproliferative activity against cell growth of human keratinocytes.' *Planta Medica* (1995, 61(1): 74–5)

[247] Syed TA, et al. 'Management of psoriasis with aloe vera extract in a hydrophilic cream: a placebo-controlled, double-blind study.' *Tropical Medicine and International Health* (1996, 1(4): 505–9)

[248] Dewsbury CE, et al. 'EPA in the treatment of psoriasis.' *British Journal of Dermatology* (1989, 120: 581–4)

[249] McGovern MC, et al. 'Reye's syndrome and aspirin: lest we forget. Aspirin is an avoidable risk factor for Reye's syndrome: heightened vigilance can prevent an increasing incidence. Clinical review.' *British Medical Journal* (2001, 322: 1591–2)

[250] Satchell AC, et al. 'Treatment of interdigital tinea pedis with 25% and 50% tea tree oil solution: a randomized, placebo-controlled, blinded study.' *Australasian Journal of Dermatology* (2002, 43(3): 175–8)

[251] Ebner F, et al. 'Topical use of dexpanthenol in skin disorders.' *American Journal of Clinical Dermatology* (2002, 3(6): 427–33)

[252] Kim HL, et al. 'St John's Wort for depression: a meta-analysis of well-defined clinical trials.' *Journal of Nervous and Mental Diseases* (1999, 187; 532–8)

[253] Wheatley D. 'Hypericum in seasonal affective disorder (SAD).' *Current Medical Research Opinions* (1999, 15: 33–7)

[254] Natta CL. 'Painful crises due to sickle-cell anaemia: effect of vitamin B6 supplementation.' *IM* (1986, 7(10):132–9)

[255] Natta CL, et al. 'Antisickling properties of pyridoxine derivatives.' *Annals of the New York Academy of Sciences* (1990, 585: 505–9)

[256] van der Dijs FP, et al. 'Optimization of folic acid, vitamin B12, and vitamin B6 supplements in pediatric patients with sickle cell disease.' *American Journal of Hematology* (2000, 69(4): 239–46)

[257] Gaby AR. 'Literature review and commentary.' *Townsend Letter for Doctors* (June 1990, 338–9)

[258] Natta CL, et al. 'A decrease in irreversibly sickled erythrocytes in sickle cell anaemia patients given vitamin E.' *American Journal of Clinical Nutrition* (1980, 33: 968–71)

[259] Ohnishi ST, Ohnishi T. 'In vitro effects of aged garlic extract and other nutritional supplements on sickle erythrocytes.' *Journal of Nutrition* (2001, 131(3): 1085–92)

[260] Westerveld GJ, et al. 'Antioxidant levels in the nasal mucosa of patients with chronic sinusitis and healthy controls.' *Archives of Otolaryngology – Head and Neck Surgery* (1997, 123(2): 201–4)

[261] Nikolaev MP, et al. 'Clinical and biochemical aspects in the treatment of acute maxillary sinusitis with antioxidants.' *Vestnik Otorinolaringologii* (1994, (1): 22–6)

[262] Sletzer A. 'Adjunctive use of bromelain in sinusitis: a controlled study.' *ENT Monthly* (1967, 46(10): 1281–8)

[263] Hada T, et al. 'Comparison of the effects in vitro of tea tree oil and plaunotol on methicillin-susceptible and methicillin-resistant strains of Staphylococcus aureus.' *Microbios* (2001, 106(2): 133–41)

[264] Zumla A, Lulat A. 'Honey – a remedy rediscovered.' *Journal of the Royal Society of Medicine* (1989, 82: 384–5)

[265] Wahdan HAL. 'Causes of the antimicrobial activity of honey.' *Infection* (1998, 26(1): 26–31)

[266] von Woedtke T, et al. 'Aspects of the

antimicrobial efficacy of grapefruit seed extract and its relation to preservative substances contained.' *Pharmazie* (1999, 54: 452–6)

[267] Grant WB. 'An estimate of premature cancer mortality in the U.S. due to inadequate doses of solar ultraviolet-B radiation.' *Cancer* (2002, 94(6): 1867–75)

[268] Burger A, et al. 'Aloe vera, renaissance of a traditional natural drug as a dermo-pharmaceutical.' *SOFW-Journal* (1994, 120(9): 526–9)

[269] Morisset R, et al. 'Evaluation of the healing activity of hydrocotyle tincture in the treatment of wounds.' *Phytotherapy Research* (1987, 117–21)

[270] Kartnig T. 'Clinical applications of Centella asiatica (L) Urb.' in *Herbs, Spices, and Medicinal Plants: Recent Advances in Botany, Horticulture, and Pharmacology*, vol. 3., eds. Craker LE, Simon JE. AZ: Oryx Press (1986, 145–73)

[271] Kaplan B. 'Homoeopathy: 2. In pregnancy and for the under-fives.' *Professional Care of Mother and Child* (1994, 4(6): 185–7)

[272] Edward B, et al. 'Cranberry Concentrate: UTI Prophylaxis.' *The Journal of Family Practice* (1997, 45(2): 167–8)

[273] Focht DR 3rd, et al. 'The efficacy of duct tape vs cryotherapy in the treatment of verruca vulgaris (the common wart).' *Archives of Pediatrics and Adolescent Medicine* (2002, 156(10): 971–4)

Chapter 1: Food fundamentals

[1] Sanchez A, et al. 'Role of Sugars in Human Neutrophilic Phagocytosis.' *American Journal of Clinical Nutrition* (1973, 26(11); 1180–4)

[2] Rinsdor E, at al. 'Sucrose Neutrophilic Phagocystosis and Resistance to Disease.' *Dental Survey* (1976, 52(12); 46–8)

[3] Goldman J, et al. 'Behavioral Effects of Sucrose on Preschool Children.' *Journal of Abnormal Child Psychology* (1986, 14: 565–77)

[4] Behar D, et al. 'Sugar Testing with Children Considered Behaviorally Sugar Reactive.' *Nutritional Behavior* (1984, 1: 277–88)

[5] Alexander Schauss. *Diet, Crime and Delinquency* (Berkeley, CA: Parker House, 1981)

[6] Cordain L, et al. 'An evolutionary analysis of the aetiology and pathogenesis of juvenile-onset myopia.' *Acta Ophthalmologica Scandinavica* (2002, 80(2): 125–35)

[7] Elliott SS, et al. 'Fructose, weight gain and the insulin resistance syndrome.' *American Journal of Clinical Nutrition* (2002, 76(5): 911–22)

[8] Jenkins DJA, et al. 'Glycemic index: overview of implications in health and disease.' *American Journal of Clinical Nutrition* (2002, 76: 266–73)

[9] Brand-Miller JC, et al. 'Glycemic index and obesity.' *American Journal of Clinical Nutrition* (2002, 76: 281–5)

[10] Nichols AB, et al. 'Daily nutritional intake and serum lipid levels. The Tecumseh study.' *American Journal of Clinical Nutrition* (1976, 29: 1384–92)

[11] Morris JN, et al. 'Diet and plasma cholesterol in 99 bank men.' *British Medical Journal* (1963, 1: 571–6)

[12] Khan HA, et al. 'Serum cholesterol: Its distribution and association with dietary and other variables in a survey of 10,000 men.' *Israel Journal of the Medical Sciences* (1969, 5: 1117–27)

[13] Ravnskov U. 'A hypothesis out-of-date: the diet-heart idea.' *Journal of Clinical Epidemiology* (2002, Nov; 55(11): 1057–63)

[14] Hooper L, et al. 'Dietary fat intake and prevention of cardiovascular disease: systematic review.' *British Medical Journal* (2001, 322: 757–63)

[15] Willett WC, et al. 'Dietary fat is not a major determinant of body fat.' *American Journal of Medicine* (2002, 30;113 9B: 47–59)

[16] Perez-Jimenez F, et al. 'Protective effect of dietary monounsaturated fat on arteriosclerosis: beyond cholesterol.' *Atherosclerosis* (2002, 163(2): 385–98)

[17] Ascherio A, Willett WC. 'Health effects of trans fatty acids.' *American Journal of Clinical Nutrition* (1997, 6(4): 1006–10)

[18] Bitterman WA, et al. 'Environmental and nutritional factors significantly associated with cancer of the urinary tract among different ethnic groups.' *Urological Clinics of North America* (1991, 18: 501–8)

[19] Wilkens LR, et al. 'Risk factors for lower urinary tract cancer: the role of total fluid consumption, nitrites and nitrosamines, and selected foods.' *Cancer Epidemiology, Biomarkers and Prevention* (1996, 5: 116–66)

[20] Shannon J, et al. 'Relationship of food groups and water intake to colon cancer risk.' *Cancer Epidemiology, Biomarkers and Prevention* (1996, 5: 495–502)

[21] Chan J, et al. 'Water, other fluids, and fatal coronary heart disease: the Adventist Health Study.' *American Journal of Epidemiology* (2002, 155(9): 827–33)

[22] Lavin JH, et al. 'The effect of sucrose- and aspartame-sweetened drinks on energy intake, hunger and food choice of female, moderately restrained eaters.' *International Journal of Obesity*

(1997, 21: 37–42)

[23] Tordoff MG, Alleva AM. 'Oral stimulation with aspartame increases hunger.' *Physiology and Behavior* (1990, 47: 555–9)

[24] Sharma RP, Coulombe RA Jr. 'Effects of repeated doses of aspartame on serotonin and its metabolite in various regions of the mouse brain.' *Food and Chemical Toxicology* (1987, 25(8): 565–8)

[25] Maher TJ, Wurtman RJ. 'Possible neurologic effects of aspartame, a widely used food additive.' *Environmental Health Perspectives* (1987, 75: 53–7)

[26] Van Den Eeden SK, et al. 'Aspartame ingestion and headaches: a randomized, crossover trial.' *Neurology* (1994, 44: 1787–93)

[27] Lipton RB et al. 'Aspartame as a dietary trigger of headache.' *Headache* (1989, 29(2): 90–2)

[28] Walton RG, et al. 'Adverse reactions to aspartame: double-blind challenge in patients from a vulnerable population.' *Biological Psychiatry* (1993, 34(1-2): 13–17)

Chapter 2: Specific foods

[1] Maynard M, et al. 'Fruit, vegetables, and antioxidants in childhood and risk of adult cancer: the Boyd Orr cohort.' *Journal of Epidemiology and Community Health* (2003, 57(3): 218–25)

[2] New SA. 'The role of the skeleton in acid-base homeostasis.' *Proceedings of the Nutrition Society* (2002, 61: 151–64)

[3] Hu FB, et al.' Frequent nut consumption and risk of coronary heart disease in women: prospective cohort study.' *British Medical Journal* (1998, 317: 1341–5)

[4] Albert CM, et al. 'Nut consumption and decreased risk of sudden cardiac death in the Physicians' Health Study.' *Archives of Internal Medicine* (2002, 24;162(12): 1382–7)

[5] Sarasua S, Savitz DA. 'Cured and broiled meat consumption in relation to childhood cancer: Denver, Colorado (United States)' *Cancer Causes Control* (1994, Mar;5(2): 141–8)

[6] Feskanich D, et al. 'Calcium, vitamin D, milk consumption, and hip fractures: a prospective study among postmenopausal women.' *American Journal of Clinical Nutrition* (2003, 77(2): 504–11)

[7] Knopp RH, et al. 'A double-blind, randomized, controlled trial of the effects of two eggs per day in moderately hypercholesterolemic and combined hyperlipidemic subjects taught the NCEP step I diet.' *Journal of the American College of Nutrition* (1997, 16(6): 551–61)

[8] Gregory, et al. 'NDNS: young people aged 4–18 years.' (2000)

[9] Armstrong LE, et al. 'Urinary indices of hydration status.' *International Journal of Sports Nutrition* (1994, 4: 265–79)

[10] Robert D, et al. 'Chlorination, chlorination by-products, and cancer: a meta-analysis.' *American Journal of Public Health* (July 1992, 82(7): 955–63)

[11] Cantor KP, et al. 'Drinking water source and chlorination by-products in Iowa. III. Risk of brain cancer.' *American Journal of Epidemiology* (1999, 150(6): 552–60)

[12] Bove FL, et al. 'Public drinking water contamination and birth outcomes.' *American Journal of Epidemiology* (1995, 143(11): 1179–80)

[13] Rondeau V, at al. 'Relation between aluminum concentrations in drinking water and Alzheimer's disease: an 8-year follow-up study.' *American Journal of Epidemiology* (2000, 152(1): 59–66)

[14] McDonagh M, et al. 'Systematic review of water fluoridation.' *British Medical Journal* (2000, 321: 855–9)

[15] Ludwig DS, et al. 'Relation between consumption of sugar-sweetened drinks and childhood obesity: a prospective, observational analysis.' *Lancet* (2001, 357: 505–8)

[16] Lubec G, et al. 'Aminoacid isomerisation and microwave exposure.' *Lancet* (1989, Dec 9;2(8676): 1392–3)

Chapter 3: Food and meal culture

[1] Neumark-Sztainer D, et al. 'Family meal patterns: associations with sociodemographic characteristics and improved dietary intake among adolescents.' *Journal of the American Dietetic Association* (2003, 103(3): 317–22)

[2] Videon TM, Manning CK. 'Influences on adolescent eating patterns: the importance of family meals.' *Journal of Adolescent Health* (2003, 32(5): 365–73)

[3] Anderson RC, et al. 'Growth in reading and how children spend their time outside of school.' *Reading Research Quarterly* (1988, 23: 286–303)

[4] Bowden BS, Zeisz JM. 'Supper's on! Adolescent adjustment and frequency of family mealtimes.' Paper presented at: 105th Annual Meeting of the American Psychological Association (1997, Chicago, Illinois)

[5] Youth Research. 'Kids make the grade: a quantitative research study on children's nutrition.' *The International Food Information Council* (1992)

[6] Gillespie AH, Achterberg CL. 'Comparison of family interaction patterns related to food and nutrition.' *Journal of the American Dietetic Association* (1989, 89: 509–12)

[7] Neumark-Sztainer D, et al. 'Family meals among

adolescents: Findings from a pilot study.' *Journal of Nutritional Education* (2000, 32: 335–340)

[8] Reviewed in Pollitt E and Mathews R. 'Breakfast and cognition: an integrative summary.' *American Journal of Clinical Nutrition* (1998, 67: 804–13)

[9] Reviewed in Pollitt E and Mathews R. 'Breakfast and cognition: an integrative summary.' *American Journal of Clinical Nutrition* (1998, 67: 804–13)

[10] Fisher JO, Birch LL. 'Restricting access to palatable foods affects children's behavioral response, food selection and intake.' *American Journal of Clinical Nutrition* (1999, 69: 1264–72)

[11] Fisher JO, Birch LL. 'Maternal restriction of young girls' food access is related to intake of those foods in an unrestricted setting.' *FASEB Journal* (1996, 10: 225)

[12] Birch LL, et al. 'Eating as the "means" activity in a contingency: effects on young children's food preference.' *Child Development* (1984, 55: 432–9)

[13] Birch LL, et al. 'The influence of social-affective context on preschoolers' food preferences.' *Child Development* (1980, 51: 856–61)

[14] Baughcum AE, et al. 'Maternal feeding practices and childhood obesity: a focus group study of low-income mothers.' *Archives of Pediatric and Adolescent Medicine* (1998, 152: 1010–16)

[15] Birch LL, et al. 'I don't like it; I never tried it: effects of exposure to food on two-year-old children's food preferences.' *Appetite* (1982, 4: 353–360)

[16] Sullivan SA, Birch LL. 'Infant dietary experience and acceptance of solid foods.' *Pediatrics* (1994, 9: 884–5)

Chapter 4: Common childhood problems

[1] Adapted from Jennie Brand-Miller and Thomas Wolever's *The Glucose Revolution: The Authoritative Guide to the Glycaemic Index* (Marlowe and Company, NY, USA)

Chapter 5: Another baby?

[1] Wang JX, et al. 'Polycystic ovarian syndrome and the risk of spontaneous abortion following assisted reproductive technology treatment.' *Human Reproduction* (2001, 16(12): 2606–9)

[2] Fedorcs P, et al. 'Obesity is a risk factor for early pregnancy loss after IVF or ICSI.' *Acta Obstetrica et Gynecologica Scandinavica* (2000, 79: 43–8)

[3] Shaw GM, et al. 'Risk of neural tube defect-affected pregnancies among obese women.' *Journal of the American Association* (1996, 275(14): 1093–6)

[4] Werler MM, et al. 'Pre-pregnant weight in relation to risk of neural tube defects.' *Journal of the American Association* (1996, 275(14): 1089–92)

[5] Galtier-Dereure F, et al. 'Weight excess before pregnancy: complications and cost.' *International Journal of Obesity and Related Metabolic Disorders* (1995, 19: 443–8)

[6] Scholl TO, et al. 'Maternal weight gain during pregnancy and the competition for nutrients.' *American Journal of Clinical Nutrition* (1991, 60: 183–8)

[7] Van der Spuy ZM, et al. 'Outcome of pregnancy in underweight women after spontaneous and induced ovulation.' *British Medical Journal* (Clin Res Ed) (1988, 296(6627): 962–5)

[8] Jacquet D, et al. 'Low birth weight: effect on insulin sensitivity and lipid metabolism.' *Hormone Research* (2003, 59(1): 1–6)

[9] Brand-Miller JC, et al. 'Glycemic index and obesity.' *American Journal of Clinical Nutrition* (2002, 76(1): 281–5)

[10] Jenkins DJ. 'Glycemic index: overview of implications in health and disease.' *American Journal of Clinical Nutrition* (2002, 76(1): 266–73)

[11] Willett WC, Leibel RL. 'Dietary fat is not a major determinant of body fat.' *American Journal of Medicine* (2002, 30;113: 47–59)

[12] MRC Vitamin Study Research Group 'Prevention of neural tube defects: results of the Medical Research Council Vitamin Study.' *Lancet* (1991, 338: 131–7)

[13] Keen CL, et al.. 'Effect of copper deficiency on prenatal development and pregnancy outcome.' *American Journal of Clinical Nutrition* (1998, 67(suppl5): 1003–11)

[14] Barrington JW, et al. 'Selenium deficiency and miscarriage: a possible link?' *British Journal of Obstetrics and Gynaecology* (1996, 103: 130–2)

[15] Czeizel A. 'Periconceptional folic acid containing multivitamin supplementation.' *European Journal of Obstetrics and Gynecology and Reproductive Biology* (1998, 78: 151–61)

[16] Olshan AF, et al. 'Maternal vitamin use and reduced risk of neuroblastoma.' *Epidemiology* (2002, 13: 575–80)

[17] Rothman KJ, et al. 'Teratogenicity of high vitamin A intake.' *New England Journal of Medicine* (1995, 333(21): 1369–73)

[18] Mills JL, et al. 'Vitamin A and birth defects.' *American Journal of Obstetrics and Gynecology* (1997, 177(1): 31–23)

[19] Miller RK, et al. 'Periconceptual vitamin A use: how much is teratogenic?' *Reproductive Toxicology* (1998, 12(1): 75–88)

[20] Godfrey KM and Barker DJ 'Foetal nutrition and adult disease.' *American Journal of Clinical Nutrition* (2000, 71(suppl): 1344–52)

[21] Mennella JA, et al. 'Prenatal and postnatal flavour learning by human infants.' *Pediatrics* (2001, 107(6): 88)

[22] Cnattingius S, et al. 'Caffeine intake and the risk of first-trimester spontaneous abortion.' *New England Journal of Medicine* (2000, 343(25): 1839–45)

[23] Wisborg K, et al. 'Maternal consumption of coffee during pregnancy and stillbirth and infant death in first year of life: prospective study.' *British Medical Journal* (2003, 22; 326:420)

[24] Hatfield D. 'Is social drink during pregnancy harmless?' *Advances in Alcohol and Substance Abuse* (1985, 5(1-2): 221–6)

[25] Kesmodel U, et al. 'Does alcohol increase the risk of preterm delivery?' *Ugeskr Laeger* (2001, 20;163(34): 4578–82)

[26] Tat-Ha C. 'Alcohol and pregnancy: what is the level of risk?' *J Toxicol Clin Ex* (1990, 10(2): 105–114)

[27] Crawford MA. 'The role of essential fatty acids in neural development: implications for perinatal nutrition.' *American Journal of Clinical Nutrition* (1993, 57(5): 703–9)

[28] Hornstra G. 'Essential fatty acids in mothers and their neonates.' *American Journal of Clinical Nutrition* (2000, 71(5): 1262–9)

[29] Olsen SF, Secher NJ. 'Low consumption of seafood in early pregnancy as a risk factor for preterm delivery: prospective cohort study.' *British Medical Journal* (2002, 324(7335): 447)

[30] Cheruku SR, et al. 'Higher maternal plasma docosahexaenoic acid during pregnancy is associated with more mature neonatal sleep-state patterning.' *American Journal of Clinical Nutrition* (2002, 76(3): 608–13)

[31] Hibbeln JR. 'Seafood consumption, the DHA content of mothers' milk and prevalence rates of postpartum depression: a cross-national, ecological analysis.' *Journal of Affective Disorders* (2002, 69(1-3): 15–29)

[32] Wynn, et al. 'Nutrition of women in anticipation of pregnancy.' *Nutrition and Health* (1991, 7: 69–88)

[33] BNF. 'Nutrition in Pregnancy.' British Nutrition Society Briefing Paper (1994)

[34] Thorsdottir I, et al. 'Weight gain in women of normal weight before pregnancy: complications in pregnancy or delivery and birth outcome.' *Obstetrics and Gynecolgy* (2002, 5 Pt 1): 799–806)

[35] Lucas, et al. 'Maternal fatness and the viscosity of preterm infants.' *British Medical Journal* (1988, 296: 1495–7)

[36] Mitchel et al. 'Weight gain and pregnancy outcome in underweight and normal weight women.' *Journal of the American Dietetic Association* (1989, 89: 634–41)

Chapter 6: Infant feeding and weaning

[1] British Nutrition Foundation BNF briefing paper 'Nutrition in infancy.' (1997)

[2] Chua S, et al. 'Influence of breastfeeding and nipple stimulation on postpartum uterine activity.' *British Journal of Obstetrics and Gynaecology* (1994, 101: 804–5)

[3] Mezzacappa ES, Katlin ES. 'Breast-feeding is associated with reduced perceived stress and negative mood in mothers.' *Health Psychology* (2002, 21(2): 187–93)

[4] Balmer SE, et al. 'Diet and faecal flora in the newborn.' *Archives of Diseases in Children* (1991, 66: 1390–4),

[5] Howie PW, et al. 'Protective effect of breast feeding against infection.' *British Medical Journal* (1990, 300: 11–16)

[6] Hanson LA, et al. 'Breastfeeding provides passive and likely long-lasting active immunity.' *Annals of Allergy, Asthma and Immunology* (1998, 81: 523–37)

[7] Lucas A, et al. 'Early diet of preterm infants and development of allergic or atopic disease: randomised prospective study.' *British Medical Journal* (1990, 300: 837–40)

[8] Saarinen UM, Kajosaari M. 'Breastfeeding as prophylaxis against atopic disease: prospective follow-up study until 17 years old.' *Lancet* (1995, 346: 1065–9)

[9] Horwood LJ, Fergusson DM. 'Breastfeeding and later cognitive and academic outcomes.' *Pediatrics* (1998, 101: 9)

[10] Mortensen EL, et al. 'The association between duration of breastfeeding and adult intelligence.' *Journal of the American Medical Association* (2002, 287: 2365–71)

[11] Armstrong J, et al. 'Breastfeeding and lowering the risk of childhood obesity.' *Lancet* (2002, 359: 2003–4)

[12] Ford RPK, et al. 'Breastfeeding and the risk of sudden infant death syndrome.' *International Journal of Epidemiology* (1993, 22: 885–90)

[13] Mitchell EA, et al. 'Four modifiable and other major risk factors for cot death: the New Zealand study.' *Journal of Paediatric Child Health* (1992, 28: 3–8)

[14] Scragg LK, et al. 'Evaluation of the cot death

prevention programme in South Auckland.' *New Zealand Medical Journal* (1993, 106: 8–10)

[15] Gerstein HC. 'Cow's milk exposure and type 1 diabetes mellitus.' *Diabetes Care* (1994, 17: 13–19)

[16] Koletzko S, et al. 'Role of infant feeding practices In development of Crohn's disease in childhood.' *British Medical Journal* (1989, 298: 1617–18)

[17] Rigas A, et al. 'Breast-feeding and maternal smoking in the etiology of Crohn's disease and ulcerative colitis in childhood.' *Annals of Epidemiology* (1993, 3: 387–92)

[18] Davis MK, etal. 'Infant feeding and childhood cancer.' *Lancet* (1988, 2: 365–8)

[19] Halken S, et al. 'Effect of an allergy prevention programme on incidence of atopic symptoms in infancy.' *Annals of Allergy, Asthma, and Immunology* (1992, 47: 545–53)

[20] Chua S, et al. 'Influence of breastfeeding and nipple stimulation on postpartum uterine activity.' *British Journal of Obstetrics and Gynaecology* (1994, 101: 804–5)

[21] Kennedy KI, Visness CM. 'Contraceptive efficacy of lactational amenorrhoea.' *Lancet* (1992, 339: 227–30)

[22] Gray RH, et al. 'Risk of ovulation during lactation.' *Lancet* (1990, 335: 25–9)

[23] Dewey KG, et al. 'Maternal weight-loss patterns during prolonged lactation.' *American Journal of Clinical Nutrition* (1993, 58: 162–6)

[24] Melton LJ, et al. 'Influence of breastfeeding and other reproductive factors on bone mass later in life.' *Osteoporosis International* (1993, 3: 76–83)

[25] Cumming RG, Klineberg RJ. 'Breastfeeding and other reproductive factors and the risk of hip fractures in elderly women.' *International Journal of Epidemiology* (1993, 22: 684–91)

[26] Rosenblatt KA, Thomas DB. 'WHO Collaborative Study of Neoplasia and Steroid Contraceptives.' *International Journal of Epidemiology* (1993, 22: 192–7)

[27] Newcomb PA, et al. 'Lactation and a reduced risk of premenopausal breast cancer.' *New England Journal of Medicine* (1994, 330: 81–7)

[28] Greer FR, et al. 'Improving the vitamin K status of breastfeeding infants with maternal vitamin K supplements.' *Pedlatrics* (1997, 99(1): 88–92)

[29] American Academy of Pediatrics Work Group on Breastfeeding. 'Breastfeeding and the Use of Human Milk (RE9729) Policy Statement.' *Pediatrics* (1997, 100: 1035–9)

[30] Setchell KD, et al. 'Exposure of infants to phyto-oestrogens from soy-based infant formula.' *Lancet* (1997, 350(9070): 23–7)

[31] Fitzpatrick M. 'Soy formulas and the effects of isoflavones on the thyroid.' *New Zealand Medical Journal* (2000, 11;113(1103): 2–6)

[32] Kankaanpaa PE, et al. 'Influence of Probiotic Supplemented Infant formula on composition of Plasma lipids in atopic infants.' *Journal of Nutritional Biochemistry* (2000, 13(6): 364–8)

[33] Lubec G, et al. 'Aminoacid isomerisation and microwave exposure.' *Lancet* (1989, Dec 9;2(8676): 1392–3)

[34] 'Development of the gastrointestinal tract.' Government Recommendations DoH (1994)

[35] Forsyth JS, et al. 'Relation between early introduction of solid food to infants and their weight and illnesses during the first two years of life.' *British Medical Journal* (1993, 306(6892): 1572–6)

[36] Wilson AC, et al. 'Relation of infant diet to childhood health: seven year follow up of cohort of children in Dundee infant feeding study.' *British Medical Journal* (1998, 316(7124): 21–5)

[37] Fergusson DM, Horwood LJ. 'Early solid food diet and eczema in childhood: a 10-year longitudinal study.' *Pediatric Allergy and Immunology* (1994, 5(6): 44–7)

[38] Beauchamp GK, et al. 'Infant salt taste: developmental methodology and contextual factors.' *Developmental Psychobiology* (1994, 27: 353–65)

[39] Birch LL. 'Psychological influences on the childhood diet.' *Journal of Nutrition* (1998, 128(2): 407–10)

[40] Jennifer O, et al. 'Children's bite size and intake of an entrée are greater with large portions than with age-appropriate or self-selected portions.' *American Journal of Clinical Nutrition* (2003, 77: 1164–70)

Useful contacts and information

Dr John Briffa can be contacted at:
Woolaston House
25 Southwood Lane
Highgate, London, N6 5ED
Tel: 020 8341 3422
Fax: 020 8340 1376
Website: www.drbriffa.com
Allergy Matters
Sells a comprehensive selection of light-emitting devices for the treatment of seasonal affective disorder (SAF).
Tel: 0800 052 8228
Website: www.allergymatters.com
BioCare
Suppliers of supplements of the BioCare range, including Pregnancy and Lactation Formula, Kids' Complete Capsule, Kids' Complete Complex, INT B1 and Strawberry Acidophilus. Available in good health food stores and also by mail order.
Tel for mail order: 0121 433 3727
Website for mail order: www.biocare.co.uk
C-Beam Developments Limited
Suppliers of KINcare head lice treatment. Send cheque for £7.50 payable to:
C-Beam Developments Ltd
PO Box 129, Urmston
Manchester M41 7WL
Cedar
Supplied of Linatox (concentrated linoleic acid supplement for the treatment of eczema).
Tel for stockists: 0161 483 1235
Website: www.cedarhealth.co.uk
Challenging Cancer and Leukaemia in Childhood (CLIC)
A national charity offering support to families in a variety of forms, including care grants and crisis breaks.
Tel: 0117 3112 600
Website: www.clic.uk.com
DDAT
A company offering assessment and treatment for conditions such as dyslexia and dyspraxia.
Tel: 0870 737 0017
Website: www.ddat.co.uk
Green People
Makers and suppliers of sunscreens based on predominantly organic ingredients. Products are available in good health food stores and some pharmacies.
Tel: 01444 401444
Website: www.greenpeople.co.uk
Healthspan
Suppliers of Vegetarian DHA (derived from algae), called Cerebrum vegetarian DHA. For details of stockists:
Tel: 0800 7312 377
Website: www.healthspan.co.uk.
The International Flower Essence Repertoire
Suppliers of a very wide range of flower essences by mail order.
Tel: 01428 741572
Website: www.ifer.co.uk
La Leche League
An organisation dedicated to breast-feeding support, information and education.
Tel: 0845 120 2918
Website: www.laleche.org.uk
Lifesource
Providers of Buteyko method educational programme on CD-rom.
Tel: 01623 490141
Website: www.lifesource.co.uk
National Childbirth Trust (NCT)
Support and advice on pregnancy, childbirth, breastfeeding and babycare.
Tel: 0870 444 8707
Website: www.nctpregnancyandbabycare.com
Nutri-Chem Pharmacies
Manufacturer and supplier of supplements specifically designed for individuals with Down's syndrome.
Tel: 001 613 820 4200
Website: www.nutrichem.com
Optima Healthcare
Manufacturers and suppliers of Allergenics, a range of skin products designed for eczema.
Tel: 02920 388422
Website: www.opitmah.com
Verity
Self-help organisation for individuals with polycystic ovarian syndrome (PCOS).
Website: www.verity-pcos.org.uk

Index